Board Review Series

MICROBIOLOGY AND IMMUNOLOGY
3rd edition

Look for all of the titles in this series:

Board Review Series

MICROBIOLOGY
AND
IMMUNOLOGY
3rd edition

Arthur G. Johnson, Ph.D.

Professor and Chairman
Department of Medical Microbiology
    and Immunology
University of Minnesota, Duluth
School of Medicine
Duluth, Minnesota

Richard J. Ziegler, Ph.D.

Professor of Microbiology
Department of Medical Microbiology
    and Immunology
University of Minnesota, Duluth
School of Medicine
Duluth, Minnesota

Omelan A. Lukasewycz, Ph.D.

Associate Professor of Microbiology
Department of Medical Microbiology
    and Immunology
University of Minnesota, Duluth
School of Medicine
Duluth, Minnesota

Louise B. Hawley, Ph.D.

Assistant Professor of Microbiology
Department of Medical Microbiology
    and Immunology
University of Minnesota, Duluth
School of Medicine
Duluth, Minnesota

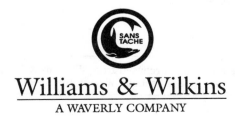

Williams & Wilkins
A WAVERLY COMPANY

BALTIMORE • PHILADELPHIA • LONDON • PARIS • BANGKOK
BUENOS AIRES • HONG KONG • MUNICH • SYDNEY • TOKYO • WROCLAW

Editor: Elizabeth Nieginski
Managing Editor: Amy Dinkel
Development Editor: Becky Krumm
Production Coordinator: Danielle Santucci
Typesetter: Maryland Composition
Printer & Binder: Mack Printing Group

Copyright © 1996 Williams & Wilkins

351 West Camden Street
Baltimore, Maryland 21201-2436 USA

Rose Tree Corporate Center
1400 North Providence Road
Building II, Suite 5025
Media, Pennsylvania 19063-2043 USA

Printed in the United States of America

Library of Congress Cataloging in Publication Data

Microbiology and immunology / Arthur G. Johnson . . . [et al.]. — 3rd
  ed.
      p.   cm. — (Board review series)
    Includes index.
    ISBN 0-683-18005-3
    1. Medical microbiology—Outlines, syllabi, etc.   2. Medical
microbiology—Examinations, questions, etc.   3. Immunology—
Outlines, syllabi, etc.   4. Immunology—Examinations, questions,
etc.   I. Johnson, Arthur G,   II. Series.
    [DNLM: 1. Microbiology—examination questions.   2. Allergy and
Immunology—examination questions.   3. Microbiology—outlines.
4. Allergy and Immunology—outlines.   QW 18.2 M623 1996]
QR46.M5387   1996
616'.01'076—dc20
DNLM/DLC
for Library of Congress   96-7007
                                                              CIP

The Publishers have made every effort to trace the copyright holders for borrowed material. If they have inadvertently overlooked any, they will be pleased to make the necessary arrangements at the first opportunity.

97 98 99
3 4 5 6 7 8 9 10

Dedication

This book is dedicated to our former colleague, and friend, Dr. Thomas J. Fitzgerald, whose untimely death following a bout with cancer was a decided loss to all of us. Tom contributed the chapter on bacteriology in earlier editions. He was a dedicated teacher and a distinguished experimental bacteriologist, specializing in sexually transmitted diseases. Students and scientists alike will miss his influential impact on their respective fields.

Contents

vii

Preface to the Third Edition

This concise review of microbiology and immunology is intended for medical and graduate students studying for the United States Medical Licensing Examination (USMLE) as well as other examinations. The third edition remains a succinct description of the most important concepts of the microbial world and the ways in which the host–parasite relationships are affected. This book is not meant to be a substitute for a major microbiology text but rather to be a review of information that has been learned in didactic courses.

Organization

The book is divided into seven chapters covering major topics of microbiology and immunology. Within each chapter, the important signs, symptoms, and etiology of diseases are described along with mechanisms of preventing infection and means of identifying and diagnosing the causative agent.

The text is presented in a tightly outlined format that facilitates rapid review of important information. Numerous tables with clinical correlations are inserted.

Each chapter is followed by review questions and answers and explanations that reflect the style and content of USMLE. A Comprehensive Examination at the end of the book serves as a practice exam and self-assessment tool to help students diagnose their weaknesses prior to reviewing microbiology and immunology.

Features of the third edition

- Updated and current information in all chapters
- Many new questions and explanations reflecting USMLE changes
- Numerous tables, including an alphabetized index of the distinguishing characteristics of the bacterial pathogens
- A comprehensive examination

Arthur G. Johnson, Ph.D.
Richard J. Ziegler, Ph.D.
Omelan A. Lukasewycz, Ph.D.
Louise B. Hawley, Ph.D.

Acknowledgments

The authors are grateful for the excellent organizational and secretarial skills of Ms. Sally Herstad, who aided the preparation of this edition. In addition, we acknowledge Mr. Mark Summers for his skillful illustrations.

1

General Properties of Microorganisms

I. The Microbial World

A. Microorganisms

–belong to the Protista biologic kingdom.

–include some eukaryotes and prokaryotes, viruses, viroids, and prions.

–are classified according to their structure, chemical composition, and biosynthetic and genetic organization.

B. Eukaryotic cells

–contain organelles and a nucleus bounded by a nuclear membrane.

–contain complex phospholipids, sphingolipids, histones, and sterols.

–lack a cell wall (plant cells have a cellulose cell wall).

–have multiple diploid chromosomes and nucleosomes.

–have relatively long-lived mRNA formed from the processing of precursor mRNA, which contains exons and introns.

1. Protozoa

–are **eukaryotic** cells.

–are classified into seven phyla; three of these phyla (Sarcomastigophora, Apicomplexa, Ciliophora) contain medically important species that are human parasites.

2. Fungi

–are **eukaryotic** cells.

–may be **monomorphic,** existing as single-celled **yeast** or multicellular, filamentous **mold.**

–may be **dimorphic,** existing as yeasts or molds, depending on temperature and nutrition.

–have both asexual and sexual reproduction capabilities.

–have a growth cycle that consists of both a vegetative and a reproductive phase.

C. Prokaryotic cells

–have no organelles, no membrane-enclosed nucleus, and no histones; in rare cases, they contain complex phospholipids, sphingolipids, and sterols.

1

–have a cell wall composed of peptidoglycan-containing muramic acid.

–are haploid with a single chromosome.

–have short-lived, unprocessed mRNA.

–have coupled transcription and translation.

1. **Bacteria**

    –are **prokaryotic** cells.

    –may be normal flora or may be pathogenic in humans.

    –do not have a sexual growth cycle; however, some can produce asexual spores.

2. **Mycoplasmas**

    –are the smallest and simplest of the bacteria that are self-replicating.

    –lack a cell wall.

    –are the only prokaryotes that contain sterols.

3. **Rickettsia**

    –are **obligate intracellular bacteria** that are incapable of self-replication.

    –depend on the host cell for adenosine triphosphate (ATP) production.

4. **Chlamydia**

    –are bacteria-like **obligate intracellular pathogens** with a complex growth cycle involving intracellular and extracellular forms.

    –depend on the host cell for ATP production.

D. **Viruses**

   –are not cells and are not visible with the light microscope.

   –are **obligate intracellular parasites.**

   –contain no organelles or biosynthetic machinery, except for a few enzymes.

   –contain either RNA or DNA as genetic material.

   –are called **bacteriophage** (or **phage**) if they have a bacterial host.

E. **Viroids**

   –are not cells and are not visible with the light microscope.

   –are **obligate intracellular parasites.**

   –are single-stranded, covalently closed, circular RNA molecules that exist as base-paired, rod-like structures.

   –cause plant diseases but have not been proven to cause human disease, although the RNA of the hepatitis D virus (HDV) is viroid-like.

F. **Prions**

   –are infectious particles associated with subacute progressive, degenerative diseases of the central nervous system (e.g., Creutzfeldt-Jakob disease).

   –copurify with a specific glycoprotein (PrP) that has a molecular weight of 27–30 kDa and are resistant to nucleases but are inactivated with proteases and other agents that inactivate proteins.

   –are altered conformations of a normal cellular protein that can autocatalytically form more copies of itself.

II. Bacterial Structure (Table 1–1)

A. Bacterial shape

–can usually be determined with appropriate staining and a light microscope.

–is usually **round** (coccus), **rod-like** (bacillus), or **spiral** with most species; cocci and bacilli often grow in doublets or chains.

–may be **pleomorphic** with some species such as *Bacteroides*.

–is used, along with other properties, to identify bacteria.

–is determined by the mechanism of cell wall assembly.

–may be altered by antibiotics that affect cell wall biosynthesis (e.g., penicillin).

B. Bacterial nucleus

–is not surrounded by a nuclear membrane, nor does it contain a mitotic apparatus.

–is generally called a **nucleoid or nuclear body.**

–consists of polyamine and magnesium ions bound to negatively charged, circular, supercoiled, double-stranded DNA, small amounts of RNA, RNA polymerase, and other proteins.

C. Bacterial cytoplasm

–contains ribosomes and various types of nutritional storage granules.

–contains no organelles.

D. Bacterial ribosomes

–have a sedimentation coefficient of 70S and are composed of 30S and 50S subunits containing 16S, and 23S and 5S RNA, respectively.

–are the sites of action of many antibiotics that inhibit protein biosynthesis.

–have proteins and RNAs that differ from those of their eukaryotic counterparts.

–form the basis for the selective toxicity of antibacterial protein synthesis–inhibiting agents, which affect 70S ribosomes (e.g., erythromycin).

–are membrane-bound if engaged in protein biosynthesis.

E. Cell (cytoplasmic) membrane

-contains the cytochromes and enzymes involved in electron transport and oxidative phosphorylation.

-contains carrier lipids and enzymes, including **penicillin-binding proteins,** involved in cell wall biosynthesis.

-contains enzymes involved in phospholipid synthesis and DNA replication.

-contains chemoreceptors.

-is responsible for selective permeability and active transport, which are facilitated by membrane-bound permeases, binding proteins, and various transport systems.

-is the site of action of certain antibiotics such as polymyxin.

F. Mesosomes

–are **convoluted invaginations** of the plasma membrane.

–function in DNA replication and cell division as well as in secretion.

–are termed **septal mesosomes** if they occur at the septum (cross-wall) or **lateral mesosomes** if they are nonseptal.

Table 1–1. Components of Microbial Cells

Structure	Composition	Fungi	Gram-Positive Bacteria	Gram-Negative Bacteria	Myco-plasmas	Chla-mydia*	Rickettsia*
Envelope capsule	Polysaccharide or polypeptide	−	+ or −	+ or −	−	−	−
Wall							
Chitin	Poly-N-acetylglucosamine	+	−	−	−	−	−
Peptidoglycan	Poly-N-acetylglucosamine-N acetylmuramic acid-tetrapeptide	−	+	+	−	−	+
Periplasm	Proteins and oligosaccharides	−	−	+	−	+	+
Lipoprotein	Lipoprotein	−	−	+	−	+	+
Outer membrane	Proteins, phospholipids, and lipopolysaccharide	−	−	+	−	+	+
Appendages							
Pili	Protein	−	+ or −	+ or −	−	−	−
Flagella	Protein	−	+ or −	+ or −	−	−	−
Cell membrane	Proteins and phospholipids	+ (plus ergosterol)	+	+	+	+	+
Cytosol							
Organelles	Protein, phospholipids, and nucleic acids	+	−	−	−	−	−
80S Ribosomes	Protein and RNA	+	−	−	−	−	−
70S Ribosomes	Protein and RNA	−	+	+	+	+	+
Genetic material							
Nucleus	Protein, phospholipids, and nucleic acids	+	−	−	−	−	−
Nucleoid	Protein and nucleic acids	−	+	+	+	+	+
Plasmids	DNA	+ or −	+ or −	+ or −	+ or −	+ or −	+ or −
Spores							
Reproductive spores	All cellular components	+	−	−	−	−	−
Endospores	All cellular components plus dipicolinic acid	−	+ or −	−	−	−	−

* Obligate intracellular pathogens because they cannot synthesize ATP

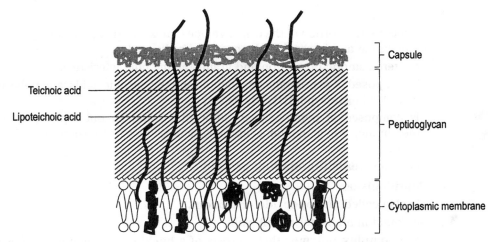

Figure 1–1. Diagrammatic representation of a gram-positive bacterial cell envelope.

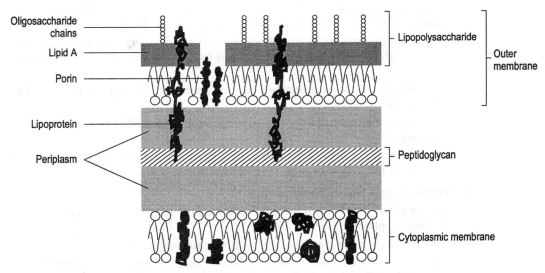

Figure 1–2. Diagrammatic representation of a gram-negative bacterial cell envelope.

G. Plasmids

–are small, circular, nonchromosomal, double-stranded DNA molecules.

–contain genes that confer protective properties such as antibiotic resistance or virulence factors or their own transmissibility to other bacteria.

H. Cell envelope (Figures 1–1 and 1–2)

–is composed of the macromolecular layers that surround the bacterium.

–always includes a cell membrane and a peptidoglycan layer.

–includes an outer membrane layer in gram-negative bacteria.

–may include a capsule, a glycocalyx layer, or both.

–contains antigens that frequently induce a specific antibody response.

1. **Cell wall**
   - refers to that portion of the cell envelope that is external to the cytoplasmic membrane and internal to the capsule or glycocalyx.
   - confers osmotic protection and gram-staining characteristics.
   - is composed of peptidoglycan, teichoic and teichuronic acids, and polysaccharides in **gram-positive bacteria.**
   - is composed of peptidoglycan, lipoprotein, and an outer phospholipid membrane, which contains lipopolysaccharide in **gram-negative bacteria.**
   - contains **penicillin-binding proteins.**

2. **Peptidoglycan**
   - is also called **mucopeptide** or **murein.**
   - is found in all bacterial cell walls.
   - is a **complex polymer** that consists of a **backbone,** which is composed of alternating N-acetylglucosamine and N-acetylmuramic acid and a set of identical tetrapeptide **side chains,** which are attached to the N-acetylmuramic acid and which are frequently linked to adjacent tetrapeptide by identical peptide **cross-bridges** or by direct peptide **bonds.**
   - contains the beta-1,4 glycosidic bond between N-acetylmuramic acid and N-acetylglucosamine, which is cleaved by the bacteriolytic enzyme **lysozyme.**
   - may contain **diaminopimelic acid,** an amino acid unique to prokaryotic cell walls.
   - is the site of action of certain antibiotics such as penicillin and the cephalosporins.
   - comprises up to 50% of the cell wall of gram-positive bacteria but only 2% to 10% of the cell wall of gram-negative bacteria.

3. **Teichoic and teichuronic acids**
   - are **water-soluble polymers,** containing a ribitol or glycerol residue linked by phosphodiester bonds.
   - are found in **gram-positive** cell walls or membranes.
   - are chemically bonded to peptidoglycan (wall teichoic acid) or membrane glycolipid (lipoteichoic acid), particularly in mesosomes.
   - contain important bacterial surface antigenic determinants, and lipoteichoic acid helps anchor the wall to the membrane.
   - may account for 50% of the dry weight of a gram-positive cell wall.

4. **Lipoprotein**
   - cross-links the peptidoglycan and outer membrane in **gram-negative** bacteria.
   - is linked to diaminopimelic acid residues of peptidoglycan tetrapeptide side-chains by a peptide bond; the lipid portion is noncovalently inserted into the outer membrane.

5. **Periplasmic space**
   - is found in **gram-negative** cells.
   - refers to the area between the cell membrane and the outer membrane.

–contains hydrated peptidoglycan, hydrolytic enzymes, and oligosaccharides.

6. Outer membrane

–is found in **gram-negative** cells.

–is a **phospholipid bilayer** in which the phospholipids of the outer portion are replaced by lipopolysaccharides.

–protects cells from harmful enzymes and prevents leakage of periplasmic proteins.

–contains embedded proteins, including matrix **porins** (nonspecific pores), some nonpore proteins (phospholipases and proteases), and transport proteins for small molecules.

7. Lipopolysaccharide

–is found in the outer leaflet of the outer membrane of **gram-negative** cells.

–consists of **lipid A,** several long-chain fatty acids attached to phosphorylated glucosamine disaccharide units, and a polysaccharide composed of a core and terminal repeating units.

–is negatively charged and noncovalently cross-bridged by divalent cations.

–is also called **endotoxin;** the toxicity is associated with the lipid A.

–contains major surface antigenic determinants, including **O antigen** found in the polysaccharide component.

8. Bayer's junction

–is found in **gram-negative** cells.

–is the region of the wall where the inner leaflet of the outer membrane is contiguous with the outer leaflet of the cell membrane.

I. External layers

1. Capsule

–is a well-defined structure of polysaccharide surrounding a bacterial cell and is external to the cell wall. The one exception to the polysaccharide structure is the poly-D-glutamic acid capsule of *Bacillus anthracis.*

–protects the bacteria from phagocytosis.

2. Glycocalyx

–refers to a loose network of polysaccharide fibrils that surrounds some bacterial cell walls.

–is sometimes called a **slime layer.**

–is associated with adhesive properties of the bacterial cell.

–is synthesized by surface enzymes.

–contains prominent antigenic sites.

J. Appendages

1. Flagella

–are protein appendages for locomotion.

–consist of a basal body, hook, and a long filament composed of a polymerized protein called **flagellin.**

–may be located in only one area of a cell (**polar**) or over the entire bacterial cell surface (**peritrichous**).

–contain prominent antigenic determinants.

2. Pili (fimbriae)

–are rigid surface appendages composed mainly of a protein called **pilin.**

–exist in two classes: **ordinary pili (adhesins),** involved in bacterial adherence, and **sex pili,** involved in attachment of donor and recipient bacteria in conjugation.

–are, in the case of ordinary pili, the colonization antigens or **virulence factors** associated with some bacterial species such as *Streptococcus pyogenes* and *Neisseria gonorrhoeae.*

–may confer antiphagocytic properties like the **M protein** of *S. pyogenes.*

K. Endospores

–are formed as a survival response to certain adverse nutritional conditions, such as depletion of a certain source.

–are metabolically **inactive bacterial cells** that are highly resistant to desiccation, heat, and various chemicals.

–possess a core that contains many cell components, a spore wall, a cortex, a coat, and an exosporium.

–contain **calcium dipicolinate,** which aids in heat resistance within the core.

–germinate under favorable nutritional conditions after an activation process that involves damage to the spore coat.

–are helpful in identifying some species of bacteria (e.g., *Bacillus* and *Clostridia*).

III. Bacterial Growth

A. General characteristics—bacterial growth

–refers to an increase in bacterial cell numbers (multiplication), which results from a programmed increase in the biomass of the bacteria.

–results from bacterial reproduction due to binary fission, which may be characterized by a parameter called **generation time** (the average time required for cell numbers to double).

–may be determined by measuring **cell concentration** (turbidity measurements or cell counting) or **biomass density** (dry weight or protein determinations).

–usually occurs asynchronously (i.e., all cells do not divide at precisely the same moment).

B. Cell concentration

–may be measured by **viable cell counts** involving serial dilutions of sample followed by a determination of colony-forming units on an agar surface.

–may be determined by **particle cell counting** or **turbidimetric density measurements** (includes both viable and nonviable cells).

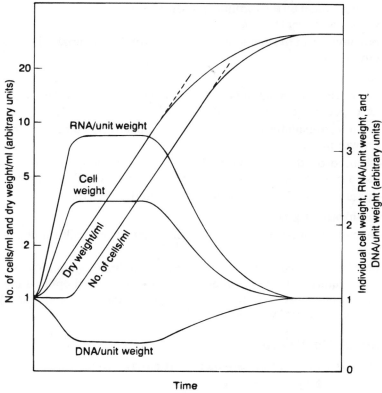

Figure 1–3. Diagram of changes in cell size and chemical composition during growth curve. Inoculum from an early stationary-phase culture. Bacterial count and dry-weight concentration on logarithmic scale (*left-hand ordinate*); average bacterial dry weight and content of RNA and DNA on arithmetic scale (*right-hand ordinate*). Initial values of all variables taken as one unit. (Reprinted with permission from Wilson GS, Miles A, eds: *Topley and Wilson's Principles of Bacteriology, Virology and Immunity,* 6th ed, vol 1. Baltimore, Williams & Wilkins, 1975, p 125.)

C. Bacterial growth curve (Figure 1–3)

–requires inoculation of bacteria from a saturated culture into fresh liquid media.

–is unique for a particular nutritional environment.

–is frequently illustrated in a plot of logarithmic number of bacteria versus time; the generation time is determined by observing the time necessary for the cells to double in number during the log phase of growth.

–consists of **four phases:**

1. **Lag**—metabolite-depleted cells adapt to new environment.

2. **Exponential or log**—cell biomass is synthesized at a constant rate.

3. **Stationary**—cells exhaust essential nutrients or accumulate toxic products.

4. **Death or decline**—cells may die due to toxic products.

D. Growth rate constant (κ)

–is the rate at which bacterial cells are reproducing.

–is determined by the formula $\kappa = Bdt/dB$, where B equals the biomass concentration and t equals time.

–is a function of the metabolic capabilities of the bacterial cell and its nutritional environment.

E. Chemostat

–is a device that maintains a bacterial culture in a specific phase of growth or at a specific cell concentration.

–is most frequently used to maintain a bacterial culture in the exponential growth phase.

–is based on the principle that toxic products and cells are removed at the same rate as fresh nutrients are added and new cells are synthesized.

–operates best if one nutrient limits bacterial growth.

F. Synchronous growth

–refers to a situation in which all the bacteria in a culture divide at the same moment.

–may be achieved by several methods, including thymidine starvation (thymidine-requiring bacteria), alternate cycles of low and optimal incubation temperatures, spore germination, selective filtration of old (large) and young (small) cells, or "trapped cell" filtration.

IV. Bacterial Cultivation

A. General characteristics—bacterial cultivation

–refers to the propagation of bacteria.

–involves specific pH, gaseous, and temperature preferences of bacteria.

–is performed in either liquid (broth) or solid (agar) growth medium.

–requires an environment that contains:

1. A carbon source

2. A nitrogen source

3. An energy source

4. Inorganic salts

5. Growth factors

6. Hydrogen donors and acceptors

B. Superoxide dismutase

–is an enzyme in aerobes and facultative and aerotolerant anaerobes that allows them to grow in the presence of the superoxide free radical (O_2^-).

–carries out the reaction $2O_2^- + 2H^+ \rightarrow H_2O_2 + O_2$.

–produces hydrogen peroxide (H_2O_2), which is toxic to cells but is destroyed by **catalase** or is oxidized by a peroxidase enzyme.

C. Oxygen requirements

1. Obligate aerobes

–refer to bacteria that require oxygen for growth.

–contain the enzyme **superoxide dismutase,** which protects them from the toxic O_2^-.

2. Obligate anaerobes

–are killed by the O_2^-; grow maximally at a pO_2 concentration of less than 0.5% to 3%.

–lack superoxide dismutase, catalase, and cytochrome C oxidase (enzymes that destroy toxic products of oxygen metabolism).

–require a substance other than oxygen as a hydrogen acceptor during the generation of metabolic energy.

–use fermentation pathways with distinctive metabolic products.

–outnumber aerobes $1000:1$ in the gut and $100:1$ in the mouth.

–comprise 99% of the total fecal flora (10^{11}/g of stool in the large bowel).

–usually cause polymicrobial infections, those involving more than one genus or species.

–are foul smelling.

–are not communicable or transmissible.

–generally are found proximal to mucosal surfaces; when this barrier is broken, anaerobes can escape into tissues.

–mucusol surfaces can be disrupted by:

a. Gastrointestinal obstruction or surgery

b. Diverticulitis

c. Bronchial obstruction

d. Tumor growth

e. Ulceration of the intestinal tract by chemotherapeutic agents

3. Facultative anaerobes

–grow in the presence or absence of oxygen.

–shift from a fermentative to a respiratory metabolism in the presence of air.

–display the **Pasteur effect,** in which the energy needs of the cell are met by consuming less glucose under a respiratory metabolism than under a fermentative metabolism.

–include most pathogenic bacteria.

4. Aerotolerant anaerobes

–resemble facultative bacteria but have a fermentative metabolism both with and without an oxygen environment.

D. Nutritional requirements

1. Heterotrophs

–require preformed organic compounds (e.g., sugar, amino acids) for growth.

2. Autotrophs

–do not require preformed organic compounds for growth because they can synthesize them from inorganic compounds.

E. Growth media

1. Minimal essential growth medium

–contains only the primary precursor compounds essential for growth.

–demands that a bacterium synthesize most of the organic compounds required for its growth.

–dictates a relatively slow generation time.

2. Complex growth medium

–contains most of the organic compound building blocks (e.g., sugars, amino acids, nucleotides) necessary for growth.

–dictates a faster generation time for a bacterium relative to its generation time in minimal essential medium.

–is necessary for the growth of fastidious bacteria.

3. Differential growth medium

–contains a combination of nutrients and pH indicators to allow visual distinction of bacteria that grow on or in it.

–is frequently a solid medium on which colonies of particular bacterial species have a distinctive color.

4. Selective growth medium

–contains compounds that prevent the growth of some bacteria while allowing the growth of other bacteria.

–uses certain dyes or sugars, high salt concentration, or pH to achieve selectivity.

V. Bacterial Metabolism

A. General characteristics

1. Bacterial metabolism

–is the sum of **anabolic processes** (synthesis of cellular constituents requiring energy) and **catabolic processes** (breakdown of cellular constituents with concomitant release of waste products and energy-rich compounds).

–is **heterotrophic** for pathogenic bacteria.

–varies depending on the nutritional environment.

2. Bacterial transport systems

–involve membrane-associated binding or transport proteins for sugars and amino acids.

–frequently require energy to concentrate substrates inside the cell.

–are usually inducible for nutrients that are catabolized; glucose, which is constitutive, is an exception.

–frequently use phosphotransferase systems when sugars are transported.

B. Carbohydrate metabolism

1. Fermentation

–is a method by which some bacteria obtain metabolic energy.

–is characterized by a **substrate phosphorylation.**

–involves the formation of **ATP** not coupled to electron transfer.

–requires an intermediate product of glucose metabolism (often pyruvate) as a final hydrogen acceptor.

–results in the synthesis of specific metabolic end products that aid in the identification of bacterial species.

2. Respiration

–refers to the method of obtaining metabolic energy that involves an **oxidative phosphorylation.**

–involves the formation of ATP during electron transfer and the reduction of gaseous oxygen.

–involves a cell membrane electron transport chain composed of cytochrome enzymes, lipid cofactors, and coupling factors.

C. Regulation

1. Regulation of enzyme activity

–may occur because enzymes are **allosteric proteins,** susceptible to binding of effector molecules that influence their activity.

–may occur by **feedback inhibition** involving the end product.

–may involve **substrate-binding enhancement** (cooperatively) of catalytic activity.

2. Regulation of enzyme synthesis

–may involve allosteric regulatory proteins that activate (**activators**) or inhibit (**repressors**) gene transcription.

–may involve **end product feedback repression** of biosynthetic pathway enzymes.

–may involve **substrate induction** of catabolic enzymes.

–may involve **attenuation control sequences** in enzyme mRNA.

–may involve the process of **catabolite repression,** which is under positive control of the **catabolite activator protein.**

3. Pasteur effect

–occurs in **facultative bacteria.**

–is caused by oxygen blocking the fermentative capacity of the bacteria.

–means that the energy needs are met by using less glucose during aerobic growth.

VI. Cell Wall Synthesis

–involves the cytoplasmic synthesis of peptidoglycan subunits, which are translocated by a membrane lipid carrier and cross-linked to existing cell wall by enzymes associated with the plasma membrane of gram-positive bacteria or found in the periplasmic region of gram-negative bacteria.

–involves the covalent linkage of teichoic acid to *N*-acetylmuramic acid residues in gram-positive cells.

–includes the addition of three components (lipoprotein, outer membrane, lipopolysaccharide), whose constituents or subunits are synthesized on or in the cytoplasmic membrane and assembled outside of it in gram-negative cells.

VII. Sterilization and Disinfection

A. Terminology

1. Sterility—total absence of viable microorganisms as assessed by no growth on any medium

2. **Bactericidal**—kills bacteria

3. **Bacteriostatic**—inhibits growth of bacteria

4. **Sterilization**—removal or killing of all microorganisms

5. **Disinfection**—removal or killing of disease-causing microorganisms

6. **Sepsis**—infection

7. **Aseptic**—without infection

8. **Antisepsis**—any procedure that inhibits the growth and multiplication of microorganisms

B. **Kinetics of killing**

   –is affected by menstruum or medium, the concentration of organisms and antimicrobial agents, temperature, pH, and the presence of spores.

   –can be exponential or logarithmic.

   –can result in a killing curve that becomes asymptotic, requiring extra considerations in killing final numbers, especially if the population is heterogeneous relative to sensitivity.

C. **Antimicrobial agents** include

   1. **Moist heat** (autoclaving at 121°C for 15 minutes at a steam pressure of 15 pounds per square inch kills microorganisms, including spore formers)

   2. **Ultraviolet radiation,** which blocks DNA replication

   3. **Chemicals**

      a. **Phenol** (Figure 1–4)

         –is used as a disinfectant standard that is expressed as a phenol coefficient, which compares the rate of the minimal sterilizing concentration of phenol to that of the test compound for a particular organism.

         –a diphenyl cationic analogue, chlorhexidine is a useful topical disinfectant.

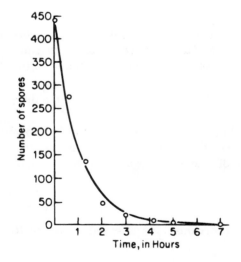

Figure 1–4. Disinfection of anthrax spores with 5% phenol at 33.3° C. The curve is drawn through a series of calculated points. The circles represent the experimental observations. (Reprinted with permission from Wilson GS, Dick HM (eds): *Topley and Wilson's Principles of Bacteriology, Virology and Immunity,* 7th ed. Baltimore, Williams & Wilkins, 1983, vol 1, p 85.)

    b. Iodine

–is bactericidal in a 2% solution of aqueous alcohol containing potassium iodide.

–acts as an oxidizing agent and combines irreversibly with proteins.

–can cause hypersensitivity reactions.

    c. Chlorine

–inactivates bacteria and most viruses by oxidizing free sulfhydryl groups.

    d. Formaldehyde

–is used as a disinfectant in aqueous solution (37%).

    e. Ethylene oxide

–is an alkylating agent that is especially useful for disinfecting hospital instruments.

–requires exposure times of 4–6 hours, followed by aeration to remove absorbed gas.

    f. Alcohol

–requires concentrations of 70%–95% to kill bacteria given sufficient time.

–isopropyl alcohol (90%–95%) is the major form in use in hospitals.

VIII. Antimicrobial Chemotherapy

A. General characteristics—antimicrobial chemotherapy

–is based on the principle of selective toxicity, which implies that a compound is harmful to a microorganism but innocuous to its host.

–involves drugs that:

1. Are antimetabolites

2. Inhibit cell wall biosynthesis

3. Inhibit protein synthesis

4. Inhibit nucleic acid synthesis

5. Alter or inhibit cell membrane permeability or transport

–includes both **bacteriostatic** (inhibit growth) and **bactericidal** (kill) drugs.

–may use synergistic combinations of bacteriostatic drugs (e.g., trimethoprim and sulfonamide).

–incorporates both **drug–parasite** relationships (e.g., location of bacteria and drug distribution) and alterations of **host–parasite** relationships (e.g., immune response and microbial flora) to be effective.

B. Drug antimicrobial activity

–is usually determined by **dilution** or **diffusion** tests.

–is quantitated by determining the minimal inhibitory concentration.

–may differ in vitro and in vivo.

–is affected by pH, drug stability, microbial environment, number of microorganisms present, length of incubation with drug, and metabolic activity of microorganisms.

–may be modified for a specific bacterium if **genetic or nongenetic drug resistance** develops.

C. Drug resistance

1. Nongenetic mechanisms of drug resistance

—may involve loss of specific target structures, such as cell wall by L forms of bacteria.

—may result from metabolic inactivity of microorganisms.

2. Genetic mechanisms of drug resistance

—may result from either chromosomal or extrachromosomal resistance.

—may involve a chromosomal mutation that alters the structure of the receptor of the drug or the permeability of the drug.

—may result from the introduction of a plasmid (R factor of R plasmid) that codes for enzymes (**beta-lactamase**) that degrade the drug or modify it (**acetyltransferase**), or from the introduction of proteins that pump it from the cell in an energy-dependent fashion.

3. R factor or R plasmid

—contains **insertion sequences** and **transposons.**

—may acquire additional resistance genes by plasmid fusion or from transposons.

—may consist of two plasmids, the **resistance transfer factor (RTF),** which codes for replication and transfer, and the **r or resistance determinant,** which contains genes for replication and resistance.

—can be transmitted from species to species.

—is responsible for the rapid development of multiple drug-resistant bacteria over the past 30 years.

D. Mechanisms of action (Table 1–2)

1. Antimetabolites

—include bacteriostatic (sulfonamide, trimethoprim, para-aminosalicylic acid) and bactericidal (isoniazid) drugs.

—are structural analogs of normal metabolites.

—may become bactericidal when used in combination (e.g., trimethoprim and sulfonamide).

—inhibit the action of specific enzymes.

2. Cell wall synthesis inhibitors

—are bactericidal.

—may inhibit transpeptidation (cross-linking) of peptidoglycan (beta-lactam drugs: penicillins, cephalosporins, and carbapenems).

—may inhibit the synthesis of peptidoglycan (cycloserine, bacitracin, vancomycin).

—may act in the cytoplasm (cycloserine), in the membrane (bacitracin), or in the cell wall (penicillins, cephalosporins, vancomycin).

—require cell wall synthesis to be effective.

—may cause bacteria to take on aberrant shapes or become **spheroplasts.**

a. Penicillins

—inhibit the transpeptidation enzymes involved in cell wall synthesis.

—are active against gram-positive bacteria and gram-negative bacteria.

Table 1–2.   Mechanisms of Action of Antimicrobial Chemotherapy

Mechanism of Action	Agent	Site of Action	Effect
Inhibitors of cell wall biosynthesis	Cycloserine	Peptidoglycan tetrapeptide side chain	Bactericidal
	Phosphomycin	Formation of N^- acetylmuramic acid	Bactericidal
	Bacitracin	Membrane carrier molecule	Bactericidal
	Penicillins	Peptidoglycan cross-linking	Bactericidal
	Cephalosporins, carbapenems	Peptidoglycan cross-linking	Bactericidal
	Vancomycin	Translocation of cell wall intermediates	Bactericidal
Inhibitors of protein biosynthesis	Streptomycin	30S ribosomal subunit	Bactericidal
	Gentamicin	30S ribosomal subunit	Bactericidal
	Tetracycline	30S ribosomal subunit	Bacteriostatic
	Spectinomycin	30S ribosomal subunit	Bacteriostatic
	Chloramphenicol	50S ribosomal subunit	Bacteriostatic
	Erythromycin	50S ribosomal subunit	Bacteriostatic
	Clindamycin	50S ribosomal subunit	Bacteriostatic
	Griseofulvin	Microtubule function	Fungistatic
Inhibitors of nucleic acid synthesis	Quinolones	DNA gyrase	Bactericidal
	Novobiocin	DNA gyrase	Bacteriostatic
	Flucytosine	Fungal thymidylate synthetase	Fungicidal
	Rifampin	DNA-dependent RNA polymerase	Bactericidal
Inhibitors of folate metabolism	Sulfonamides	Pteroic acid synthetase	Bacteriostatic
	Trimethoprim	Dihydrofolate reductase	Bacteriostatic
Inhibitor of mycolic acid synthesis	Isoniazid	Mycobacterial mycolic acid biosynthesis	Bactericidal
Alteration of cytoplasmic membrane	Polymyxins	Bacterial membrane permeability	Bactericidal
	Polyenes	Fungal membrane permeability	Fungicidal
	Azoles	Fungal ergosterol biosynthesis	Fungicidal

–react with penicillin-binding proteins.

–have a beta-lactam ring structure that is inactivated by beta-lactamases (penicillinases), which are genetically coded in some bacterial DNA or some R plasmids.

b. Cephalosporins

–have a mechanism of action similar to that of penicillin.

–are active against both gram-positive and gram-negative bacteria.

–contain a beta-lactam ring structure that is inactivated by some beta-lactamases.

–are frequently used to treat patients who are allergic to penicillins.

c. Carbapenems

–have a mechanism similar to that of penicillin.

–have a beta-lactam ring fused to a five-carbon ring and are resistant to beta-lactamases.

3. Protein synthesis inhibitors

–include, for example, the aminoglycosides and lincomycins.

–are frequently known as broad-spectrum antibiotics.

–require bacterial growth for their effect.

a. Aminoglycosides

–include streptomycin, neomycin, kanamycin, and gentamicin.

–are bactericidal for gram-negative bacteria and bind to the 30S ribosomal subunit.

–are not active against anaerobes or intracellular bacteria.

–may irreversibly block initiation of translation or cause mRNA misreading (or both).

–have a narrow effective concentration range before toxicity occurs, causing renal damage and eighth cranial nerve damage (hearing loss).

–may be modified (acetylation) and rendered inactive by enzymes contained in R plasmids.

b. Tetracyclines

–include tetracycline, oxytetracycline, and chlortetracycline.

–are bacteriostatic, bind to the 30S ribosomal subunit, and prevent binding of aminoacyl tRNA to the acceptor site.

–may be deposited in teeth and bones, which can cause tooth staining and structural problems in the bones of children.

–are transported out of or bound to a plasmid-derived protein in cells containing specific tetracycline R plasmids.

c. Chloramphenicol

–is bacteriostatic for gram-positive and gram-negative bacteria, rickettsia, and chlamydia.

–binds to the 50S ribosomal subunit and inhibits peptide-bond formation.

–may be inactivated by the enzyme chloramphenicol acetyltransferase, which is carried on an R plasmid.

d. Griseofulvin

–is a fungistatic drug that is active against fungi with chitin in their cell walls.

–inhibits protein assembly, which interferes with cell division by blocking microtubule assembly.

e. Macrolides and lincomycins

–include erythromycin (macrolide), and lincomycin and clindamycin (lincomycins).

– are bacteriostatic.

–bind to the 23S RNA in the 50S ribosomal subunit and block translocation.

–are rendered ineffective in bacteria that have a mutation in a 50S ribosomal protein or that contain an R plasmid with genetic information, which results in methylation of 23S RNA and which inhibits drug binding.

4. **Nucleic acid synthesis inhibitors**

   −can inhibit DNA (quinolones, derivatives of nalidixic acid) or RNA (rifampin) synthesis.

   −are generally bactericidal and are quite toxic to mammalian cells.

   −bind to strands of DNA (actinomycin and mitomycin) or inhibit replication enzymes. Nalidixic acid inhibits DNA gyrase activity; rifampin inhibits DNA-dependent RNA polymerase.

5. **Mycolic acid synthesis inhibitor—isoniazid**

   −is a bactericidal drug that inhibits mycobacterial mycolic acid biosynthesis.

6. **Cytoplasmic membrane inhibitors**

   −alter the osmotic properties of the plasma membrane (polymyxin and polyenes) or inhibit fungal membrane lipid synthesis (azoles: miconazole and ketoconazole).

   −are used in the treatment of some gram-negative (polymyxin) and sterol-containing mycoplasma and fungal (polyenes: nystatin and amphotericin B) infections.

   −can react with mammalian cell membranes and are therefore toxic.

   −are primarily used as a topical treatment or with severe infections.

IX. Toxins

A. Definition

−toxins are broadly defined as microbial products that damage host cells or host tissues.

B. Classification

−toxins are generally classified into two groups: **exotoxins** and **endotoxins**.

−Table 1–3 lists the groups and the properties of each group.

Table 1–3. Properties of Exotoxins and Endotoxins

Property	Exotoxin	Endotoxin
Organisms	Gram-positive and gram-negative	Gram-negative
Composition	Proteins	Lipopolysaccharides
Released by organisms	Yes	No
Heat sensitivity	Labile	Stable
Toxoids (vaccines)	Yes	No
Neutralization by antitoxin	Yes	No
Degree of toxicity	Very potent	Less potent
Specificity for target cells	High	Low

C. Mechanism of action

–many toxins possess an **A and a B polypeptide fragment.**

1. **The A (active) subunit** enters the cell and exerts its toxic effect.

2. **The B (binding) subunit** is responsible for initial attachment of the toxin to the specific target tissue.

3. **Antitoxin** interacts only with the B subunit to block its attachment; once toxin is bound, the antitoxin is ineffective.

D. Toxins composed of A and B polypeptides

1. *Corynebacterium diphtheriae*—exotoxin that inhibits protein synthesis by catalyzing transfer of the adenosine diphosphate (ADP) release moiety of nicotinamide adenine dinucleotide to tRNA elongation factor 2 (EF-2), which disrupts protein synthesis.

2. *Pseudomonas aeruginosa*—exotoxin A that also inhibits protein synthesis via the tRNA EF-2 factor.

3. *Shigella dysenteriae*—shiga neurotoxin that inhibits synthesis via the 60S ribosomal unit by RNase action on 28S ribosomal RNA.

4. *Vibrio cholerae*—choleragen enterotoxin binds to Gm^-1 ganglioside and transfers ADP-R to guanosine 5′ triphosphate, which stimulates adenylate cyclase to overproduce cyclic adenosine monophosphate (cyclic AMP) and induce loss of fluids and electrolytes.

5. *Escherichia coli*—heat-labile enterotoxin similar to choleragen that also stimulates adenylate cyclase to overproduce cyclic AMP and induce loss of fluids and electrolytes.

6. *Campylobacter jejuni*—an enterotoxin also similar to choleragen.

7. *Bordetella pertussis*—ADP-ribosylation of a G protein, which increases adenylate cyclase activity by preventing its inactivation.

8. *Clostridium tetani*—tetanospasm exotoxin that acts on synaptosomes; gangliosides bind the toxin and block the release of glycine, which obliterates the inhibitory reflex response of nerves, causing uncontrolled spastic impulses (hyperreflexia of skeletal muscles).

9. *Clostridium botulinum*—botulinum exotoxin that acts on myoneural junctions; cholinergic nerve fibers are paralyzed, which suppresses the release of acetylcholine, causing flaccid paralysis.

E. Toxins composed of a single polypeptide

1. *Clostridium perfringens*—alpha-toxin that is an enzyme phospholipase C; it disrupts cellular and mitochondrial membranes.

2. *Escherichia coli*—heat-stable enterotoxin that stimulates guanylate cyclase to overproduce cyclic guanosine monophosphate, which impairs chloride and sodium absorption.

3. *Salmonella*—enterotoxin that stimulates cyclic AMP.

4. *Staphylococcus aureus*—exfoliative toxin that disrupts the stratum granulosum in the epidermis.

5. *Streptococcus pyogenes*—erythrogenic and pyrogenic exotoxins that act

as T-cell super antigens, stimulating release of tumor necrosis factor and interleukin-1.

X. Bacteriophages

A. General characteristics—bacteriophages

–are bacterial viruses that are frequently called **phages.**

–are obligate intracellular parasites.

–are host-specific infectious agents for bacteria.

–are called bacteriophage virions when they are complete (genetic material and capsid) infectious particles.

–contain protein and RNA or DNA as major components.

B. Morphologic classes of bacteriophages

1. Polyhedral phages

–are usually composed of an outer polyhedral-shaped protein coat (capsid), which surrounds the nucleic acid.

–may contain a lipid bilayer between two protein capsid layers (PM-2 phage).

–have either circular double-stranded (PM-2) or single-stranded DNA (ϕX174 and M-12) or linear single-stranded RNA (MS2 and Qβ) as their genetic material, although one phage (ϕ6) that has three pieces of double-stranded RNA has been described.

2. Filamentous phages

–have a filamentous protein capsid that surrounds a circular single-stranded DNA genome (f1 and M13).

–are male bacteria–specific in that infection occurs through the pili, which are only present on male bacteria.

–do not lyse their host cells during the replication process.

3. Complex phages

–have a protein polyhedral head containing linear double-stranded DNA and a protein tail and other appendages.

–include the T and lambda phages of *E. coli.*

C. Genetic classes of bacteriophages

1. RNA phages

–refer to all phages with RNA as their genetic material.

–are specific for bacteria with male pili (male-specific).

–contain single-stranded RNA (except for ϕ6, see X B 1), which can act as polycistronic mRNA.

2. DNA phages

–refer to all phages with DNA as their genetic material.

–contain nucleic acid bases that are frequently glucosylated or methylated.

–may contain some unusual nucleic acid bases, such as 5-hydroxymethyl cytosine or 5-hydroxymethyl uracil.

–are classified as **virulent** or **temperate,** depending on whether their pattern of replication is strictly lytic (virulent) or alternates between lytic and lysogenic (temperate).

D. Bacteriophage replication

–requires that the phage use the biosynthetic machinery of the host cell.

–follows a basic sequence of events, which includes adsorption; penetration; phage-specific transcription, translation, or both; assembly; and release.

–is initiated by interaction of phage receptors and specific bacterial surface receptor sites.

–involves the injection of the phage genome into the host cell (filamentous phages are the exception).

–follows one of two types of patterns, **lytic** or **lysogenic,** for DNA phages.

–is usually complete in 30 to 60 minutes for virulent phages.

1. Lytic replication cycle

–occurs with virulent phage (*E. coli* T phages) and results in **lysis of the host cell.**

–is the basis for **phage-typing** of bacteria, which can identify strains of bacteria based on their lysis by a selected set of phages.

–may be analyzed in an experimental situation using a **one-step growth curve.**

a. One-step growth curve

–is the result of an experimental situation in which one cycle of lytic phage replication is monitored.

–is a plot of infectious virus produced versus time after infection.

–involves the use of a **plaque assay,** which is an infectious-center assay in which counts are made of focal areas of phage-induced lysis on a lawn of bacteria.

b. Data obtained from one-step growth curve
(1) Replication time
–is the average time necessary for a phage to replicate within a specific host cell and be released from that cell.
(2) Burst size
–is the number of infectious phages produced from each infecting phage.
(3) Eclipse period
–is the time from infection to the synthesis of the first intracellular infectious virus.

2. Lysogenic replication cycle

a. General characteristics—lysogenic replication

–may occur only with temperate phages (*E. coli* phage lambda).

–involves limited phage-specific protein synthesis, because of the synthesis of a phage-specific **repressor protein** that inhibits phage-specific transcription.

–includes the incorporation of **prophage** (phage DNA) into specific attachment sites in the host cell DNA.

–confers immunity to infection by phages of a type similar to the infecting phage.

–results in passage of the prophage to succeeding generations of the bacteria.

–can revert to lytic replication if the phage repressor is destroyed.

–can result in the generation of **specialized or restricted transducing phages.**

–may result in **lysogenic phage conversion.**

b. **Lysogenic phage conversion**

–refers to a change in the phenotype of the bacteria as a result of limited expression of genes within a prophage.

–occurs in *Salmonella* polysaccharides as a result of infection with the epsilon prophage.

–is the genetic mechanism by which nontoxigenic strains of *C. diphtheriae* are converted to toxin-producing strains.

–results in the conversion of nontoxigenic *C. botulinum* types C and D to toxin-producing strains.

Review Test

Directions: Each of the numbered items or incomplete statements in this section is followed by answers or by completions of the statement. Select the **one** lettered answer or completion that is **best** in each case.

1. Which of the following enzymes would be most likely to affect sugar transport into bacteria?

(A) Acetyltransferase
(B) Neuraminidase
(C) Oxidase
(D) Phosphotransferase

2. Polymers of *N*-acetylglucosamine and *N*-acetylmuramic acid are found in which one of the following chemical structures?

(A) Teichoic acid
(B) Cell wall
(C) Glycocalyx
(D) Lipopolysaccharide

3. Which of the following bacterial structures is most involved in adherence?

(A) Capsule
(B) Lipopolysaccharide
(C) Ordinary pili
(D) O-specific side-chain

4. Which of the following characteristics applies to cephalosporin antibiotics?

(A) Are bacteriostatic
(B) Inhibit protein biosynthesis
(C) Treat fungal infections
(D) Treat patients allergic to penicillin

5. Which one of the following statements applies to bacteria that contain superoxide dismutase?

(A) Need superoxide to grow
(B) Are frequently obligate anaerobes
(C) Grow slowly in the presence of CO_2
(D) Produce hydrogen peroxide from hydrogen ion and the superoxide free radical (O_2^-)

6. Which of the following statements describes lysogenic phage conversion?

(A) The transformation of a virulent phage to a lysogenic phage
(B) A change in bacterial phenotype due to the presence of a prophage
(C) The conversion of a prophage to a temperate phage
(D) The incorporation of a prophage into the bacterial chromosome

7. Which of the following types of media would best be used to isolate bacteria capable of growth in a high salt concentration?

(A) Minimal growth media
(B) Complex growth media
(C) Differential growth media
(D) Selective growth media

8. Which of the following characteristics applies to bacteriostatic antibiotics?

(A) Are effective when used in combination with bactericidal antibiotics to obtain a synergistic effect
(B) Include all the antimetabolites
(C) Are effective against bacteria in all phases of growth
(D) Include some broad-spectrum antibiotics

9. Which of the following statements concerning prokaryotic cells is true?

(A) They have coupled transcription and translation.
(B) They have processed mRNAs.
(C) They generally have exons and introns.
(D) They transfer secretory proteins into the Golgi apparatus before secretion.

10. Which of the following statements applies to the regulation of enzyme activity in bacterial cells?

(A) Can be coupled to the binding of effector molecules
(B) Can be controlled by a catabolite activator protein (CAP)
(C) May occur via attenuation sequences
(D) Can involve inducer molecules

Directions: Each of the numbered items or incomplete statements in this section is negatively phrased, as indicated by a capitalized word such as NOT, LEAST, or EXCEPT. Select the **one** lettered answer or completion that is **best** in each case.

11. All of the following characteristics are associated with the outer membrane EXCEPT it

(A) contains matrix porins.
(B) includes endotoxin.
(C) is a structure found in gram-negative bacteria.
(D) contains the enzymes involved in bacterial oxidative phosphorylation.

Directions: Each group of items in this section consists of lettered options followed by a set of numbered items. For each item, select the **one** lettered option that is most closely associated with it. Each lettered option may be selected once, more than once, or not at all.

Questions 12–15

Match each characteristic with the type of microorganism to which it pertains.

(A) Viruses
(B) Fungi
(C) Prions
(D) Bacteria
(E) Viroids

12. Contain RNA or DNA as a genetic material

13. Are dimorphic

14. May be inactivated by RNAses with endonuclease activity

15. Have a nuclear membrane

Questions 16–18

Match each metabolic feature with the appropriate bacterial type.

(A) Heterotrophs
(B) Obligate anaerobes
(C) Aerobes
(D) Facultative anaerobes
(E) Autotrophs

16. Synthesize organic compounds from inorganic compounds

17. May display the Pasteur effect

18. Lack superoxide dismutase

Questions 19–21

Match each characteristic with the appropriate type of phage.

(A) Prophage
(B) Virulent phage
(C) Temperate phage
(D) Filamentous phage

19. Used in phage typing

20. Not inactivated by proteases

21. Exemplified by phage lambda

Questions 22–24

Match each characteristic to the toxin that it best describes.

(A) *Escherichia coli* heat-labile toxin
(B) *Clostridium tetani* exotoxin
(C) *Corynebacterium diphtheriae* exotoxin
(D) *Pseudomonas aeruginosa* exotoxin
(E) *Clostridium perfringens* alpha-toxin

22. Has phospholipase C activity

23. Acts on synaptosomes

24. Induces electrolyte loss as a result of over-production of cyclic adenosine monophosphate.

Answers and Explanations

1–D. The transport of sugar into a bacterium frequently involves the transfer of a phosphate group to the sugar molecule.

2–B. *N*-acetylglucosamine and *N*-acetylmuramic acid are polymerized to form the peptidoglycan backbone of the cell wall.

3–C. Ordinary pili and the glycocalyx are the two bacterial structures that are involved in adherence.

4–D. Patients who are allergic to the various penicillins are frequently given one of the cephalosporins.

5–D. Superoxide dismutase is found in aerobic and facultative anaerobic bacteria. It protects them from the toxic free radical (O_2^-) by combining it with hydrogen ion to form hydrogen peroxide, which is subsequently degraded by peroxidase.

6–B. Lysogenic phage conversion refers to a change in bacterial phenotype resulting from the presence of a lysogenic prophage of a temperate phage.

7–D. A selective growth medium that contains a high salt concentration would permit bacterial growth.

8–D. The broad-spectrum antibiotics—tetracycline, chloramphenicol, the macrolides, and the lincomycins—are bacteriostatic. They are not effective against stationary phase bacteria and do not give a synergistic effect with bactericidal drugs.

9–A. Prokaryotic cells differ from eukaryotic cells in that the former have coupled transcription and translation of mRNA in the cytoplasm.

10–A. The biochemical activity of an enzyme may be regulated by binding of effector molecules or by biosynthetic pathway end-product feedback inhibition. Enzyme synthesis may be controlled by inducers, attenuation sequences, or catabolite activator protein.

11–D. The plasma membrane contains the enzymes involved in oxidative phosphorylation.

12–A. Viruses are the only entities that contain either RNA or DNA as genetic material. Fungi and bacteria have DNA, viroids have RNA, and the genetic material of prions is unknown.

13–B. Fungi are dimorphic; that is, they have two morphologic forms.

14–E. Viroids are single-stranded, covalently closed, circular RNA molecules that may be degraded by endonucleases.

15–B. Fungi are eukaryotic cells and, therefore, have a distinct nuclear membrane as part of the cellular structure.

16–E. Autotrophic bacteria do not require organic compounds for growth because they synthesize them from inorganic precursors.

17–D. Facultative anaerobes shift from a fermentative to a respiratory metabolism in the presence of air because the energy needs of the cell are met by consuming less glucose (Pasteur effect) under respiratory metabolism.

18–B. Superoxide dismutase, which is present in aerobes and facultative anaerobe organisms, protects them from the toxic O_2^- radical. This enzyme is not present in obligate anaerobes.

19–B. Phage typing is useful for identifying certain types of bacteria and depends on bacterial lysis by a selected set of virulent phages.

20–A. A prophage is the intracellular DNA of a phage and is, therefore, resistant to protease degradation.

21–C. *Escherichia coli* phage lambda is a prototypic temperate bacteriophage.

22–E. The phospholipase C activity of the alpha-toxin of *Clostridium perfringens* disrupts cellular and mitochondrial membranes.

23–B. *Clostridium tetani* exotoxin acts on synaptosomes, thereby causing hyperreflexia of skeletal muscles.

24–A. Both *Escherichia coli* heat-labile toxin and *Vibrio cholerae* choleragen stimulate the overproduction of cyclic adenosine monophosphate, resulting in fluid and electrolyte loss.

2

Bacterial Genetics

I. Organization of Genetic Information—General concepts

A. Deoxyribonucleic acid (DNA)

–stores genetic information as a sequence of nucleotide bases (adenine, thymine, guanosine, cytosine).

–is generally double-stranded, composed of complementary base pairs (A-T or G-C) joined by hydrogen bonds.

B. Ribonucleic acid (RNA)

–transcribes and translates DNA-bound genetic instructions for protein synthesis.

–is generally single-stranded.

–substitutes uracil for the thymine base used by DNA; the complementary base pairs for RNA are A-U or G-C.

–is found in three types:

1. Messenger RNA (mRNA)

–is the template that carries DNA gene sequences to ribosomes, the site of protein synthesis.

2. Ribosomal RNA (rRNA)

–is a structural component of ribosomes.

–acts as a substrate for protein synthesis.

3. Transfer RNA (tRNA)

–carries specific amino acids to the triplet-encoded, mRNA-borne message that translates the message into the amino acid structure of proteins.

II. Comparison of Prokaryotic and Eukaryotic Genomes

A. Eukaryotic genome

1. Structure

a. Except in some fungi, eukaryotes are **diploid** with two homologous copies of each chromosome.

b. Virtually all genetic information is contained in two or more linear chromosomes located within a membrane-bound nucleus.

c. Unlike prokaryotes and viruses, eukaryotic genomes contain **introns** (DNA sequences not translated into gene products) and redundant genetic information.

29

      d. Certain eukaryotic organelles (mitochondria, chloroplasts) contain a self-replicating, circular, double-stranded DNA molecule (**plasmid**) relating to their intracellular function.

  2. Replication

    –begins at several points along the linear DNA molecule.

    –is regulated by specific gene inducer or repressor substances.

    –involves a specialized structure, the **spindle,** which pulls newly formed chromosomes into separate nuclei during mitosis.

B. Prokaryotic genome

  1. Structure

    a. Most prokaryotes are **haploid** (single chromosome).

    b. Genes essential for bacterial growth are carried on a **single, circular chromosome** encoding generally several thousand genes; they are not enclosed in a membrane-circumscribed nucleus.

    c. Many bacteria contain additional, specialized genes on smaller **extrachromosomal plasmids.** Prokaryotic plasmids exist in transmissible and non-transmissible forms and may be integrated into the bacterial chromosome.

    d. Specialized information may also be carried on **transposons,** moveable genetic elements that cannot self-replicate. Transposons contain **insertion sequences** and can transfer their information by inserting themselves into other loci in the same or other genetic elements (e.g., plasmids, chromosomes, viral DNA).

  2. Replication

    a. Replicons

      –is a general term for double-stranded DNA circles (chromosomes, plasmids) capable of self-replication. Plasmid replication is independent of chromosome replication.

      –replicate bidirectionally (5′ PO_4 to 3′ OH) from a fixed origin.

      (1) The replicon attaches to a projection of the cell membrane (**mesosome**), which acts as the replication origin site, and one of the DNA strands is broken.

      (2) The 5′ end of the broken strand attaches to a new membrane site.

      (3) Elongation of the cell membrane via localized membrane synthesis pulls the broken strand through the mesosomal attachment site, where replication takes place.

      (4) Replication is completed, and the free ends of the new replicon are joined.

    b. Transposons

      –are replicated, along with the code of the host, after insertion into a replicon.

C. Viral genome

  1. Structure

    a. Genetic information may be coded as DNA or RNA and in double-stranded or single-stranded form.

b. The viral genome may contain exotic bases.

2. Replication

–takes place only after successful infection of an appropriate host.

–proceeds when the injected viral genome subverts normal replicative processes of the host, producing new virus particles.

3. Bacteriophage types

–may be discerned by their mode of propagation.

a. Lytic phages quickly produce many copies of themselves as they kill the host.

b. Temperate phages can lie seemingly dormant in the host (**prophage state**), timing replication of prophage genetic material to replication of the host cell. Various activation signals trigger the prophage to enter a lytic cycle, resulting in host death and the release of new phages.

III. Gene Transfer Between Organisms

–maintains genetic variability in microbes through the **exchange and recombination** of allelic forms of genes.

–is most efficient between cells of the same species.

–may also occur as the crossing over of homologous chromosomes or by nonhomologous means (e.g., movement of plasmids or transposons, insertion of viral genes).

–can result in the acquisition of new characteristics (e.g., antigens, toxins, antibiotic resistance).

–occurs via three mechanisms: conjugation, transduction, and transformation (Figure 2–1).

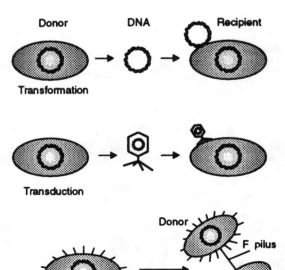

Figure 2–1. Three major mechanisms of genetic transfer in bacteria. In transformation, naked DNA is taken up directly by the recipient cell. During transduction, host DNA is transferred attached to viral DNA via bacteriophage. In conjugation, donor DNA is transferred via a conjugative plasmid (F pilus) to a recipient cell by physical contact. (Adapted with permission from Atlas RM: *Microbiology: Fundamentals and Application,* 2nd ed. New York, Macmillan, 1988, p 215.)

A. Conjugation

–is a one-way transfer of genetic material (usually plasmids) from donor to recipient by means of physical contact.

–typically involves three types of plasmids:

1. F$^+$ Cell

–possesses a fertility plasmid (F), mediating the creation of a sex pilus necessary for conjugal transfer of the F plasmid to the recipient.

–can integrate into chromosomal DNA, creating **high-frequency recombination (Hfr)** donors from which chromosomal DNA is readily transferred.

2. R factors

–contain genes conferring **drug resistance.** Frequently, the resistance genes are carried on transposons.

–express resistance phenotype through natural selection.

3. F′ and R′

–are recombinant **fertility or resistance plasmids** in which limited regions of chromosomal DNA can be replicated and transferred by conjugation independently of the chromosome.

B. Transduction (Figure 2–2)

–is **phage-mediated transfer** of host DNA sequences.

–can be performed by temperate phages and, under special conditions, by lytic phages.

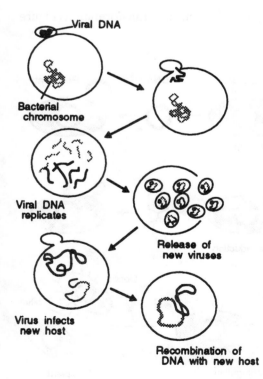

Viral DNA

Bacterial chromosome

Viral DNA replicates

Release of new viruses

Virus infects new host

Recombination of DNA with new host

Figure 2–2. Transduction of genes from one bacterium to another. Viral DNA enters the bacterial cell after attachment of bacteriophage. As it replicates, fragments of host DNA are incorporated into the viral DNA. Newly formed virus leaves the infected cell with new, altered DNA, infects a new host bacterium, and recombines with DNA of the latter cell, thereby transducing genes from one bacterium to another. (Adapted with permission from Atlas RM: *Microbiology: Fundamentals and Application*, 2nd ed. New York, Macmillan, 1988, p 215.)

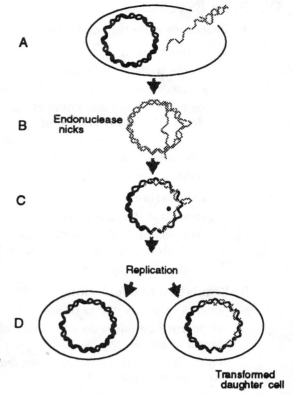

Figure 2–3. Sequential steps during bacterial transformation. *(A)* Double-stranded DNA enters the bacterial cell where an exonuclease converts the transforming DNA into a single strand. *(B)* A heteroduplex forms when transforming DNA pairs with complementary host DNA. *(C)* A ligase completes the integration of transforming DNA. *(D)* One daughter cell is a mutant, like the recipient cell, and one other is transformed. (Adapted with permission from Atlas RM: *Microbiology: Fundamentals and Application*, 2nd ed. New York, Macmillan, 1988, p 216.)

–occurs in two forms:

1. In **generalized transduction,** the phage randomly packages host DNA in a bacteriophage coat and may transfer any gene. The transducing particle contains only host DNA.

2. In **specialized transduction,** the lysogenic phage favors the transfer of host DNA segments near the site of prophage integration. Specialized transducing phages contain both viral and host genes.

C. **Transformation** (Figure 2–3)

–is the **direct uptake** and recombination of naked DNA fragments through the cell wall by competent bacteria. Natural occurrence of this process is uncommon.

–is sometimes mediated by surface **competence factors** (DNA receptor enzymes) produced only at a specific point in the bacterial growth cycle.

–can sometimes be forced by treatment with calcium chloride and temperature shock.

–is used in recombinant DNA research and commercially to introduce human genes via vectors into bacteria for rapid and large-scale production of human gene production.

IV. Gene Expression

A. Processes affecting expression

1. Transcription

–is the transfer of DNA-bound protein synthesis instructions to mRNA.

–is mediated in bacteria by **RNA polymerase.**

–is initiated by the binding of **sigma factor,** a subunit of RNA polymerase, to the **promoter region** of the DNA molecule.

–involves the unwinding of a short sequence of DNA bases and alignment of complementary ribonucleotide bases onto the DNA template.

–occurs in a $5'$ PO_4 to $3'$ OH direction.

2. Translation

–occurs at the ribosomes.

–is accomplished by the tRNA-mediated linkage of amino acids, in accordance with the triplet-encoded mRNA transcript.

–is the assembly of polypeptide chains from the mRNA transcript.

B. Regulation of expression

–occurs primarily during transcription.

–is determined partly by the ability of the DNA promoter region to bind with sigma factor.

–can be facilitated or blocked by regulator proteins binding to operator sequences near the promoter.

–typically affects an **operon,** a group of genes under the control of one operator controlled by the action of regulatory proteins.

1. Negative control

–is inhibition of transcription by the binding of a repressor protein.

–is exemplified by:

a. The *lac* operon

–controls expression of three structural genes for **lactose metabolism** via a repressor protein.

–transcription is induced by the presence of lactose (allolactose), which binds to the repressor protein and frees the *lac* operator.

b. The *trp* operon

–controls **tryptophan synthesis.**

–synthesis of tryptophan is halted by the binding of a repressor protein (tryptophan complex) to the *trp* operator when excess tryptophan is available.

2. Positive control

–is the initiation of transcription in response to the binding of an activator protein, for example:

a. Expression of the *ara* operon proceeds only when arabinose binds to a special protein, forming an activator compound necessary for the transcription of the *ara* operon.

    b. Cyclic adenosine monophosphate (cyclic AMP) binding protein, when bound to a specific DNA sequence near the promoter, enhances the expression of many genes associated with fermentation. Cyclic AMP enhances RNA polymerase activity.

V. Mutation

  –occurs approximately once for any gene in every 1 million cells.

  –is an induced or spontaneous heritable alteration of the DNA sequence.

  –introduces variability into the gene pool and changes in the phenotype.

  –may be caused by various mutagens, including ultraviolet light, acridine dyes, base analogues, and nitrous acid.

A. Mutation types

1. Nucleotide substitutions

  –arise from mutagenic activity or the mispairing of complementary bases during DNA replication.

  –often do not significantly disrupt the function of gene products.

2. Frameshift mutations

  –result from the insertion or deletion of one or two base pairs, disrupting the phase of the triplet-encoded DNA message.

3. Deletions

  –are usually large excisions of DNA, dramatically altering the sequence of coded proteins.

  –may also result in frameshift mutations.

4. Insertions

  –change genes and their products by integration of new DNA via transposons.

B. Results of mutation

1. Missense mutations

  –result in the substitution of one amino acid for another.

  –may be without phenotypic effect (silent mutation).

2. Nonsense mutations

  –terminate protein synthesis and result in truncated gene products.

  –usually result in inactive protein products.

C. Reversions

  –function lost to mutation may be regained in two ways:

1. Genotypic (true) reversion

  –is restoration at the site of DNA alteration.

2. Phenotypic (suppression) reversion

  –is restoration of an activity lost to mutation, often by a mutation at a second site (**suppressor mutation**).

Review Test

Directions: Each of the numbered items or incomplete statements in this section is followed by answers or by completions of the statement. Select the **one** lettered answer or completion that is **best** in each case.

1. Bacterial antibiotic resistance is frequently conveyed by

(A) a temperate bacteriophage.
(B) an R factor plasmid.
(C) a replicon.
(D) a lytic bacteriophage.
(E) an intron.

Directions: Each of the numbered items or incomplete statements in this section is negatively phrased, as indicated by a capitalized word such as NOT, LEAST, or EXCEPT. Select the **one** lettered answer or completion that is **best** in each case.

2. All of the following statements concerning the expression of the *lac* operon are true EXCEPT it

(A) must be initiated by the binding of an inducer protein.
(B) involves the synthesis of a regulatory gene protein.
(C) involves the synthesis of three structural genes.
(D) must have a functional promoter region.

Directions: Each group of items in this section consists of lettered options followed by a set of numbered items. For each item, select the **one** lettered option that is most closely associated with it. Each lettered option may be selected once, more than once, or not at all.

Questions 3–7

For each statement about genetic transfer among bacteria, select the term that most closely describes or defines it.

(A) Transformation
(B) Conjugation
(C) Transduction
(D) Transcription
(E) Recombination
(F) Translation

3. Requires cell–cell contact

4. Mediated by a bacteriophage that carries host-cell DNA

5. Exchange of allelic forms of genes

6. Involves synthesis of RNA from a DNA template

7. Creates high-frequency recombination (Hfr) donors

Answers and Explanations

1–B. R factor (resistance) plasmids contain genes for proteins that degrade antibiotics or alter antibiotic transport, thus conferring antibiotic resistance. They also carry transfer genes, which facilitate their intercellular transfer to other genomes.

2–A. The transcription of the *lac* operon is under negative control. Initiation depends on the binding of allolactose to a repressor protein. This reaction prevents the repressor from binding to the operator region, thus allowing RNA polymerase to bind and transcription to proceed.

3–B. Conjugation involves the transfer of genetic information from a donor to a recipient cell during physical contact.

4–C. Bacteriophages containing portions of host-cell DNA can introduce this genetic material into new host cells via the process of transduction.

5–E. DNA or genetic recombination is the general term used to describe the exchange of allelic forms of genes in bacteria or eukaryotic cells.

6–D. The synthesis of mRNA from DNA by DNA-dependent RNA polymerase is called transcription.

7–E. Hfr donors, which result from the integration of a fertility (F) factor into chromosomal DNA, are created by recombination.

3
Bacteriology

In this chapter, the medically important pathogens are described in association with the major organ system that they affect. Because several organ systems may be affected by the same or different species from the same genera, their relevance in other systems is only highlighted.

Upper Respiratory Infections

I. *Streptococcus pyogenes* (Group A)

  A. **General characteristics—*Streptococcus pyogenes***

   –occurs as single, paired, or chained gram-positive cocci, depending on the environment.

   –is a facultative anaerobe.

   –attaches to epithelial surfaces via the lipotechoic acid portion of fimbriae (pili).

  B. **Classification—*Streptococcus pyogenes***

   –is classified as **group** A of the 21 Lancefield groups of streptococci, which are distinguished serologically by slight differences in specific **cell wall carbohydrates.**

   –contains group A–specific carbohydrate and several antigenic proteins (**M, T, and R antigens**) in the cell wall.

   –is subdivided into more than 80 types based on antigenic differences in the M protein (e.g., *S. pyogenes* type 12 is a nephritogenic strain).

   –is classified into the β-hemolytic group of the three types of enzymatic hemolysis of red blood cells produced by streptococci on blood agar plates:

   1. **Alpha (α)-hemolytic group** is characterized by incomplete lysis, with green pigment surrounding the colony.

   2. **Beta (β)-hemolytic group** is characterized by total lysis and release of hemoglobin and a clear area around the colony.

   3. **Gamma (γ)-hemolytic group** is characterized by absence of lysis.

   –is **sensitive to bacitracin,** an antibacterial polypeptide, in contrast to other streptococci.

39

Table 3–1. Streptococcal Groups and Their Associated Diseases and Distinguishing Features

Group	Associated Diseases	Distinguishing Features
Group A (prototype: *Streptococcus pyogenes*)	Pharyngitis	Contains M protein
	Scarlet fever	Bacitracin-sensitive
	Impetigo	Catalase-negative
	Cellulitis and erysipelas	β-hemolytic
	Rheumatic fever	Produces erythrogenic exotoxins
	Acute glomerulonephritis	Produces streptolysins S and O
	Endocarditis	
Group B (prototype: *Streptococcus agalactiae*)	Neonatal sepsis (early and late onset)	Part of normal oral and vaginal flora
	Meningitis	Hydrolyzes hippurate
		Has five serotypes
		Bacitracin-resistant
		Sialic acid capsule
		β-hemolytic
Group D (enterococci and nonenterococcal organisms)	Endocarditis	Part of normal oral and intestinal flora
	Urinary tract infections	Causes variable hemolysis
	Septicemia	Bacitracin-resistant
		Grow in 40% bile or pH 9.6
		Killed by penicillin
Streptococcus viridans (no group classification)	Endocarditis	Part of normal oral flora
	Dental caries	α-Hemolytic
		Not inhibited by optochin
		Differentiate from pneumococci
Streptococcus pneumoniae	Pneumonia	Large polysaccharide capsule
		Antiphagocytic
		Sensitive to optochin
		Lysed by bile

(handwritten note in Group A cell: C rxnse)

   –is catalase negative.

   –rarely becomes resistant to penicillin.

   –can be detected by throat smears on blood agar, latex agglutination tests, or rapid (10-minute) test using a fluorescein-labeled monoclonal antibody.

   –is compared with other serogroups in Table 3–1.

C. **Attributes of pathogenicity—*Streptococcus pyogenes***

   –possesses M proteins, **a potent virulence factor** found on fimbriae that interferes with phagocytosis.

   –has **a nonantigenic, antiphagocytic hyaluronic acid capsule** that promotes invasiveness.

   –secretes three serologic types of **erythrogenic exotoxins** that require lysogenic phage for production and cause the rash in scarlet fever.

–produces two hemolysins: **streptolysin S** (a leukocidal protein responsible for β-hemolysis on blood agar plates) and **streptolysin O** (an oxygen-sensitive leukocidal protein).

–possesses multiple other enzyme systems (e.g., hyaluronidase, streptokinase, streptodornase, nicotinamide adenine dinucleotidase).

D. Clinical diseases

1. Streptococcal pharyngitis

–is characterized by sore throat, fever, headache, nausea, cervical lymphadenopathy, and leukocytosis.

–can result in complications (e.g., tonsillar abscesses, mastoiditis, septicemia, osteomyelitis, rheumatic fever).

–is differentiated from viral infections and infectious mononucleosis by **intense pharyngeal redness,** edema of the mucous membranes, and a purulent exudate.

–is treated with penicillin, preferably one that is effective for 3 weeks.

2. Scarlet fever

–exhibits symptoms resembling those of streptococcal pharyngitis.

–is accompanied by a rash caused by erythrogenic toxins.

3. Rheumatic fever

–follows group A streptococcal throat infection in genetically predisposed individuals; however, 20% of patients may show no early signs or symptoms.

–results in a systemic inflammatory process involving the connective tissue, heart, joints, and central nervous system (CNS).

–may lead to progressive chronic debilitation.

–may **damage heart muscle and valves,** with **mitral stenosis** as a lesion hallmark.

–is presumed to result from antistreptococcal antibodies cross-reacting with sarcolemmal muscle and kidney, leading to a damaging inflammatory process.

–should be treated promptly with penicillin, which should be continued prophylactically to prevent recurring infections and increased damage.

II. *Haemophilus influenzae*

A. General characteristics—*Haemophilus influenzae*

–is an organism that colonizes the upper respiratory tract and, in unvaccinated young children, may cause **otitis media, meningitis, epiglottitis, cellulitis, bronchitis, bacteremia, arthritis, osteomyelitis,** and **conjunctivitis.**

–Most normal flora are nonencapsulated and cause most otitis media, sinusitis, and bronchitis infections, whereas serious disease is usually caused by encapsulated forms, most commonly type B.

–*Haemophilus parainfluenzae* can cause the same spectrum of infection.

–is a gram-negative pleomorphic rod and contains endotoxin.

–requires the X (hemin) and V (NAD) factors, which, although found in blood, must be released by lysis. (Therefore, it is cultured on chocolate agar or seen as satellite growth near *Staphylococcus aureus* on blood agar.)

B. Attributes of pathogenicity

1. Polysaccharide capsule (polyribitol phosphate)

–antibodies to the capsule relate to immune status. Little or no antibody exists in unvaccinated children age 3 months to 2 years, the period of the highest incidence of meningitis. In unvaccinated individuals beyond 5 years old, increasing antibody titers appear and infection incidence decreases.

–anticapsular antibodies promote phagocytosis and resultant killing of the organism.

2. IgA protease

–facilitates upper respiratory tract colonization.

C. Clinical disease

1. Common infections

a. Chronic otitis media, sinusitis, and bronchitis occur in older children and adults (unencapsulated strains).

b. Acute bacterial meningitis (see Central Nervous System Infections)

2. Rare infections

a. Acute bacterial epiglottitis in young children (usually caused by capsule type B) is rapidly progressive. Severe problems occur within 2 hours; death may occur within 24 hours. Microabscesses and edema restrict breathing, causing respiratory arrest.

b. Pneumonia (see XI B)

D. Laboratory diagnosis

1. Specimens. Otitis media is generally not cultured. Posterior pharynx cultures in epiglottitis should not be done. Blood and direct aspirates are cultures taken for other respiratory infections.

2. Cultures on chocolate agar speciate using requirement for X and V factor.

E. Control

1. Treatment. Beta-lactamase production is seen in 20% to 30% of strains.

2. Prevention

a. Vaccination with conjugate vaccine reduces the incidence of type B infections.

b. This vaccine and other important bacterial vaccines are listed in Table 3–2.

III. *Corynebacterium diphtheriae*

A. General characteristics—*Corynebacterium diphtheriae*

–is a gram-positive club-shaped rod (called a coryneform) often occurring in V- and L-shaped arrangements or clumps sometimes called "Chinese characters."

Table 3–2. Bacterial Vaccines

Organism	Component	Mechanism of Protection	Use
Streptococcus pneumoniae	23 Capsular polysaccharides	Antibodies to capsule	Elderly; compromised patients
Neisseria meningitidis	Capsular polysaccharides (A, C, W135, Y)	Antibodies to capsule	Infants; military settings
Haemophilus influenzae	Capsular polysaccharide conjugated to diphtheria toxoid or to *N. meningitidis* outer membrane protein	Antibodies to capsule	Infants
Bordetella pertussis	Inactivated whole organism for primary series Acellular for boosters	Antibodies and cell-mediated immunity	Infants
Corynebacterium diphtheriae	Diphtheria toxoid	Antibodies to toxin	Infants
Clostridium tetani	Tetanospasmin toxoid	Antibodies to toxin	Infants

   –causes diphtheria through upper respiratory colonization and elaboration of
   a potent exotoxin. (In immunized persons, this occurs without significant
   disease.)

B. Classification—*Corynebacterium diphtheriae*

   –is related to the nocardia and mycobacteria.

C. Attributes of pathogenicity—diphtheria exotoxin

   –is a potent A-B ("two component") exotoxin, with the B component binding
   to specific cell membrane receptors required to trigger uptake of the A-B
   component by the cell. Primary target cells include upper respiratory tract,
   heart, and nerve cells.

   –is produced only in strains of *C. diphtheriae*, which are stably infected (lysoge-
   nized) by *β*-corynephage. The DNA of the bacteriophage resides in the bacterial cell (*tox +* cells) and directs the synthesis of the toxin. Toxin production
   occurs at low iron concentrations.

   –component A is an enzyme (ADP ribosyl transferase) which ADP ribosylates
   elongation factor 2 (EF2) inhibiting nascent peptide chain movement, thus
   shutting down protein synthesis. Estimates suggest the enzymic activity of
   one molecule of toxin can effectively shut down an entire cell.

   –in its inactivated form (toxoid), is a component of the diphtheria and tetanus
   toxoids and pertussis (DTP) vaccine.

D. Clinical disease—respiratory tract diphtheria (membranous pharyngitis)

–is rare ($<$ 5 cases/year in the United States since 1983).

–begins as a mild pharyngitis with slight fever and chills.

–spreads up to the nasopharynx or down to the larynx and trachea. The bacteria themselves do not disseminate but elaborate the diphtheria exotoxin, which circulates and causes additional symptoms such as hoarseness and stridor.

–results in a firmly adherent, dirty gray, spreading pseudomembrane, composed of inflammatory necrosis, fibrin, epithelial cells, neutrophils, monocytes, and bacteria.

–causes cervical adenitis and edema, which, in severe cases, may produce the characteristic "bull neck" appearance.

–has the following complications:

   –asphyxiation from the pseudomembrane

   –myocarditis and, occasionally, more severe cardiotoxicity

   –paralysis of the soft palate and more severe neuropathies

E. Laboratory diagnosis

–yields the highest success rate when rapid presumptive clinical diagnosis permits a rapid therapeutic start, which is supported later by laboratory identification.

–requires notification of laboratory and culture on two special media:

   –Löffler's coagulated serum medium on which *C. diphtheriae* produces many metachromatically staining volutin granules.

   –tellurite-containing differential medium. *C. diphtheriae* imports and reduces tellurite, turning the colonies gray to black.

–requires demonstration of toxin production, which is generally done with the agar diffusion Elek test, in which filter paper strips containing diphtheria antitoxin are perpendicular to streaks of the patient's strain and known toxin-producing and non–toxin-producing strains. Where antigen (the toxin produced by the growth) and antibody meet at optimal concentration, a precipitin line is seen in the agar.

F. Control

1. **Treatment** is with antitoxin and antibiotics.

2. **Prevention** is by proper vaccination with toxoid in DTP followed by Td (tetanus and diphtheria toxoids) boosters. Vaccination does not prevent colonization but has resulted in greatly reduced colonization rates.

IV. *Fusobacterium nucleatum*

A. General characteristics—*Fusobacterium nucleatum*

–are gram-negative, polymorphic, long, slender filaments and fusiform rods.

–are non–spore-forming anaerobes killed by oxygen.

–occur normally in the mouth and occasionally in the stool.

–prompt local anaerobic growth when oxygen is used by oral aerobic or facultative microorganisms, thereby lowering the redox potential.

–anaerobes outnumber aerobes 100:1 in the mouth.

–attributes of pathogenicity have not been clearly identified.

B. Infections—*Fusobacterium nucleatum*

–acts synergistically with oral spirochetes, resulting in an ulcerating, necrotizing gingivitis (Vincent's angina, or trench mouth).

–is responsible for head, neck, and chest infections, and is a common microorganism isolated from brain abscesses.

C. Treatment is with penicillin and cephalosporin (penicillin G is preferred).

Lower Respiratory Tract Infections

I. *Streptococcus pneumoniae*

A. General characteristics—*Streptococcus pneumoniae*

–is part of the **normal oropharyngeal flora** in 40% to 70% of human beings.

–is a gram-positive, α-hemolytic, lancet-shaped diplococcus.

–possesses a group-specific carbohydrate common to all pneumococci, which can be precipitated by a C-reactive protein found in the plasma during an inflammatory response.

–quantitation of precipitate is a clinical laboratory index of the extent of inflammation, not an antigen–antibody reaction.

–experimental injection of relatively large amounts of capsular polysaccharide leads to tolerance rather than immunity.

–possesses a type-specific polysaccharide capsule with more than 80 different antigenic types.

–types are differentiated by swelling of the capsule in the presence of type-specific antiserum (**quellung reaction**).

–should be differentiated from nonpathogenic *Streptococcus viridans* because the latter also is gram-positive, is usually diplococcal, is found in the pharynx and sputum, and produces α-hemolysis on blood agar.

–is differentiated from other streptococci by:

1. Sensitivity to the quinine derivative ethyl hydrocuprine (**optochin**)

2. Sensitivity to bile, which solubilizes pneumococci by increasing an autolytic amidase

3. Fermentation of inulin

B. Attributes of pathogenicity

1. Little evidence exists for production of toxins; disease probably occurs through multiplication.

2. Virulence is attributed to the antiphagocytic capacity of the capsule.

C. Clinical disease

1. **Pneumococcal pneumonia** seldom occurs as a primary infection.

2. Pathogenicity is associated with disturbances of normal defense barriers of the respiratory tract.

3. Infants, elderly, immunosuppressed persons, and chronic alcoholics are most vulnerable.

4. Self-infection can occur by aspiration after epiglottal reflexes have been slowed due to chilling, anesthesia, morphine use, alcohol use, virus infection, or increased pulmonary edema.

5. Classic manifestations include an abrupt onset, fever, chills, chest pain, and productive cough, followed by a crisis on days 7 to 10 after infection.

6. In 50% to 70% of untreated cases, **recovery** is associated with the appearance of an anticapsular antibody.

7. Two thirds of deaths occur in the first 5 days of infection.

8. The disease is identified by **culture of lung sputum** (not saliva), followed by typing via the quellung reaction.

9. **Otitis media** and **septicemia** occur in infants older than 2 months of age.

10. Pneumococcal pneumonia is a leading cause of bacterial meningitis (see Central Nervous System Infections).

D. **Treatment**

1. Penicillin or other appropriate antibiotics are used; however, penicillin-resistant strains are emerging.

2. An effective vaccine for adults, which contains at least 23 different type-specific polysaccharides, is available; the vaccine is poorly immunogenic in infants.

II. *Mycoplasma pneumoniae*

A. **General characteristics—***Mycoplasma pneumoniae*

–is the smallest and simplest of the self-replicating prokaryotes.

–lacks a cell wall (unique for bacteria) and should not be confused with bacterial L forms, which lack a cell wall in the presence of antibiotics. (L forms revert back to cell wall forms after the antibiotic is removed.)

–requires cholesterol (unique for bacteria).

–is a mucous membrane pathogen that does not invade other tissues.

B. **Classification**

1. *Mycoplasma pneumoniae* [also termed pleuropneumonia-like organism (PPLO)], or Eaton agent causes respiratory tract infections.

2. *Mycoplasma hominis* and *Ureaplasma urealyticum* (*T-strain mycoplasma*) appear to be involved in genital tract infections.

C. **Attributes of pathogenicity—***Mycoplasma pneumoniae*

–organisms possess a lipopolysaccaride, LPS, different from that of gram-negative bacteria.

–has a glycolipid fraction that may play a role in autoimmune-like reactions.

–releases hydrogen peroxide, which may damage epithelial cells.

D. **Clinical manifestations—***Mycoplasma pneumoniae*

–causes primary atypical pneumonia, sometimes called **walking pneumonia.**

–causes a slow onset of fever, throbbing headache, malaise, and nonproductive cough; over several weeks, interstitial or bronchopneumonic pneumonia develops; radiographs reveal segmental lobar pneumonia.

–has its highest incidence in children age 5 to 15 years.

–accounts for one third of all cases of pneumonia in teenagers.

E. Laboratory diagnosis

1. Identification

a. In vitro culture is not routinely attempted; identification is based on clinical presentation and serology.

b. Culture is performed on PPLO agar; colonies may not form for 2 to 3 weeks; colonies exhibit a characteristic "fried egg" appearance.

c. Giemsa stain on cultured organisms reveals small pleomorphic bacteria.

d. DNA probes are under development.

2. Clinical specimens include the following:

a. Acute and convalescent sera; complement fixation test and cold agglutinin reaction

b. Nasopharyngeal secretions

F. Control

1. Treatment is with tetracycline or erythromycin over a prolonged period to help resolve manifestations; *M. pneumoniae* is still shed by treated patients.

2. Prevention. Reinfections with *M. pneumoniae* are common.

III. *Legionella pneumophila*

A. General characteristics—*Legionella pneumophila*

–is a poorly staining, gram-negative, rod-shaped bacterium that may form longer filaments.

–stains well only with Dieterle's silver stain.

–is a facultative, intracellular parasite.

–has a high density of cellular branched fatty acids.

–is catalase positive; most strains are weakly oxidase positive.

–hydrolyzes hippurate (unlike other species of *Legionella*).

–is a stream bacterium that contaminates air-conditioning cooling towers.

–is frequently harbored by amoeba.

B. Classification—*Legionella pneumophila*

–is classified in a new family and genus of **aquatic organisms.**

–is the major causative agent of **legionnaires' disease.**

C. Attributes of pathogenicity—*Legionella pneumophila*

–grows **intracellularly** and fails to activate the alternate complement pathway.

–produces cytotoxin, a small peptide, interfering with oxygen-dependent processes of phagocytosis.

–produces β-lactamases to inactivate cephalosporins and penicillins.

–produces an endotoxin.

D. Clinical disease

1. Pneumonia (legionnaires' disease)

–is acquired by **inhalation** of the organism from environmental sources.

–is most common in smokers and in the presence of an organ transplant, T-cell defect, or chronic lung disease.

–starts with abrupt onset of fever and chills, an initially nonproductive cough, headache (frequently accompanied by mental confusion), diarrhea, microscopic hematuria, and proteinuria.

–peaks in frequency from July to October (air-conditioning cooling towers are more susceptible to bacterial growth in hot months).

–often occurs in clusters.

–is not transmitted by person-to-person contact.

2. Pontiac fever

–is a mild disease consisting of headache, fever, and myalgia without pneumonia.

–is caused by *L. pneumophila.*

E. Laboratory diagnosis—*L. pneumophila*

–is often diagnosed by direct fluorescent antibody staining of specimens or by demonstration of Dieterle's silver-stained rods in a specimen demonstrated to be negative by Gram stain.

–may be grown and identified on buffered charcoal yeast extract agar (which provides the required cysteine and iron).

–may also be identified by an increase in antibody titer.

F. Control

1. Treatment

–is with erythromycin.

–is given concomitantly with rifampin therapy to immunocompromised patients.

2. Prevention. Contaminated sources, cooling towers, shower heads, and nebulizers should be decontaminated with hyperchlorination, other disinfectants, or heat.

IV. *Bordetella pertussis*

A. General characteristics—*Bordetella pertussis*

–is a strict aerobic, gram-negative coccobacillus.

–causes whooping cough, predominantly in children younger than 1 year of age.

–is part of the highly effective DTP vaccine.

–is a classic example of the need for continued vaccination; 2000 to 5000 cases occur yearly in the United States, despite a high rate of vaccination; in countries where vaccine compliance waned, major outbreaks followed within 5 years.

B. Classification

1. *Bordetella pertussis* causes classic **whooping cough.**

2. *Bordetella parapertussis* causes a mild form of whooping cough.

3. *Bordetella bronchiseptica* is primarily an animal pathogen that occasionally causes a mild whooping cough in humans.

C. Attributes of pathogenicity

    1. Pertussis toxin (A-B type) is a single antigen causing local tissue damage associated with inflammation.

    2. Hemagglutinin (adhesins) are responsible for specific attachment to the cilia of the upper respiratory tract epithelium.

    3. An **undefined cough toxin** is probably active neurologically; the cough persists for weeks after organisms are killed by erythromycin.

D. Clinical manifestations—*Bordetella pertussis*

    –is localized only in the respiratory tract and is highly contagious.

    –is characterized by a **paroxysmal cough.**

    –is associated with a variety of symptoms; generally, the younger the patient, the more severe the disease.

    –is associated with the following prognosis: one third of patients recover without problems, neurologic problems develop in one third, and one third exhibit severe neurologic deficits (coma, convulsions, blindness, and paralysis, probably associated with anoxia).

    –occurs in three distinct stages:

        1. Catarrhal stage: mild upper respiratory tract infection with sneezing, slight cough, low fever, and runny nose (lasts 1 to 2 weeks)

        2. Paroxysmal stage: extends to the lower respiratory tract, with severe cough (5 to 20 forced hacking coughs per 20 seconds); little time to breathe causes anoxia and vomiting; tissue damage predisposes the patient to secondary bacterial infections and pneumonia (lasts 1 to 6 weeks)

        3. Convalescent stage: less severe cough that may persist for several months

E. Laboratory diagnosis

    –relies primarily on clinical manifestations.

    –reveals lymphocytosis.

    –is made using laboratory specimens obtained with posterior nasopharyngeal swabs.

    –has the best chance for a positive specimen to be obtained during the catarrhal stage; organisms are rarely isolated after 1 to 3 weeks of the paroxysmal stage.

    –requires plating on charcoal blood agar with cephalexin.

    –must be performed by inoculating agar immediately because organisms die rapidly.

    –uses immunofluorescence, either directly on the patient specimen or after in vitro growth.

F. Treatment

    –is with erythromycin to eradicate *B. pertussis.*

    –is with other antibiotics to prevent secondary bacterial infection; 30% of patients develop pneumonias attributable to other organisms.

    –is with supportive measures (e.g., secretions are removed, oxygen and humidity are provided, electrolytes and nutritional status are monitored).

–is not necessarily a failure when cough persists after erythromycin therapy (due to residual toxins).

G. Prevention

1. The disease is most contagious in the catarrhal stage when the highest concentration of organisms is present; the patient should be isolated (especially from infants age 1 year or younger) for 4 to 6 weeks.

2. The attack rate is 90% in persons who are nonimmune to *B. pertussis*.

3. Immune contacts who are younger than age 4 years should be boosted with vaccine, and prophylactic erythromycin should be given.

4. Nonimmune contacts should be given erythromycin only (it is too late to give vaccine).

5. Vaccination should be started with the killed whole organism at age 2 months, and three boosters should be given (maternal antibodies do not provide protection).

6. Occasional severe adverse reactions to vaccine involve encephalopathy, CNS abnormalities, convulsions, and brain damage in 1 in 300,000 to 5,000,000 recipients; mild adverse reactions of tenderness and fever routinely occur.

7. A newer, less toxic acellular vaccine has been approved for booster injections.

8. A low rate of severe adverse reactions dictates continued routine use of the vaccine.

V. *Chlamydia psittaci*

A. General characteristics—*Chlamydia psittaci*

–is an **obligate intracellular pathogen** (cannot synthesize adenosine triphosphate).

–has a cell wall, but the cell wall lacks peptidoglycan.

–resembles gram-negative bacteria.

–exists in two forms:

1. An **elementary body,** which is infectious

2. A **reticular body,** which is the intracellular reproductive form

B. Attributes of pathogenicity

1. Some toxic effects of antigens kill the host cell.

2. The reticular body divides by binary fission in an intracellular vacuole.

3. The pathogen usually causes subclinical infections in the natural host.

C. Clinical disease

–is a natural disease of birds (ornithosis), particularly psittacine birds such as parrots.

–is a zoonotic human disease of the lower respiratory tract that ranges from subclinical to fatal pneumonia.

–is an occupational disease associated with the raising and processing of poultry.

   D. Laboratory diagnosis

   –is usually made on the basis of patient history and clinical symptoms.

   –may be aided by fluorescent monoclonal antibody staining of elementary bodies in exudates.

   E. Control

      1. Treatment is with tetracycline.

      2. Prevention is by improved hygienic standards.

VI. *Chlamydia pneumoniae*

   A. General characteristics—*Chlamydia pneumoniae*

   –was formerly known as the TWAR agent.

   –has the same general characteristics as those listed for *C. psittaci.*

   B. Attributes of pathogenicity. Some toxic effects of antigens kill the host cell.

   C. Clinical disease

   –causes various lower respiratory infections, including bronchitis and pneumonia.

   –causes "walking pneumonia" in young adults.

   D. Laboratory diagnosis requires organism isolation accompanied by fluorescent antibody staining or complement fixation testing for antibody.

   E. Control is with tetracycline.

VII. *Mycobacterium tuberculosis*

   A. General characteristics—*Mycobacterium tuberculosis*

   –is a slender, slightly curved rod; the waxy arabinogalactan cell wall layer (known as Wax D) is an active immunoadjuvant in complete Freund's adjuvant.

   –has a complex peptidoglycan–arabinogalactan mycolate cell wall that is approximately 60% lipid.

   –stains poorly with Gram stain but has a highly cross-linked peptidoglycan and no endotoxin.

   –is an acid-fast bacillus that retains the carbol fuchsin even when decolorized by acid alcohol (because of long-chain fatty acids called **mycolic acids** in the cell wall).

   –is resistant to acid and alkali, which allows treatment of sputum to reduce normal contaminating bacteria before culture.

   –is a slow grower because it has single copies of ribosomal genes.

   –is resistant to drying and to many disinfectants.

   –stimulates a strong cell-mediated immune response in a healthy host.

   B. Classification

      1. Mycobacteria are related to the *corynebacterium, actinomyces,* and *nocardia.*

      2. *M. tuberculosis* is distinguished from other mycobacteria by substantial niacin production.

C. **Attributes of pathogenicity**

1. **Sulfatides** (sulfur-containing glycolipids) potentiate the toxicity of cord factor and promote **intracellular survival** by inhibiting the phagosome–lysosome fusion and suppressing superoxide formation.

2. **Cord factor** (a trehalose mycolate) disrupts mitochondrial membranes, interfering with respiration and oxidative phosphorylation.

   a. Cord factor inhibits neutrophil migration and causes the organism to grow in a cord or serpentine fashion in culture.

   b. Cord factor is associated with **granuloma formation.**

D. **Clinical disease—tuberculosis**

   –is caused by *M. tuberculosis* and *Mycobacterium bovis.*

   –is more common in persons of lower socioeconomic class, recent immigrants, and persons infected with the human immunodeficiency virus.

   –exposure occurs most commonly through inhalation of organisms in **droplet nuclei** from another individual or through ingestion of contaminated food.

1. **Infection** begins in the **lungs;** in immunologically naive individuals, it begins with a mild inflammatory reaction.

   a. The phagocytosed organisms replicate rapidly.

   b. A small **Ghon lesion** forms in the lung and regional lymph nodes (a combination termed the **Ghon complex**).

   c. **Clinical findings** usually are insignificant at this stage.

2. When cell numbers are relatively small and the cell-mediated response is high, tissue response (lymphocytes, macrophages, Langhans' giant cells, fibroblasts, and capillaries) produces granulomas containing the infection.

3. When cell numbers are large and cell-mediated immunity (CMI) is high, there is an exudative and gaseous response that may result in cavitary disease and bronchogenic spread.

4. In an **immunologically incompetent individual,** the infection spreads either hematogenously, resulting in **miliary tuberculosis,** or by coalescence.

5. In an **untreated primary infection,** the infection may be reactivated later (in the elderly or by conditions of immunosuppression).

   a. Called secondary or postprimary tuberculosis, **reactivation** occurs only in previously sensitized individuals.

   b. **Necrosis** is a prominent finding.

E. **Laboratory diagnosis—tuberculosis** is diagnosed (in addition to symptoms of cough and an abnormal chest radiograph) by:

1. Demonstration of **acid-fast bacteria** in sputum, induced sputum, or gastric washings.

   a. The specimen is first screened with auramine-rhodamine fluorescent stain and read with fluorescent microscope.

   b. Positive specimens are confirmed with Ziehl-Neelsen acid-fast stain (Table 3–3).

Table 3–3. Ziehl-Neelsen Acid-Fast Stain

Steps	Color at End of Each Step	
Reagent	**Acid-fast Bacteria**	**Non–acid-fast Bacteria***
Carbol fuchsin with heat†	Red (hot pink)	Red (hot pink)
Acid alcohol	Red	Colorless
Methylene blue (pale blue)‡	Red	Blue

* *Mycobacterium* is acid fast; *Nocardia* is partially acid fast. Most bacteria are non–acid fast.
† Without heat, the dye would not enter mycobacterial cells.
‡ Sputa and human cells appear blue.

2. **Culture** of *M. tuberculosis* or *M. bovis* from specimens on Lowenstein-Jensen medium or in a radiometric test demonstrating the metabolism of ^{14}C-labeled palmitic acid with release of $^{14}CO_2$.

3. **Skin testing** with a purified protein derivative (PPD) of *M. tuberculosis*.

    a. A positive test result indicates infection at some time but not necessarily current disease. (Disease is indicated by clinical symptoms and positive cultures.)

    b. Individuals with known tuberculous disease and a negative PPD test are **anergic** to the antigen (a poor prognostic sign).

F. **Control**

  –is prophylactic using **isoniazid** in individuals with known exposure to tuberculosis and conversion of the skin test to positive, or in anyone with a positive skin test who is younger than 35 years old.

  –for uncomplicated pulmonary tuberculosis in a previously untreated, cooperative patient is with isoniazid, rifampin, pyrazinamide, and ethambutol for 2 months followed by 4 months of isoniazid and rifampin (unless susceptibilities indicate drug resistance).

  –is hampered by resistant strains that are emerging.

VIII. *Mycobacterium avium-intracellulare* (MAI or MAC for *M. avium* complex)

A. **General characteristics**—*Mycobacterium avium-intracellulare*

  –is a *Mycobacterium;* thus it is acid-fast with a cell wall similar to that of *M. tuberculosis.*

  –does not produce niacin nor reduce nitrate.

  –is generally nonchromogenic but strains from acquired immune deficiency syndrome (AIDS) patients may produce the carotenoid pigments.

  –is an environmental organism found in water, soil, birds, and other animals.

B. **Attributes of pathogenicity**—*Mycobacterium avium-intracellulare*

  –is an opportunist rather than a pathogen, causing diseases resembling tuberculosis in compromised patients.

  –is not considered contagious.

  –is an intracellular organism.

C. **Clinical disease**

–occurs as chronic bronchopulmonary pulmonary disease in adults with preexisting chronic pulmonary problems.

–occurs as an overwhelming disseminated infection in AIDS patients with low CD4+ counts. (This condition is common in AIDS patients and is an AIDS-defining condition with a poor prognosis.) It is characterized by fever, night sweats, anorexia, weight loss, and diarrhea. Although the lungs are involved, the gastrointestinal tract may be the initial site of infection.

D. **Laboratory diagnosis** is with blood cultures using a variety of procedures, including radiometric techniques with probes for rapid identification of growth.

E. **Control**

1. Treatment response in AIDS patients is poor because of their compromised immune status.

2. The organism has underlying drug resistance.

IX. *Nocardia*

A. **General characteristics—*Nocardia***

–is a filamentous soil **bacterium** that fragments into rods.

–is gram-positive and partially acid-fast.

–is aerobic.

–grows relatively slowly.

–is related to *Corynebacterium*, *Mycobacterium*, and *Actinomyces* (Table 3–4).

B. **Clinical manifestations—pulmonary infection**

–from inhalation of *Nocardia* organisms is **acute** in children and compromised adults and is **chronic** in other adults.

–may **metastasize** to the brain.

C. **Laboratory diagnosis**

–is often made at autopsy.

–tests include gastric washings, lung biopsy, and brain biopsy with culture and cytologic testing.

D. **Control** is by surgically draining abscesses, removing necrotic tissues, and administering **sulfonamides.**

Table 3–4. Characteristics of Mycobacteria and Related Organisms

Genus	Anaerobic	Acid Fast	Morphologic Features
Actinomyces	Yes	No	Rods, filaments, some branching
Corynebacterium	No	No	Rods
Mycobacterium	No (obligate aerobe)	Yes	Rods (slightly curved or straight)
Nocardia	No	Partially	Filaments fragmenting into rods

X. *Prevotella melaninogenica* (formerly *Bacteroides melaninogenicus*)

   A. General characteristics—Prevotella melaninogenica

      –is a small gram-negative coccobacillus with occasional long forms.

      –has a distinctive black colonial appearance on agar.

      –is mainly a part of the normal flora of the mouth; saliva has 10^9 anaerobes/ mL.

      –is found in low numbers in the gastrointestinal and genitourinary tracts.

   B. Attributes of pathogenicity—*Prevotella melaninogenica*

      –possesses a potent endotoxin and a collagenase.

   C. Infections—*Prevotella melaninogenica*

      –causes lung abscesses; putrid sputum is a clue to anaerobic lung infection.

      –causes infections of the female genital tract.

   D. Treatment is with metronidazole and clindamycin. Carbapenems are the most potent beta-lactam.

XI. OTHER

   A. *Staphylococcus aureus* pneumonia

      –has a high mortality rate.

      –is rare except as a secondary infection following influenza (mostly in patients younger than 1 year of age) or in severely immunocompromised patients.

      –has a patchy pattern on radiograph with necrotic focal lesions consisting of multiple abscesses.

   B. *Haemophilus influenzae* pneumonia

      –occurs in the elderly, particularly those with chronic pulmonary disease, or in alcoholics or infants.

      –increased incidence is seen following viral influenza outbreaks.

   C. *Pseudomonas aeruginosa* pneumonia

      –mucoid strains colonize the lungs of patients with cystic fibrosis and cause repeated infections.

      –may occur in patients exposed to high levels of *Pseudomonas* organisms in contaminated inhalation therapy equipment.

      –often results in mental confusion, gram-negative septic shock, and cyanosis of increasing severity.

Gastrointestinal Tract Infections

I. Enterobacteriaceae Family (Enterics)

   A. General characteristics—Enterobacteriaceae family

      –is composed of hundreds of closely related species and strains inhabiting the large bowel of humans and animals.

      –plasmids and DNA are exchanged frequently, resulting in new strains.

–includes the medically important tribes of Escherichieae, Serratieae, Salmonelleae, Klebsielleae, Proteeae, and Yersinieae.

–is characterized by gram-negative, non–spore-forming rods (generally facultative anaerobes) that ferment glucose to acid and reduce nitrates to nitrites.

–may be differentiated according to genera and species by antigens (serology), biochemical fermentations, carbohydrate fermentation, or growth on differential and selective media.

–causes two major disease syndromes: **nosocomial infections** and **gastrointestinal disturbances.**

B. **Identification of pathogens among normal flora**

–is difficult because the normal flora in the intestine vastly outnumber any pathogen.

–is aided by the knowledge that most pathogens, except *Escherichia coli*, do not ferment lactose.

–is facilitated by the use of differential or selective media tailored to the pathogen.

1. **Examples of differential media** include:

   a. **Eosin methylene blue**

      –differentiates *E. coli* as metallic green colonies, whereas pathogenic, non–lactose fermenting *Salmonella* and *Shigella* organisms are translucent.

      –inhibits gram-positive organisms via aniline dyes.

   b. **MacConkey agar**

      –differentiates lactose fermenters such as *E. coli* colonies (which appear pink) from non–lactose fermenting pathogenic colonies (which appear translucent).

      –inhibits other organisms by its content of bile salts and crystal violet.

2. **Examples of selective media** include:

   a. **Hektoen enteric media**

      –inhibits gram-positive and many commensal nonpathogenic organisms.

      –permits direct plating of feces and growth of pathogen.

      –differentiates lactose fermenting from non–lactose fermenting organisms.

   b. **Salmonella–Shigella agar** contains a high concentration of bile salts and sodium citrate, which inhibit gram-positive and many gram-negative bacteria, including coliforms.

3. **Other differential tests** include:

   a. **Fluorescent antibody**

   b. **Agglutination**

   c. **Packaged systems** containing multiple carbohydrates and other biochemicals to detect differential fermentations

C. **Antigenic structure**

1. **Capsular (K) antigens**

   –are generally polysaccharide in nature.

   –are exemplified by *Klebsiella pneumoniae* and *Salmonella typhi.*

2. **Flagellar (H) antigens** are proteins with antigenically specific and non-specific phase variations.

3. **Fimbriae (pili)** are responsible for attachment and colonization of the organism.

4. **Somatic (O) antigens**

    —are lipopolysaccharides, with the terminal sugars as the dominant, determinant group in serologic classification.

    —can be classified within the Salmonelleae tribe into a wide variety of serotypes by the Kauffmann-White schema.

D. **Attributes of pathogenicity**

1. **The capsule** suppresses phagocytosis.

2. **Enterotoxins (exotoxins)**

    —cause transduction of fluid into the ileum.

    —both a heat-labile and heat-stable exotoxin occur under the genetic control of a transmissible plasmid produced by *E. coli* (and *Vibrio cholerae*). The **heat-labile toxin** has two subunits, A and B.

    a. **Subunit B** binds to the G_{M1} ganglioside at the brush border of small intestinal epithelial cells, facilitating entrance of subunit A.

    b. **Subunit A** activates adenylate cyclase, which increases cyclic adenosine monophosphate (cyclic AMP).
        (1) Hypersecretion of water and chloride and inhibition of sodium resorption lead to **electrolyte imbalance.**
        (2) The gut lumen becomes distended with fluid, causing hypermotility and diarrhea.

    —the **heat-stable toxin** activates guanylate cyclase in epithelial cells, stimulating fluid secretion via cyclic guanosine monophosphate (cyclic GMP, or cGMP).

3. **Endotoxins** are an LPS complex in the outer membrane, which differs serologically in terminal end sugars (O antigen) but has a common toxic lipid A core, causing:

    a. **Hypotension** from release of endogenous hypotensive agents from platelets and other cells, mainly tumor necrosis factor, interleukin 1 (IL-1), and interleukin 6 (IL-6)

    b. **Fever** because minute amounts (micrograms) induce IL-1 and IL-6 in humans

    c. **Hemorrhage** in the adrenal glands, intestine, heart, and kidney, which is produced experimentally in animals in two ways:
        (1) **Local Shwartzman reaction,** in which two injections of endotoxin are given (the first given intradermally, followed in 16 to 36 hours by the second given intravenously)
            —results in hemorrhage at the intradermal site of first injection. Capillaries become plugged with a thrombus of platelets, white blood cells, and fibrinoid material.
            —resembles hemorrhage seen in humans during gram-negative bacteremia.

(2) **Generalized Shwartzman reaction,** in which two injections of endotoxin are given intravenously, 16 to 36 hours apart

–results in **bilateral renal cortical necrosis** resembling disseminated intravascular coagulation (DIC).

–may act by the following mechanism: the first injection causes conversion of fibrinogen to fibrin; the second injection inhibits phagocytosis of fibrin, and fibrin deposits interrupt circulation in the kidney.

–may be produced by only one exposure to endotoxic bacteria during pregnancy or cortisone treatment.

d. **Adjuvant action** on the immune response by increasing antibody response to unrelated antigens and stimulating B cells as a mitogen

e. **Increased resistance** to other infectious agents and tumors by causing secretion of protective cytokines

f. **Mediator release,** in which many diverse, physiologically active molecules are released from macrophages and other cells under varying conditions

E. Disease syndromes

1. Nosocomial (hospital-acquired) infections

–occur frequently, affecting approximately 2 million people yearly, or 5% to 10% of the hospital population.

–can cause bacteremia, which frequently results in shock.

–have a high fatality rate (40% to 60%) because many of these organisms are relatively resistant to antibiotics.

–are normally noninvasive in healthy individuals; however, patients who are immunocompromised (such as those with cancer or heart or lung disease) or immunosuppressed are at particular risk.

–have outcomes dependent on the extent of preexisting debilitating disease.

2. Gastrointestinal disturbances

–are usually due to enterotoxins secreted by Enterobacteriaceae organisms.

–must be differentiated from gastrointestinal upsets caused by staphylococci, which have a shorter incubation period (6 hours); Enterobacteriaceae organisms generally have an incubation period of 1 to 2 days.

–caused by *E. coli* may cause three distinct disease syndromes: **enterotoxigenic syndrome** (traveler's diarrhea), **enteropathogenic syndrome** (occurs in infants), and **enteroinvasive syndrome** (dysentery).

II. *Salmonella*

A. General characteristics—*Salmonella*

–have a **wide host range,** including humans, animals, and birds.

–are gram-negative motile rods indistinguishable microscopically from other Enterobacteriaceae organisms.

–are categorized into more than 1800 serotypes; most human disease results from *Salmonella typhi, Salmonella enteritidis, Salmonella typhimurium, Salmonella paratyphi A, Salmonella schottmuelleri,* or *Salmonella choleraesuis.*

–do not ferment lactose, but many species are identified by production of acid, gas, and hydrogen sulfide from glucose.

B. Classification—*Salmonella*

–may possess a **capsular (K) antigen,** exemplified by the virulence (Vi) antigen of *S. typhi.*

–are grouped via the Kauffmann-White schema into more than 40 groups based on differences in the oligosaccharide ligands (determinant groups) of the somatic (O) antigens found in the outer membrane.

  1. Assignment of an organism to a particular group is based on the common possession of a major O antigen, which is identified by an Arabic numeral.

  2. For example, *S. typhi* 9 and 12 and *S. enteritidis* 1, 9, and 12 are assigned to Group D because they possess the major antigen, number 9.

–are identified further by the presence of different **flagellar (H) antigens.**

C. Attributes of pathogenicity—*Salmonella*

–possess an endotoxin that causes diverse toxic manifestations, including fever, leukopenia, hemorrhage, hypotension, shock, and DIC.

–may possess an exotoxin (enterotoxin).

–are aided by antiphagocytic activity of the capsule.

–can survive within macrophages by an unknown means.

D. Clinical disease

  1. Enterocolitis (gastroenteritis or food poisoning)

    –is the most common form of salmonella infection in the United States (approximately 2 million cases per year).

    –occurs in multiple **sources of contamination,** including food (most commonly poultry and poultry products), human carriers (particularly food handlers), and exotic pets (turtles and snakes).

    –is commonly caused by *S. typhimurium* and *S. enteritidis,* which usually require a high infecting dose with an 8- to 48-hour incubation period.

    –is a **self-limiting illness** manifested by fever, nausea, vomiting, and diarrhea.

    –may have an increased carrier rate with antibiotic therapy.

    –is usually characterized by the following pattern:

    a. Ingestion of organisms in contaminated food

    b. Colonization of the ileum and cecum

    c. Penetration of epithelial cells in the mucosa and invasion, resulting in acute inflammation and ulceration

    d. Release of prostaglandin by enterotoxins, resulting in activation of adenyl cyclase and increased cyclic AMP

    e. Increased fluid secretion in the intestines

2. Septicemic (extraintestinal) disease

–is an acute illness most often of nosocomial origin, with abrupt onset and early invasion of the bloodstream.

–is characterized by a precipitating incident that introduces bacteria (e.g., catheterization, contaminated intravenous fluids, abdominal or pelvic surgery), followed by a triad of chills, fever, and hypotension.

–may cause local abscesses, osteomyelitis, and endocarditis if the organisms are disseminated widely.

–may be caused by many *Salmonella* species as well as other Enterobacteriaceae organisms.

–has a high mortality rate (30%–50%), depending on the degree of preexisting debilitation.

3. Enteric fevers

–are produced mainly by *S. typhi* (typhoid fever) and, to a lesser degree, by *S. paratyphi* and *S. schottmuelleri*, all of which are strictly human pathogens.

–occur through ingestion of food or water, usually contaminated by an unknowing carrier.

–are highly infective even with small numbers of bacteria (e.g., 200).

–progress as follows:

a. During an incubation period of 7 to 14 days, the organisms multiply in the small intestine, enter the intestinal lymphatics, and are disseminated via the bloodstream to multiple organs.

b. Blood cultures then become positive and the patient experiences malaise, headache, and gradual onset of a fever that increases during the day, reaching a plateau of 102°F to 105°F each day.

c. Multiplication takes place in the reticuloendothelial system and lymphoid tissue of the bowel, producing hyperplasia and necrosis of the lymphoid Peyer's patches.

d. A characteristic rash ("rose spots") may appear in the second to third week.

e. Typically, the disease lasts 3 to 5 weeks; the major complications are gastrointestinal hemorrhage and bowel perforation with peritonitis.

f. After recovery, 3% of patients become carriers; the organism is retained in the gallbladder and biliary passages, and cholecystectomy may be necessary.

E. Laboratory diagnosis

1. Enterocolitis. Blood cultures are usually negative, and agglutination reactions are not helpful.

2. Septicemic disease. Diagnosis is usually by blood culture because the organisms do not localize in the bowel and stool cultures are often negative.

3. Enteric fevers

a. Diagnosis is usually by isolation of the organism from the blood or stool after 1 to 2 weeks by plating onto differential media, selective media, or both.

         b. Diagnosis by serology, showing increasing titers of O antibody, is of lesser significance.

F. Control

1. Enterocolitis

–requires no specific therapy except replacement of fluid loss.

–antibiotic therapy may increase the carrier rate.

2. Septicemic disease

–has no specific therapy other than maintenance.

–can be controlled with antibiotics.

3. Enteric fevers.
Chloramphenicol is usually the drug of choice, but ampicillin is also effective against most strains.

III. *Shigella*

A. General characteristics—*Shigella*

–is a gram-negative, facultative anaerobic, nonmotile rod.

–species are pathogenic in small numbers for humans.

–species have no known animal reservoir and are not found in soil or water unless contaminated with human fecal material.

–causes perpetuated disease largely because of unrecognized clinical cases and because carriers are convalescent or healthy carriers (<1% of carriers are under the care of a physician).

–disease spreads through poor sanitation and is readily transmitted from person to person via food, touch, feces, and flies.

–species ferment glucose with acid, but rarely with gas; only *Shigella sonnei* ferments lactose.

B. Classification.
Shigella is classified into four groups based on differences in somatic (O) antigens:

1. Group A, *Shigella dysenteriae* (rarely found in the United States, unless imported)

2. Group B, *Shigella flexneri* (common in the United States)

3. Group C, *Shigella boydii* (rarely found in the United States)

4. Group D, *Shigella sonnei* (the most common cause of shigellosis in the United States)

C. Virulence attributes

1. All shigellae contain an endotoxic LPS.

2. *S. dysenteriae* type 1 secretes a potent, heat-labile protein exotoxin (Shiga toxin) that causes diarrhea and acts as a neurotoxin.

3. Organisms possess the capacity to multiply intracellularly, resulting in focal destruction and ulceration.

D. Clinical disease

1. **Shigellosis** (bacillary dysentery) is characterized by acute inflammation of the wall of the large intestine and terminal ileum; bloodstream invasion is rare.

2. **Complications** include necrosis of the mucous membrane, ulceration, and bleeding.

3. Disease is characterized by a sudden onset after a short incubation period (1–4 days), with **abdominal pain, cramps, diarrhea, and fever.**

4. Stools are liquid and scant; after the first few bowel movements, they contain mucus, pus, and occasionally blood.

E. Laboratory diagnosis

–is made from stool culture of the organism onto differential and selective media.

–cannot be made by using serology and blood culture.

F. Control

1. Only *S. dysenteriae* infections require antibiotic therapy; however, resistance to antibiotics has been developing.

2. **Fluid replacement** is the most important therapy.

3. **Vaccines** are under development.

4. Epidemiologic control by isolation of carriers, disinfection of excrement, and proper sewage disposal can be effective.

IV. *Escherichia coli*

A. General characteristics—*Escherichia coli*

–is a gram-negative short rod.

–is a facultative anaerobic member of the Enterobacteriaceae family.

–is present without incident in high concentrations (10^8/g) in normal human feces.

B. Attributes of pathogenicity—*Escherichia coli*

–can result in serotypic changes and associated pathogenicity through plasmid exchange of virulence (toxin) genes.

–can cause damage to intestinal epithelium after adherence through pili.

C. Clinical disease—diarrhea

–is caused by four different strains:

1. **Enteropathogenic *E. coli* (EPEC)**

–is nontoxigenic; adhesion to enterocytes damages villi.

–affects mainly infants and children.

2. **Enterohemorrhagic *E. coli* (EHEC)**

–occurs as contaminant in undercooked meats.

–has a dominant serotype of 0157:H7, with cattle being the main reservoir.

–secretes a Shiga-like toxin (a cytotoxin also called verotoxin) responsible for inflammation of the colonic mucosa, resulting in bloody diarrhea.

3. **Enteroinvasive *E. coli* (EIEC)**

–causes bloody diarrhea in children similar to shigellosis.

–rarely occurs in the United States.

4. **Enterotoxigenic *E. coli* (ETEC)**

–causes "traveler's diarrhea" in all age-groups.

–spreads through contaminated food and water.

-adheres to small intestine via pili.

-secretes a heat-labile (LT) and a heat-stable (ST) exotoxin.

    a. LT toxin is an A-B toxin acting similarly to cholera toxin (see Table 1–3); it catalyzes ADP ribosylation, increasing adenylate cyclase activity and resulting in increased cyclic AMP and loss of water and ions into the intestinal lumen.

    b. ST toxin activates guanylate cyclase, increasing cGMP and resulting in hypersecretion of fluids and electrolytes.

D. Treatment is with antibiotics; selection depends on site of infection and age of patient.

V. *Vibrio cholerae*

A. General characteristics—cholera

-is one of the most devastating pandemic diseases.

-outbreaks of small, sporadic nature have been linked to ingestion of contaminated seafood along the coast of the Gulf of Mexico in the United States.

-occurs in individuals who are predisposed to the infection by poor nutrition and debilitation.

-is a prototype of an enterotoxin-induced diarrhea.

-is endemic in several countries.

B. Classification

    1. *V. cholerae* causes classic cholera; most epidemics are due to biotypes cholerae, El Tor, and 0139.

    2. *Vibrio parahaemolyticus* causes relatively mild gastroenteritis.

C. Attributes of pathogenicity

    1. Almost all pathology is attributed to **choleragen,** a protein enterotoxin.

    2. Choleragen has an A fragment (toxic action) and a B fragment (binding to cells); it specifically attaches to epithelial cells of microvilli at the brush borders of the small intestine.

    3. Choleragen stimulates adenyl cyclase to overproduce cyclic AMP, which upsets the fluid and electrolyte balance; this causes hypersecretion of chloride and bicarbonate.

    4. Choleragen is similar to *E. coli* LT toxin.

D. Clinical manifestations

-result from ingestion of contaminated water or food.

-have an abrupt onset of **intense vomiting and diarrhea** as the key finding.

-**copious fluid** loss (15–20 L /day) leads to rapid metabolic acidosis and hypovolemic shock.

-occur as sunken eyes and cheeks with diminished skin turgor.

-result in remission or death after 2 or 3 days.

E. Laboratory diagnosis

    1. Identification

        a. Diagnosis relies on clinical manifestations, combined with a history of residence in or recent visit to an endemic area.

    b. Gram-negative, short-curved ("comma-shaped") rods appear in the stool specimen.

    c. A fluorescent antibody test should be performed on the stool specimen.

    d. Culture the selective medium; then a fluorescent antibody or slide agglutination test should be performed on organisms from isolated colonies.

  2. Clinical specimens

    a. Stool specimens are clear and watery (**"rice-water" stools**).

    b. Organisms are sensitive to acid pH; therefore, stools should be cultured immediately.

F. Treatment

  1. The key is **prompt replacement of fluids and electrolytes;** the patient should appear healthier within 1 to 3 hours.

  2. Fluids should initially be administered intravenously; as the patient responds, they should be administered orally.

  3. Fluid and electrolyte therapy reduces the fatality rate from 60% to 1%.

  4. Tetracycline should be given to prevent the patient from infecting others; if antibiotics are not given, the patient will recover but will shed organisms for 1 year.

G. Prevention

–is by **adequate sewage disposal** and **water purification.**

–is by hospitalizing the patient (rice-water stools are highly contagious).

–is by identifying and treating carriers with **tetracycline.**

VI. *Staphylococcus aureus*

A. General characteristics—*Staphylococcus aureus*

–causes "food poisoning" rather than infection.

–is a β-hemolytic, catalase-positive, gram-positive coccus.

B. Clinical disease

–is associated with food poisoning by **toxin** production **in improperly refrigerated high-protein foods** (custard-filled pastries, potato salad, ham) contaminated by *Staphylococcus* from nares or cutaneous lesion of food preparer.

–toxin has a short incubation time, producing abdominal cramping, vomiting, and diarrhea in 2 to 6 hours.

–symptoms resolve quickly (generally in less than 24 hours).

C. Control

  1. No treatment is generally necessary.

  2. Prevention is by properly refrigerating foods and by preventing contamination of foods through glove use.

VII. *Campylobacter jejuni*

A. General characteristics—*Campylobacter jejuni*

–is a gram-negative, oxidase-positive, and catalase-positive curved rod with polar flagella.

–is microaerophilic.

–is sometimes seen in "nose-to-nose" pairs with extending polar flagella described as having the appearance of "seagull's wings."

–has an incidence as high as that of both salmonella and shigella infections.

–is found in a wide variety of wild and domestic animals and is transmitted to humans most commonly through dogs or by poultry products. Outbreaks have been caused by unpasteurized milk and contaminated rural wells.

B. Classification. *Campylobacter jejuni* is related to *Vibrio* species and was previously classified as such.

C. Attributes of pathogenicity

–include tissue invasion.

–include flagellated forms, which are more virulent than nonflagellated forms.

–include an enterotoxin and cytotoxin but the role of either is unclear.

D. Clinical disease. Acute enteritis results from oral ingestion of the organism, leading to colonization and invasion of the intestinal lining and "inflammatory diarrhea."

E. Laboratory diagnosis—*Campylobacter jejuni*

–is found in the stool as numerous darting, motile organisms along with blood and neutrophils.

–is isolated on special agar (Campy or Skirrow's agar) grown at 42°C (which suppresses most of the growth of other gastrointestinal tract flora) under microaerophilic conditions.

F. Control

   1. Treatment in severe cases is with erythromycin, but the disease is generally self-limiting (lasts less than 1 week).

   2. Prevention is by sanitation and pasteurization.

VIII. *Helicobacter pylori*

A. General characteristics—*Helicobacter pylori*

–is associated with gastritis, gastric and duodenal ulcers, and gastric carcinomas.

–is gram-negative; oxidase-, catalase-, and urease-positive; motile with corkscrew motility.

B. Classification. *H. pylori* is a relative of *Vibrio* and *Campylobacter*.

C. Attributes of pathogenicity—*Helicobacter pylori*

–produces urease to neutralize stomach acid in the near vicinity.

–produces a mucinase, which improves penetration of the mucous layer.

–adheres to fucose-containing receptors; these may be the ABO(H) and Lewis blood group antigens that are expressed on the gut epithelia, possibly explaining the increased incidence of ulcers in Lewis and type O individuals. Pili appear involved in adherence.

D. Clinical disease occurs as epigastric pain, sometimes with nausea, vomiting, anorexia, and gas production.

E. Laboratory diagnosis

–is by biopsy with microscopy and culture on *Campylobacter* medium. (However, culture is not very reliable.)

–is by demonstration of antibodies.

–is by breath test to reveal urease activity.

F. Control. Treatment is generally with a triad of antibiotics using bismuth subsalicylate, metronidazole, and tetracycline or amoxicillin or using clarithromycin and omeprazole.

IX. *Clostridium botulinum*

A. General characteristics—*Clostridium botulinum*

–is a gram-positive, spore-forming anaerobic rod.

–requires a low redox potential within tissues; clostridia cannot infect healthy tissues.

–spores are ubiquitous in soil and are highly resistant to environmental conditions.

B. Attributes of pathogenicity—*Clostridium botulinum*

–produces a potent exotoxin that acts at the myoneural junction to produce flaccid muscle paralysis due to suppression of acetylcholine release from the axon terminals of peripheral nerves.

–is compared with other clostridial toxins in Table 3–5.

C. Clinical manifestations. *C. botulinum* causes two types of infection:

1. **Food poisoning** follows ingestion of the preformed toxin in contaminated food. **Clinical findings** include nausea, vomiting, dizziness, cranial palsy, double vision, swallowing and speech problems, muscle weakness, respiratory paralysis, and death (in 20% of cases).

2. **Intestinal (infant) botulism** occurs in infants after spore ingestion and subsequent germination in the gastrointestinal tract.

   a. The exotoxin disseminates, causing constipation, generalized weak-

Table 3–5. Clostridia

Organism	Toxin	Mechanism of Action
Clostridium tetani	Tetanospasm exotoxin	Obliterates inhibition reflex response at synaptosomes of brain stem and spinal cord
Clostridium botulinum	Botulinum exotoxin	Paralysis of cholinergic nerve fibers at myoneural junction suppresses acetylcholine release
Clostridium difficile	Enterotoxin, cytotoxin	Gastrointestinal distress, kills mucosal cells
Clostridium perfringens	α-toxin (11 other toxins)	Lecithinase, destroys cell membranes

ness, and loss of head and limb control (resulting in a floppy appearance).

    b. This type of infection rarely is fatal.

  3. In rare cases, **wound infection** occurs, with manifestations similar to those of soft-tissue wounds.

D. Laboratory diagnosis. The presence of the toxin in food, stool, blood, and vomitus is demonstrable by injection of sample into mice; protection from death is with botulinum antitoxin.

E. Treatment

  –for food poisoning give antitoxin and supportive measures for respiratory control, stomach lavage, and enemas. Antibiotics should not be given and the caregiver should act rapidly.

  –for **intestinal botulism** in infants only supportive care is needed; there should be complete recovery without deficits.

F. Prevention

  –give antitoxin to all persons who ate contaminated food, even if symptoms have not developed.

  –heat food to 80°C–100°C for 10 minutes to inactivate the toxin (but not the spores).

  –use proper sterilization techniques for home canning.

  –refrain from giving honey, which may contain organisms, to infants younger than 1 year old.

X. *Clostridium difficile*

A. General characteristics—*Clostridium difficile*

  –is a gram-positive, spore-forming, anaerobic rod.

  –is a component of the normal intestinal flora of infants and some adults.

  –contamination of hospitals and hospital personnel persists via asymptomatic carriers.

B. Attributes of pathogenicity—*Clostridium difficile*

  –has many strains that are resistant to antibiotics relative to other members of the gut flora.

  –antibiotic treatment kills organisms normally restricting growth of *C. difficile*, resulting in overgrowth of the latter.

  –produces two toxins: an enterotoxin that causes gastrointestinal upset and a cytotoxin that kills mucosal cells.

C. Clinical manifestations occur as severe gastroenteritis, termed **pseudomembranous colitis** or **antibiotic-associated** colitis, and follows antibiotic therapy to treat other bacterial infections.

D. Treatment is with vancomycin or metronidazole and fluid and electrolyte status should be monitored.

XI. *Bacteroides fragilis*

A. General characteristics—*Bacteroides fragilis*

  –is a gram-negative, anaerobic rod, usually pleomorphic, with vacuoles and swelling.

Table 3–6. Properties of Non–spore-forming Anaerobic Bacteria

Organism	Distinguishing Bacteriologic Feature	Habitat	Clinical Correlation	Treatment
Bacteroides fragilis	Pleomorphism	Gut; female genital tract	Brain abscess; gastrointestinal abscess; pelvic inflammatory disease; cellulitis	Débridement and drainage; metronidazole (clindamycin as second-line agent)
Prevotella melaninogenica	Black colonies on agar; putrid sputum	Mouth; gastrointestinal and genitourinary tracts (occasionally)	Lung abscess; female genital tract infections	Débridement and drainage; metronidazole (clindamycin as second-line agent)
Fusobacterium nucleatum	Cigar shape	Mouth	Necrotizing gingivitis; head, neck, and chest infections	Penicillin; cephalosporin

–grows rapidly under anaerobic conditions and is stimulated by bile.

–contains levels of superoxide dismutase and catalase, which make it somewhat resistant to short exposure to oxygen.

–accounts for 1% of gut anaerobes, most of which are bacteroides.

–is found in the female genital tract but rarely in the oral cavity.

–usually causes **polymicrobic infections,** involving more than one genus or species; consequently, therapy with several antibiotics may be necessary.

–is compared with other non–spore-forming anaerobes in Table 3–6.

B. Attributes of pathogenicity—*Bacteroides fragilis*

–possesses a **capsule** that inhibits phagocytosis.

–has a weak endotoxin (in contrast to *Prevotella*) and no exotoxin.

–also possesses a collagenase and hyaluronidase, which aids its spread.

C. Infections

–are a frequent cause of gastrointestinal **abscesses** after damage to mucosal barriers.

–are foul smelling.

–are the leading cause of pelvic inflammatory disease.

–are a frequent cause of brain abscesses and cellulitis.

–are not communicable or transmissible.

D. Treatment

–with tetracyclines is generally ineffective because most organisms are resistant; they possess a beta-lactamase that destroys penicillins and cephalosporins.

–is with metronidazole; clindamycin, kanamycin, and chloramphenicol also are suggested as therapeutic agents for this relatively resistant organism.

Genitourinary Tract Infections

I. *Escherichia coli*

A. General characteristics—*Escherichia coli*

–is discussed under Gastrointestinal Tract Infections.

–is the most common infection of the urinary tract.

–occurs after contamination of the genital area with feces.

–is more common in women due to shortness of the urethra and its proximity to the anal area.

B. Attributes of pathogenicity

1. Organisms adhere readily to the mucosa via pili, causing damage.

2. Endotoxin (LPS) induces inflammation.

3. Host factors include obstructions, sexual intercourse, catheters, diaphragms, and voiding impairment.

C. Clinical diseases

1. **Cystitis** is characterized by painful frequent urination, hematuria, and urgency.

2. **Pyelonephritis** infection of the kidneys follows ascending urinary tract infection; it is characterized by fever, flank pain, and tenderness and may lead to endotoxin shock.

3. **Prostatitis** can occur in older men.

D. Treatment is with an appropriate antibiotic. Most *E. coli* strains are susceptible to penicillin and ciprofloxacin.

II. *Staphylococcus saprophyticus*

A. General characteristics—*Staphylococcus saprophyticus*

–belongs to the genus *Staphylococcus*, which are all catalase-positive, gram-positive cocci usually arranged in clusters (singles, diplococci, and short chains in tissues).

–is nonhemolytic, coagulase-negative, novobiocin-resistant, culture on blood agar.

–lacks protein A.

B. Attributes of pathogenicity. *S. saprophyticus* adheres to uroepithelial cells.

C. Clinical disease. Urinary tract infections occur in sexually active young women ("honeymoon cystitis").

III. *Proteus mirabilis*

A. General characteristics—*Proteus mirabilis*

–is a gram-negative, motile short rod.

–produces a typical "swarming" growth on blood agar.

–is primarily an opportunist, transmitted via catheters.

B. **Attributes of pathogenicity—*Proteus mirabilis***

–produces a powerful urease that hydrolyzes urea to ammonia and CO_2.

–results in stones and calculi, leading to urinary tract obstruction.

C. **Clinical disease.** Infection is a major cause of urinary tract infections, both community acquired and nosocomial.

D. **Treatment** is with ampicillin and cephalosporin; the organism is resistant to tetracyclines.

IV. *Enterococcus faecalis*

A. **General characteristics—*Enterococcus faecalis***

–was formerly classified as group D streptococci.

–occurs as part of the normal intestinal and oral flora in humans and animals.

–is a facultative anaerobic, gram-positive coccus.

–produces β-hemolysis on blood agar; other strains exhibit variable hemolysis, but most are alpha- or gamma-hemolytic.

–can be differentiated by reactivity with antiserum, bacitracin resistance, and growth in 40% bile, pH 9.6 or 6.5% salt solution.

B. **Attributes of pathogenicity**

1. Attributes of pathogenicity have not been identified.

2. Organisms are generally noninvasive opportunists; however, they are a leading cause of nosocomial infections.

3. Clinical significance needs to be established over mere contamination.

C. **Clinical disease** includes urinary tract infections, septicemia, and associated endocarditis.

D. **Treatment**

1. Antibiotic sensitivity should be tested to determine appropriate treatment.

2. The organism is relatively **resistant to many antibiotics;** it is inhibited but not killed by penicillin.

V. *Neisseria gonorrhoeae*

A. **General characteristics—*Neisseria gonorrhoeae***

–is an oxidase-positive, gram-negative diplococcus with a "kidney bean" morphologic appearance.

–is **epidemic,** with the highest incidence in the most sexually active group (age 15–25 years).

B. **Classification**

1. *N. gonorrhea* does not use maltose, which distinguishes it from *Neisseria meningitidis.*

2. Differentiation is by **auxotyping** (nutritional requirements) or **colonial morphology** (types 1 and 2 are virulent; types 3, 4, and 5 are much less virulent).

C. **Attributes of pathogenicity—*Neisseria gonorrhoeae***

–produces IgAase that degrades IgA_1; this antibody probably plays a key early role in mucosal infections. (IgAase is also found in *Haemophilus* and streptococcal organisms.)

–possesses a plasmid that codes for penicillinase production.

–possesses pili, which are protein surface fibrils that mediate attachment to the mucosal epithelium.

  1. Pili undergo phase variation (on/off switch of pili production). Nonpiliation greatly reduces virulence.

  2. Pili also exhibit antigenic variation and have the capacity to produce millions of variants, which is partly responsible for the lack of protection against subsequent infections.

–possesses outer membrane proteins that form porins (PI and PIII) and that determine clumping (PII) or opacity. PII$^-$ strains are isolated from disseminated forms. Pili and PII play major roles in adherence.

–possesses endotoxin activity that damages mucosal cells. Unlike most LPSs, *N. gonorrhea* lacks lengthy O-antigenic side chains and is termed lipo-oligosaccharide (LOS).

D. Clinical disease

–results in **mucous membrane infections,** primarily in the anterior urogenital tract.

–is **absent** in 20% to 80% of infected women and 10% of infected men; these asymptomatic carriers may transmit the bacteria to consorts, causing **symptomatic gonorrhea.**

–is compared with other sexually transmitted diseases in Table 3–7.

–repeated infection may cause scarring with subsequent **sterility** in either gender and may predispose women to ectopic pregnancy.

Table 3–7. Bacterial Sexually Transmitted Diseases

Organism	Prominent Clinical Feature	Complication	Complications in Pregnancy
Neisseria gonorrhoeae	Urethritis	Pelvic inflammatory disease; arthritis	Newborn conjunctivitis (severe)
Chlamydia trachomatis serotypes D–K	Urethritis	Pelvic inflammatory disease	Newborn pneumonia or conjunctivitis
Chlamydia trachomatis (lymphogranuloma venereum)	Regional adenopathy	Genital fistulas, ulcers, and elephantiasis	. . .
Treponema pallidum	Hard chancre, primary stage	Nerve; aorta; brain damage of tertiary stage	Congenital infection causing stillbirth or birth defects
Haemophilus ducreyi	Soft chancre with multiple ulcers	. . .	. . .
Group B streptococci	Mild genital tract infection	. . .	Fulminant meningitis in baby

–reflects various types of infections including:

1. **Urethritis** in men is characterized by thick, yellow, purulent exudate containing bacteria and numerous neutrophils; frequent, painful urination; and possibly an erythematous meatus. Complications include epididymitis and prostatitis in males.

2. **Endocervicitis or urethritis** in women is characterized by a purulent vaginal discharge, frequent, painful urination, and abdominal pain. Approximately 50% of cases go undiagnosed. Complications include arthritis, pelvic inflammatory disease, and sterility.

3. **Rectal infections** (prevalent in homosexual males) are characterized by painful defecation, discharge, constipation, and proctitis.

4. **Pharyngitis** is characterized by purulent exudate; the mild form mimics viral sore throat, whereas the severe form mimics streptococcal sore throat.

5. **Disseminated infection** (bloodstream invasion) is infection in which organisms initially localize in the skin, causing **dermatitis** (a single maculopapular, erythematous lesion), then spread to the joints, causing overt, painful arthritis of the hands, wrists, elbows, and ankles.

6. **Infant eye infection (ophthalmia neonatorum),** which is contracted during passage through the birth canal, is characterized by severe, bilateral purulent **conjunctivitis** that may rapidly lead to blindness.

E. **Laboratory diagnosis**

1. **Identification**

   a. Organisms are gram-negative, intracellular and extracellular diplococci. Numerous neutrophils appear in purulent exudate in men. Because of endocervical localization, a characteristic Gram stain of organisms is less likely in females.

   b. Culture should be immediately placed on warm Thayer-Martin chocolate agar in a candle jar.

   c. Oxidase test is positive.

   d. Organisms utilize glucose but not maltose.

   e. Newer techniques involve immunofluorescence, enzyme-linked immunosorbent assay (ELISA) on gene probes on a clinical swab.

2. **Clinical specimens**

   a. In women, both genital and rectal cultures should be obtained.

   b. If a speculum or anoscope is used, lubricant should not be used because it kills many organisms and reduces the chance for a successful culture.

   c. The organisms are labile, and specimens should be plated immediately.

   d. If disseminated gonorrhea is present, blood and synovial fluid should be cultured; culture of skin lesions is rarely successful.

F. **Control**

1. **Treatment**

   a. Ceftriaxone should be given, followed by a tetracycline to treat possible chlamydial infection.

     b. In approximately 50% of cases, pelvic inflammatory disease is severe enough to warrant hospitalization.

     c. Pelvic inflammatory disease predisposes the patient to repeated episodes caused by other bacteria and to ectopic pregnancy.

  2. Prevention

     a. The patient's sexual partners should be treated and **condom** use should be encouraged.

     b. Asymptomatic patients should be identified by culture and treated.

     c. To prevent neonatal gonococcal conjunctivitis, topical silver nitrate or tetracycline should be used; the antibiotic is preferred because it also kills *Chlamydia trachomatis,* if present.

VI. *Treponema pallidum*

A. General characteristics—*Treponema pallidum*

–is a corkscrew-shaped, motile organism with unusual morphologic appearance of the outer envelope, three axial filaments, a cytoplasmic membrane–cell wall complex with endotoxin, and a protoplasmic cylinder.

–causes chronic, painless infections that may last 30 to 40 years if untreated.

–decreases in number as host defenses are stimulated, causing disappearance of symptoms; subsequently, organisms multiply and symptoms reappear.

B. Classification

  1. Subspecies *pallidum* causes **syphilis,** which is sexually transmitted, epidemic worldwide, and may affect any tissue.

  2. Subspecies *pertenue* causes **yaws** (seen in hot tropical climates, not in the United States). Yaws involves bone and soft tissues.

  3. Subspecies *carateum* causes **pinta** (seen in Central and South America). Pinta involves the skin only.

  4. All three subspecies are morphologically and antigenically identical; differentiation is based solely on clinical manifestations.

C. Attributes of pathogenicity. Immunosuppressive treponemal components are responsible for the chronic nature of syphilis and for subsequent emergence of different stages.

D. Clinical disease—syphilis

  1. Vascular involvement leads to endarteritis and periarteritis, resulting in inhibited blood supply and necrosis.

  2. Lymphocyte and plasma cell infiltration occurs at sites of infection.

  3. The pathogenesis of syphilis varies considerably. It may involve many tissues of the body and is generally divided into three stages:

     a. Primary—localized infection with erythema, induration with a firm base (a **hard chancre**), and ulceration

     b. Secondary—disseminated infection with lesions in almost all tissues; mucocutaneous rash; may recur if untreated

     c. Tertiary—aortitis and CNS problems may be fatal

4. **In utero infection** has severe manifestations, including abortion, still-birth, birth defects, or latent infection (most common) with the snuffles (rhinitis) followed by a rash and desquamation.

E. **Laboratory diagnosis**

1. **Identification**

   a. Syphilis is identified partly on the basis of **clinical manifestations.**

   b. **Darkfield microscopy** of lesion exudate may demonstrate **cork-screw-shaped spirochetes** (the organisms are too thin to identify by Gram stain).

   c. **Serology.** Two antibodies are produced in response to *T. pallidum* infection:

      (1) Nontreponemal (reaginic) antibodies (these are not IgE)
      –are nonspecific (positive in many related or chronic diseases) but economical as a screening test.
      –are identified by other screens: Venereal Disease Research Laboratory (VDRL) test, rapid plasma reagin (RPR) card test, or automated reagin test (ART).
      –titers are decreased in tertiary syphilis (even if untreated). If treated, a positive reagin test after 1 year suggests persistent infection, reinfection, or a false-positive result.

      (2) Specific treponemal antibodies
      –are more specific, but tests are costly and are used only to confirm a positive reagin test.
      –are screened for by fluorescent treponemal antibody absorption (FTA-abs) test, *T. pallidum* hemagglutination (TPHA) test, and the rarely used *T. pallidum* immobilization (TPI) test.
      –titers remain positive in most people even with proper treatment.
      –biologic false-positive results may confuse the diagnosis (positive serology in the absence of treponemal disease).

2. **Clinical specimens**

   a. Lesion exudate should be obtained from a pustule or an ulcer for darkfield microscopy.

   b. The organism cannot be grown in vitro.

F. **Control**

1. **Treatment**

   a. Long-acting **penicillin** should be given.

   b. **Jarisch-Herxheimer** reaction immediately after antibiotic therapy for secondary syphilis involves intensification of manifestations for 12 hours; this indicates that penicillin is effective.

   c. With treatment, reagin-based serologic tests become negative 6 months after primary syphilis and 12 months after secondary syphilis; beyond the secondary stage, the patient may remain seropositive for years.

   2. **Prevention**

      a. Use of a **condom** minimizes transmission.

      b. **All sexual contacts** should be treated prophylactically with **penicillin.**

      c. In **pregnant patients,** serologic syphilis tests should be performed during the first and third trimesters.

VII. *Chlamydia trachomatis*

   A. **General characteristics—*Chlamydia trachomatis***

      –is differentiated into 15 serotypes.

      –has characteristics similar to *C. psittaci* (see Lower Respiratory Tract Infections V).

   B. **Attributes of pathogenicity.** Toxic effects of antigens kill host cells.

   C. **Clinical disease**

      1. **Subtypes D–K**

         –cause a **sexually transmitted disease** that may involve an associated inclusion conjunctivitis.

         –are a prominent cause of **nongonococcal urethritis** in men and urethritis, cervicitis, salpingitis, and **pelvic inflammatory disease** in women.

         –produce a relatively high incidence of asymptomatic or relatively inapparent infections.

         –can produce a self-limiting **inclusion conjunctivitis in neonates** delivered through an infected birth canal.

         –may cause neonatal pneumonia.

      2. **Subtype L1, L2, L3**

         –causes a sexually transmitted disease called **lymphogranuloma venereum,** which is characterized by a suppurative inguinal adenitis.

         –may cause **lymphadenitis** to progress to lymphatic obstruction and rectal strictures if the disease is untreated.

   D. **Laboratory diagnosis**

      –is frequently made by direct staining of genital tract specimen with fluorescence-conjugated monoclonal antibodies.

      –is made by enzyme immunoassays for chlamydial antigens and nonradioisotope probes for 16s RNA sequences.

   E. **Control**

      1. **Treatment** is with doxycycline or erythromycin.

      2. **Prevention** is by diagnosing mothers of infected neonates and urging standard control measures (e.g., use of condoms) to help prevent sexual transmission.

VIII. *Bacteroides fragilis*

      –is a leading bacterial cause of pelvic inflammatory disease.

      –is characterized as described in Gastrointestinal Tract Infections.

Central Nervous System Infections

I. *Streptococcus agalactiae*

A. General characteristics—*Streptococcus agalactiae*

–occurs frequently as part of the normal vaginal and oral flora in adult women.

–colonization of the female genital tract predisposes newborns to infection, sepsis, and meningitis.

–occurs as five serotypes (Ia, Ib, Ia/c, II, and III) based on antigenic differences in capsular polysaccharides.

–is a β-hemolytic, gram-positive coccus.

–can be differentiated from other streptococci with group B antiserum, sodium hippurate hydrolysis, and resistance to bacitracin.

–acts synergistically with a staphylococcal hemolysin.

B. Attributes of pathogenicity

1. A capsule is the major virulence component.

2. Polymorphonuclear influx can be negated by peptidase inactivation of C′5a.

3. An anticapsular antibody is protective in the presence of competent phagocytic cells and complement.

C. Clinical disease

1. **Early onset neonatal sepsis** (birth to 7 days)

   –occurs readily in newborns, but only 1 in 100 infected newborns becomes clinically ill.

   –is associated with obstetric complications, premature birth, and respiratory distress.

   –has a fatality rate of more than 50%.

2. **Late onset neonatal sepsis** (7 days to 4 months)

   –is characterized by meningitis.

   –commonly leads to permanent neurologic damage.

   –is caused mainly by serotype III.

   –has a fatality rate of 15% to 20%.

D. Treatment

1. Penicillin G generally is given.

2. Vaccine use is limited because of poor response of children to polysaccharide antigens.

II. *Neisseria meningitidis*

A. General characteristics—*N. meningitidis*

–is a gram-negative, oxidase-positive bacterium with the ability to use both glucose and maltose.

–causes a highly fulminant but generally sporadic disease prevalent at age 6 months to 2 years, with occasional outbreaks in military recruit settings.

–colonizes upper respiratory membranes before causing **meningococcemia.**

B. Classification. There are nine different capsular serogroups of *N. meningitidis;* most infections are caused by the B and Y serogroups.

C. Attributes of pathogenicity—*N. meningitidis*

–possesses a capsular polysaccharide that inhibits phagocytosis.

–possesses an LPS, causing extensive tissue necrosis, hemorrhage, circulatory collapse, intravascular coagulation, and shock.

–possesses IgAase that degrades IgA_1; this is probably important because infections begin on mucosal membranes (streptococci and *Haemophilus* organisms also have this enzyme).

D. Clinical manifestations

1. The disease begins as **mild pharyngitis** with occasional slight fever.

2. In the susceptible age-group, organisms disseminate to most tissues (especially the skin, meninges, joints, eyes, and lungs), resulting in a **fulminant meningococcemia** that can be fatal in 1 to 5 days.

3. Initial signs and symptoms are fever, vomiting, headache, and stiff neck.

4. A **petechial eruption** then develops that progresses from erythematous macules to frank purpura; **vasculitic purpura** is the hallmark.

5. The LPS of the organism causes intravascular coagulation, circulatory collapse, and shock.

6. Death may occur with or without spread to the meninges.

7. **Waterhouse-Friderichsen syndrome** is fulminating meningococcemia with hemorrhage, circulatory failure, and adrenal insufficiency.

8. Sequelae after recovery involve eighth-nerve deafness, CNS damage (learning disabilities and seizures), and severe skin necrosis that may warrant skin grafting or amputation.

E. Laboratory diagnosis

1. **Identification**

   a. Gram-negative diplococcus are identified by Gram stain of cerebrospinal fluid (CSF) and skin lesion aspirates.

   b. Identification should be rapid; countercurrent immunoelectrophoresis or agglutination reactions detect capsular polysaccharide in blood and CSF.

   c. Nutrient broth (blood and CSF) or Thayer-Martin chocolate agar (skin lesion or pharyngeal swab) should be inoculated and incubated in high CO_2.

   d. Meningococcus is oxidase positive.

   e. *N. meningitidis* uses glucose and maltose; *N. gonorrhoeae* uses only glucose.

2. **Clinical specimens**

   a. Organisms are delicate and must be transported to the laboratory and processed quickly.

   b. For Gram stain of CSF, centrifuging may be needed to concentrate organisms.

F. Control

1. Treatment

–is with **early diagnosis** and **prompt hospitalization** based primarily on the petechial rash; problems with differential diagnosis may occur because the rash resembles those caused by Rocky Mountain spotted fever, secondary syphilis, rubella, and rubeola.

–is with **high-dosage intravenous penicillin,** which passes through the inflamed blood–brain barrier.

–is with **supportive measures** against shock and intravascular coagulation.

2. Prevention

–is by giving **rifampin** to the patient (following penicillin) and to all family members and close contacts to eradicate the carrier state.

–is with vaccine, which is a capsular polysaccharide from A, C, W-135, and Y serogroups (B serogroup polysaccharide is poorly immunogenic). The major problem is vaccine failure in the target group (age 6 months to 2 years) in whom most infections occur. Infants are not routinely vaccinated in the United States. The vaccine is used routinely in the military, in asplenic individuals, and in individuals deficient in late complement components (C5–C8).

III. *Clostridium tetani*

A. General characteristics—*Clostridium tetani*

–is a gram-positive, spore-forming anaerobe.

–possesses a terminal spore, resulting in a characteristic "tennis racquet" morphologic appearance.

–spores are ubiquitous in soil.

–is of major concern during wars.

B. Attributes of pathogenicity

1. Toxigenicity is mediated by a large plasmid.

2. The organism secretes an exotoxin (tetanospasmin) that acts as synaptosomes to obliterate the inhibitory reflex response of nerve fibers, thus producing uncontrolled spasms; its main action is against the brain stem and anterior horns of the spinal cord. Release of acetylcholine is also impaired.

3. Tetanus toxin and botulinum toxin are two of the most potent toxins known.

C. Clinical disease

1. Infection follows minor trauma (such as a laceration or puncture) or occurs as umbilical cord stump infection in a neonate.

2. Manifestations include muscle stiffness, **tetanospasms** of **lockjaw** and back arching, and short, frequent spasms of voluntary muscles.

3. Death occurs after several weeks from exhaustion and respiratory failure.

D. Control

1. Treatment

a. The patient should be hospitalized and treatment begun without waiting for definitive diagnosis.

b. Antitoxins are effective only if toxins have not yet bound to tissues; therefore, administration should not be delayed.

c. Antitoxin and penicillin should be given, tissue should be débrided, a tracheotomy should be performed to aid breathing, and a quiet, dark environment should be provided to minimize external stimuli that can induce spasms.

2. Prevention

a. The **toxoid** is a component of the DTP vaccine. A booster should be given every 10 years; for major trauma, a booster should be given if the patient has not had one within the last 5 years.

b. Boosters should be given to pregnant women to stimulate maternal antibodies that will protect the newborn.

IV. Other

A. *Escherichia coli*

–is a common cause of meningitis in newborns and is similar to group B streptococcus.

–infection generally occurs from the vaginal tract during childbirth.

–causative strains are generally encapsulated.

–is counteracted by the following drugs of choice: penicillin, third-generation cephalosporin, imipenem cilastatin, or ciprofloxacin.

B. *Haemophilus influenzae*

–is a gram-negative, fastidious rod requiring the X and V factors and grown on chocolate agar (see Upper Respiratory Infections).

1. Clinical disease—meningitis

–occurs primarily in unvaccinated children 3 months to 2 years of age.

–is rapidly progressive; CNS deficits result in one third of cases (hydrocephalus, mental retardation, paresis, and speech and hearing problems).

2. Diagnosis.
Rapid diagnosis can be made by identifying the polyribitol phosphate (PRP) capsular antigen in CSF using latex particle agglutination (latex beads coated with specific anti-*Haemophilus* capsular antibodies) or counter-immunoelectrophoresis along with Gram stain of CSF sediment. Antibiotic susceptibilities are difficult to identify.

3. Control

a. **Treatment** is with ceftriaxone or cefotaxime (both used with dexamethasone) for meningitis.

b. **Vaccination** with conjugated vaccine (capsular PRP linked to protein, either diphtheria toxoid or *N. meningitidis* outer membrane protein) has been 95% effective in preventing meningitis and has caused reduced colonization rates as well.

c. **Prophylaxis** of unvaccinated, close contacts younger than 5 years old is with rifampin.

C. *Streptococcus pneumoniae* is a common cause of meningitis, particularly in aging individuals, following pneumococcal pneumonia.

D. *Bacteroides fragilis*

–is a pleomorphic **anaerobe.**

–is a frequent cause of brain abscesses.

–virulence factors include a polysaccharide capsule and an endotoxin.

–is usually associated with mixed infections.

–is resistant to penicillin; contains a beta-lactamase.

–is sensitive to metronidazole.

E. *Fusobacterium nucleatum*

–is a common **anaerobe** isolated from brain abscesses and anaerobic meningitis.

–is associated with mixed infections.

–is sensitive to penicillin in contrast to *Bacteroides.*

F. *Listeria monocytogenes*

–causes meningitis and septicemia in immunocompromised patients, particularly in renal transplant patients.

––may cause diarrhea in immunocompetent patients.

–causes clinical infections in pregnant patients, which may result in fetal meningitis or systemic disease.

–is characterized under Multisystem Infections.

Cardiovascular Infections

I. Viridans streptococci

A. **General characteristics—viridans streptococci**

–predominate in the normal human oral cavity.

–unlike other streptococci, cannot be classified by group-specific antigens.

–include 19 species differentiated by biochemical tests; most common species are *Streptococcus salivarius, Streptococcus mutans, Streptococcus mitis,* and *Streptococcus sanguis.*

–are alpha-hemolytic, are uninhibited by optochin, and are not bile soluble. The latter two properties differentiate them from *S. pneumoniae.*

B. **Attributes of pathogenicity**

1. No attributes of pathogenicity have been identified.

2. Organisms are generally noninvasive opportunists, commonly disseminated intravascularly by dental or other oral manipulation.

3. Secreted biotins promote adherence.

C. **Clinical disease**

1. On access to the bloodstream, these organisms are the most frequent cause of subacute bacterial endocarditis, which can result from inflammation

induced by deposition of viridans streptococci or any of several other bacterial genera on heart valves damaged by previous group A streptococcal (or congenital) disease.

2. Viridans streptococci are a major cause of dental caries.

D. Treatment

–is with penicillin, which generally is effective; resistant strains require an aminoglycoside as well.

–requires prophylactic penicillin in dental patients or other patients with preexisting valvular damage.

II. Enterococci

–are a common nosocomial cause of subacute bacterial endocarditis in a manner similar to viridans streptococci.

–are exemplified under Genitourinary Tract Infections.

III. *Staphylococcus aureus*

A. General characteristics—*Staphylococcus aureus*

–is a β-hemolytic, catalase-positive, gram-positive coccus.

–is characterized under Skin and Soft Tissue Infections.

–causes bacterial endocarditis, usually acute, often in "normal" heart.

–like many streptococci, has properties that allow it to adhere to heart valves as well as prosthetic replacement valves.

B. Clinical Disease—*S. aureus* bacterial endocarditis

–occurs sometimes with native valves not known to be damaged.

–infection rapidly damages the heart. Responsible toxins include coagulase, which allows formation of platelet and fibrin clots and reduces access of phagocytic cells to *S. aureus* and cytolytic toxins that damage cells.

–occurs in intravenous drug abusers because of increased *S. aureus* colonization of skin; infections are not as virulent but may be drug resistant.

IV. *Staphylococcus epidermidis*

A. General characteristics—*Staphylococcus epidermidis*

–is a coagulase-negative *Staphylococcus* that is sensitive to novobiocin.

–has a remarkable ability to adhere to artificial materials in the body (e.g., prosthetic heart valves).

B. Clinical disease—bacterial endocarditis

–occurs generally with prosthetic valves.

–is generally a chronic infection.

V. *Pseudomonas aeruginosa*

–causes endocarditis in intravenous drug abusers as a result of *Pseudomonas* contaminating drug paraphernalia or drug diluents.

–in most cases, affects the tricuspid valve.

Skin and Soft Tissue Infections

I. *Staphylococcus aureus*

A. General characteristics—*Staphylococcus aureus*

–is a catalase-positive, gram-positive coccus arranged in clusters.

–is the only coagulase-positive and β-hemolytic *Staphylococcus*.

–may be part of the normal flora of carriers, usually in the nares or perineum. Carriage rate is 25% to 75%, with hospital staff having the higher carriage rates and being more likely to carry drug-resistant strains. Surgical staff is an important source of staphylococci in surgical infections. Food handlers who sneeze or who have staphylococcal hand lesions are the major source infecting food that may lead to staphylococcal food poisoning.

–is a major cause of infections in hospitalized patients and patients with chronic granulomatous disease, indwelling catheters, surgery, etc.

–has a high incidence of drug resistance, with methicillin-resistant strains resistant to β-lactams and most other antibiotics.

–is controlled primarily by phagocytic destruction (a major problem in chronic granulomatous disease).

–infection is enhanced in the presence of artificial materials in the body (e.g., sutures, tampons, surgical packing, intravenous catheters).

B. Classification

1. Staphylococci are catalase positive whereas streptococci are catalase negative.

2. *S. aureus* (β-hemolytic and coagulase positive) is distinguished from the coagulase-negative staphylococci, which are nonhemolytic.

C. Attributes of pathogenicity

1. Coagulase enhances fibrin deposition and abscess formation. There is also a surface clumping factor that coats the cell with fibrin.

2. Cytolytic toxins (alpha, beta, delta, gamma, and leukocidin) are all hemolytic (except leukocidin) and destroy cellular membranes.

3. Enterotoxins secreted by some strains are fast acting, producing gastrointestinal symptoms in 2 to 6 hours. They are heat and acid resistant and bind to neural receptors causing vomiting.

4. TSST-1, formerly termed enterotoxin F, is a superantigen and toxin produced under certain environmental conditions, most commonly associated with tampon use and surgical packing. TSST-1 reduces liver clearance of endogenous endotoxin.

5. Exfoliatins produced by phage group II *S. aureus* cause surface cell layers of the skin to separate (probably through disruption of intracellular junctions) leading to desquamation.

6. Protein A (a surface protein) is antiphagocytic (binding to the Fc portion of antibody, making it unavailable to attach to phagocytes).

7. Teichoic acids aid in attachment and stimulate the inflammatory response when complexed with peptidoglycan.

D. Clinical disease

1. **Skin infections** include impetigo (often bullous), folliculitis of the bearded region, boils (furuncles), carbuncles (more extensive), styes, and surgical wound, burn, or traumatic-lesion infections.

2. Scalded skin syndrome, with its characteristic bullae and desquamation of body surfaces, occurs most commonly in children younger than 5 years old, sometimes with fairly minor infections but circulating exfoliatins.

3. Other *S. aureus* infections include toxic shock syndrome, food poisoning, pneumonia, osteomyelitis, and endocarditis.

E. Laboratory diagnosis—*Staphylococcus aureus*

–is a gram-positive coccus found in tissue infections in pairs and short chains (clusters typical of solid media growth) with numerous neutrophils.

–is the only *Staphylococcus* to grow on **mannitol salt agar** with fermentation of the mannitol and production of acid. (This is a surveillance medium.)

–grows with β-hemolysis on blood agar.

–is catalase positive (as are all staphylococci) and coagulase positive.

–was formerly phage typed for epidemiologic identification of strains; newer methods such as plasmid typing and ribotyping are replacements.

F. Control

1. **Treatment**

   a. Drainage of lesions is important along with antibiotic treatment.

   b. Antibiotic susceptibilities must be determined.

   c. Nonpenicillinase producers are treated with penicillin G.

   d. Penicillinase (plasmid-mediated) producers are treated with a penicillinase-resistant penicillin.

   e. Methicillin-resistant staphylococci strains have a mutated (chromosomal) penicillin-binding protein, making them resistant to all beta-lactam drugs and must be treated with vancomycin or vancomycin plus other antibiotics.

   f. Penicillin-tolerant strains fail to stimulate autolysis.

   g. Drug resistance is often transferred by transduction.

2. **Prevention**

   –disrupt transmission (hand washing, effective disinfectants), reduction of *Staphylococcus* on sheets and clothing (>70°C or dry cleaning).

   –reduce carriage.

   –use brief, high-dose perioperative antibiotics.

II. *Clostridium perfringens*

A. General characteristics—*Clostridium perfringens*

–is an **anaerobic**, spore-forming, large gram-positive rod.

–spores can be central or subterminal and are relatively heat resistant.

–produces 12 exotoxins causing food poisoning.

–has soil as a natural habitat; contamination can occur in home-canned goods, smoked fish, and honey.

–has germination of spores and emergence of vegetative cells as being necessary for toxin production.

B. **Attributes of pathogenicity—*Clostridium perfringens***

–produces **alpha toxin,** a potent lecithinase that damages cellular membranes and is identified in vitro by the Nagler reaction.

–produces 11 other toxins or enzymes that damage eukaryotic cells.

–produces an enterotoxin associated with food poisoning.

C. **Clinical manifestations.** *C. perfringens* causes two types of infection:

1. **Soft tissue (muscle) wound** infection following severe trauma (gunshot, car and industrial accidents, compound fractures, septic abortion, hypothermia); organisms elaborate toxins and enzymes to produce gas, edema, and impaired circulation; vascular destruction and lactic acid accumulation lower the redox potential, with two consequences:

   a. **Anaerobic cellulitis,** causing destruction of traumatized tissue only

   b. **Myonecrosis** (gas gangrene) or destruction of traumatized tissue and surrounding healthy tissue; progresses rapidly to shock and renal failure; is fatal in 30% of cases

2. **Food poisoning** following ingestion of contaminated food containing a **preformed enterotoxin;** abdominal pain with severe cramps and diarrhea occur for 1 day.

D. **Treatment**

1. For **anaerobic cellulitis,** penicillin and additional antibiotics are given to prevent secondary bacterial infections; necrotic tissue should be débrided.

2. For **myonecrosis,** penicillin and antitoxin are given and necrotic tissue is débrided. Surgery is likely. Bandages should not be too tight. Hyperbaric oxygen may be helpful.

3. For **food poisoning,** treatment usually is not necessary because the infection is self-limiting.

III. *Pseudomonas aeruginosa*

A. **General characteristics—*Pseudomonas aeruginosa***

–is a small, polarly flagellated, gram-negative rod with pili.

–is a nonfermentative, oxidase-positive bacterium.

–is a ubiquitous environmental organism found in water and soil and widely distributed on plants. It can grow in both distilled or tap water overnight to large numbers.

–may form a mucoid polysaccharide glycocalyx or slime layer, particularly in lung colonization of cystic fibrosis patients.

–often produces pigments that may be clinically useful, such as fluorescein (pyoverdin), a greenish fluorescent pigment, and pyocyanin, a blue-green pigment. Blue-green pus is a classic sign of *P. aeruginosa* burn infection.

B. Classification. *P. aeruginosa* is only one of a large number of pseudomonads (many of which also cause opportunistic infections) which are typed by ribosomal RNA and DNA homology into five groups.

C. Attributes of pathogenicity

1. Invasive factors include:

a. Pili, which adhere

b. A polysaccharide slime layer, which increases adherence to tissues, making them less susceptible to phagocytosis; particularly prominent in cystic fibrosis

2. Virulence factors include:

a. Exotoxin A, an ADP-ribose transferase similar to diphtheria toxin, which inactivates the tRNA elongation factor (EF-2), halts protein synthesis, and causes liver necrosis

b. Exoenzyme S, an ADP-ribose transferase capable of inhibiting eukaryotic protein synthesis

c. Lipopolysaccharide

d. Phospholipase C, which damages membranes causing tissue damage

e. Elastase and other proteolytic enzymes, which damage elastin, human IgA, IgG, complement components, and collagen

D. Clinical manifestations

1. Cellulitis

–occurs in patients with burns, wounds, or neutropenia.

–is indicated by blue-green pus and a grape-like, sweet odor.

–may be highly necrotic.

2. Septicemia

–results from hematogenous spread of the infection from local lesions or gastrointestinal tract and causes gram-negative shock.

–may result in a distinctive skin lesion, **ecthyma gangrenosum,** when dermal veins and tissue are invaded. These lesions become necrotic.

E. Laboratory diagnosis

–is most commonly made by clinical suspicion (grape-like odor, blue-green pus, or ecthyma gangrenosum) and confirmed by culture.

–shows β-hemolysis on blood agar with pigment production for most strains.

–shows nonfermentation on MacConkey agar, blue-green pigment, grape-like odor, and oxidase positivity.

F. Treatment

1. Control

–is difficult because of frequent resistance to antibiotics.

–requires **combination therapy** (aminoglycoside) and an antipseudomonal beta-lactam agent until drug susceptibilities are determined.

2. Prevention is difficult, but the incidence of infection can be reduced by careful sanitization of drains, aerators, and whirlpools in burn units, by a hospital ban on plants and raw vegetable foods for burn patients, and by pasteurization of respiratory therapy equipment.

IV. *Streptococcus pyogenes* (see Upper Respiratory Infections)

A. Impetigo

–is an easily spread exudative infection of the epidermis occurring primarily in children.

–may result in nephritis as a complication.

–should be treated with penicillin and scratching should be prevented.

B. Cellulitis and erysipelas

–are initiated by infection through a small break in the skin.

–the term **cellulitis** applies if the lesion is confined; **erysipelas** applies if the lesion spreads, primarily through the lymphatics.

C. Fasciitis

–is a rapidly spreading, dangerous infection of the fascia.

–tends to occur in diabetic patients who are particularly susceptible.

–infections necessitates rapid surgical débridement of necrotic tissue followed by therapy with antibiotics.

V. *Bacteroides fragilis* (see Gastrointestinal Tract Infections)

–causes cellulitis and necrotizing fasciitis, especially in diabetic patients, similar to group A streptococci.

–infection is treated with surgical débridement and drainage, followed by treatment with metronidazole.

VI. Other organisms

A. *Actinomyces*

–is a gram-positive, anaerobic filamentous bacterium that causes a variety of soft tissue infection.

–invades bone and disseminates (rarely) to the brain.

–is characterized under Multisystem Infections.

B. Cutaneous diphtheria (see Upper Respiratory Infections)

–occurs in tropics and hot arid regions.

–occurs as grayish skin ulcers started typically with an insect bite and perhaps superinfected by streptococci or *S. aureus*.

–rarely results in toxic damage to heart or nerves but may spread to other persons, causing **pharyngeal diphtheria**.

Eye and Ear Infections

I. *Chlamydia trachomatis*

A. General characteristics (see Genitourinary Tract Infections)

B. Attributes of pathogenicity. Some toxic effects of antigens kill host cells.

C. **Clinical diseases**

1. **Subtypes A–C**

–cause a **chronic keratoconjunctivitis (trachoma)** that can progress to conjunctival and corneal scarring and blindness.

–are frequently accompanied by a concomitant secondary bacterial infection.

–cause neonatal pneumonia.

2. **Subtypes D–K** can be self-inoculated from genital secretion into eye, resulting in an inclusion conjunctivitis.

D. **Laboratory diagnosis** is similar to that for genital infections with this agent.

E. **Control. Treatment** is with doxycycline or erythromycin.

II. *Neisseria gonorrhoeae* (see Genitourinary Tract Infections)

–causes **gonococcal ophthalmia.**

–is generally apparent in the first 5 days of life.

–is a purulent conjunctivitis.

–if not treated promptly, leads to blindness.

III. *Haemophilis influenzae* (see Central Nervous System Infections)

–**biotype** *aegyptius* causes bacterial **"pinkeye."**

–is an epidemic, purulent conjunctivitis.

–occurs often in school-age children but also spreads to adults.

IV. *Streptococcus pneumoniae* (see Lower Respiratory Tract Infections)

–is the most common cause of otitis media in infants older than 2 months of age.

–is treated with penicillin, although there are resistant strains.

V. *Haemophilus influenzae*

–is the second most common causative agent of **otitis media** in children, after *S. pneumonia.*

–has a tendency to recur.

–is most commonly unencapsulated.

VI. *Pseudomonas aeruginosa*

–causes **otitis externa** ("swimmer's ear"), sometimes along with normal flora.

–causes **chronic otitis media** with mixed flora.

–causes **malignant otitis externa,** an invasive pseudomonad infection that is generally found in diabetic patients and may be life threatening.

Multisystem Infections

I. *Listeria monocytogenes*

A. **General characteristics—*Listeria monocytogenes***

–is a gram-positive club-shaped bacillus that has tumbling motility at room temperature and is a psycrophile, growing in cooler temperatures.

Table 3-8. Important Bacterial Zoonoses

Organism	Spread to Humans	Site of Infection	Most Prominent Clinical Problem
Listeria monocytogenes	Birds, fish, mammals, food	Mononuclear phagocytes	Granulomas, especially in newborns and compromised adults
Yersinia pestis	Rat fleas	Monocytes	Vascular collapse; disseminated intravascular coagulation
Francisella tularensis	Rabbits, rodents	Mononuclear phagocytes	Granulomas; necrosis
Brucella species	Livestock	Reticuloendothelial system	Granulomas (generalized symptoms)
Bacillus anthracis	Sheep, cattle	Generalized toxemia	Necrosis, shock, respiratory distress

—causes zoonosis in vertebrate animals (birds, fish, and mammals) and can infect humans (see Table 3-8).

B. Attributes of pathogenicity

1. *L. monocytogenes* takes up intracellular residence within mononuclear phagocytes and epithelial cells.

2. *Listeria* "reorganizes" host cell actin, and these form actin trails as *Listeria* moves directly into other cells, avoiding the extracellular environment.

3. **Listeriolysin O** is required for the rapid egress of *Listeria* from the initial membrane-bound (phagosomal) state into the cytoplasm, allowing protected intracellular replication.

C. Clinical manifestations

1. **Infections in pregnant women** result in flu-like symptoms with potential to pass *Listeria* to the fetus transplacentally or during birth to the neonate.

2. **Granulomatosis infantiseptica** (from in utero infection) results in widely distributed abscesses and granulomas in the fetus. Fatality rate is 30% to 100%.

3. **Meningoencephalitis** occurs in neonates (acquired during passage through an infected birth canal), patients with malignancy, immunocompromised patients (particularly renal transplant patients), and adults older than 40 years. This disease has become the most common meningitis to occur in immunocompromised patients but is recognized also in patients with no known compromising conditions.

4. **Septicemia** occurs in the same population as for meningoencephalitis.

5. **Focal lesions** result from direct contact, generally as eye or skin lesions.

D. Laboratory diagnosis

1. Identification

   –is by identification of gram-positive coccobacillus (intracellular and/or extracellular).

   –is by culture on blood agar and demonstration of β-hemolysis.

   –is by identifying characteristic "tumbling motility" in 25°C broth cultures.

   –is by identifying the organism as catalase positive; in addition, it does not produce H_2S on triple sugar iron medium.

2. Clinical specimens

   –are obtained from CSF, blood, amniotic fluid from the newborn, or the genital tract of the mother.

   –**cold enrichment** (storage of specimen at 4°C with weekly 37°C cultures) may be necessary if *Listeria* is in mixed culture with normal flora that will overgrow it. (The other organisms die at 4°C.) Gene probe methods are replacing this method.

E. Control

1. Treatment

   a. Ampicillin should be given intravenously.

   b. The prognosis is poor, with a high fatality rate in newborns.

2. Prevention

   a. **Animal reservoirs** are a major problem.

   b. Milk pasteurization kills the organisms.

   c. Infections in pregnant women should be treated immediately, but recognizing the infection may be difficult when symptoms are mild.

II. *Yersinia pestis*

A. General characteristics—*Yersinia pestis*

   –is a gram-negative Enterobacteriaceae (oxidase negative, catalase positive, fermentor of glucose) and a nonfermentor of lactose.

   –is the causative agent of **plague,** one of the most devastating diseases in humans. It is rapidly progressive and still has a death rate of approximately 20%.

   –is endemic in the United States in the southwestern desert in wild rodents and langomorphs (e.g., ground squirrels, rats, rabbits, mice, prairie dogs) and is spread to humans by flea bite.

B. Attributes of pathogenicity

1. **Coagulase** plays a role in transmission.

2. **F1 protein** capsule is major virulence factor inhibiting phagocytosis.

3. **V and W surface antigens** are also considered virulence factors.

4. **Endotoxin.**

5. *Y. pestis* is a **facultative intracellular organism.**

C. **Clinical disease**

1. **Bubonic plague** begins as a flea bite with regional lymph node swelling caused by infection, necrosis, and suppuration to produce a bubo.

2. **Fever, bubos, and conjunctivitis** are the hallmark symptoms. The organism may spread to lungs (through pulmonary emboli) to produce pneumonia (5% of cases), which is highly contagious.

3. **Pneumonic plague** occurs with respiratory exposure to *Y. pestis*. This is a rapidly necrotic pneumonia, with death occurring within days.

D. **Laboratory diagnosis**

1. Cultures are hazardous and the organism grows on common laboratory media (e.g., MacConkey agar). The laboratory should be warned if *Y. pestis* is suspected.

2. Distinctive bipolar staining (Wayson's stain or Gram stain) gives a safety-pin appearance under microscopy.

3. Immunofluorescence test (reference laboratory) gives a rapid diagnosis.

E. **Control**

1. **Treatment** is with streptomycin.

2. **Prevention** is with vaccine for individuals at high risk.

III. *Borrelia burgdorferi*

A. **General characteristics—*Borrelia burgdorferi***

–is a large motile **spirochete.**

–is carried by the *Ixodes* tick:

1. *Ixodes dammini* (*I. scapularis*) in the northeastern and central United States

2. *Ixodes pacificus* in the northwestern United states

–usually infects people by **nymph** stage biting from **May to September.**

–mates on **deer,** which are important to its life cycle. Larvae feed on the **white-footed mouse,** the most important source of *B. burgdorferi,* before developing into nymphs.

B. **Classification—*Borrelia burgdorferi***

–is taxonomically related to *Treponema;* there are some parallels between syphilis and Lyme disease in terms of spread, stages, and crossing of both the placenta and the blood–brain barrier.

–is related to *Borrelia recurrentis* (louse borne) and the other *Borrelia* species (tick borne), which cause relapsing fever. *B. burgdorferi* shares with them the tendency for **antigenic variation.**

C. **Attributes of pathogenicity** include:

–production of blebs containing DNA and surrounded by cell envelope containing antigens, peptidoglycan, and outer membrane

–antigenic variation

–invasiveness

D. Clinical manifestations—Lyme disease

–is a **bloodstream infection** that seeds other tissues, especially the brain, heart, and joints.

–manifestations are protean; like syphilis, this disease has been termed "the great imitator."

1. **Stage 1.** The hallmark is **erythema (chronicum) migrans (EM),** a circular rash that spreads out from the site of the tick bite. It may last for several weeks and enlarge to several inches in diameter; additional EMs may appear. Malaise, fatigue, headache, fever, chills, stiff neck, aches, and pains occur for several weeks.

2. **Stage 2.** Neural and heart problems arise, including meningitis, cranial neuropathy, radiculoneuropathy, and some cardiac dysfunction; follows stage 1 by weeks to months.

3. **Stage 3.** Joint problems occur, especially in large joints, producing oligoarthritis. Bouts of arthritis last for 3 to 7 years. Neural dysfunction leads to dementia and paralysis; it follows stage 1 by months to years.

E. Laboratory diagnosis—Identification

1. The organism is difficult to culture but may be seen in skin biopsy with Giemsa stain.

2. The key to diagnosis is recognition of clinical manifestations along with tick bite. (Tick attachment may be missed by patients because the ticks inject an antihistamine, anesthetic, and anticoagulant.) EM may be missing in 25% of cases.

3. Several antibody (both IgM and IgG) tests are available but may be falsely negative in serious infection with such high levels of antigen that there may be no free antibody to measure.

4. Lyme urine antigen capture tests identify **antigens.**

5. **Polymerase chain reaction** is being used on joint fluid and CSF to detect the presence of organisms.

F. Control

1. **Treatment**

   a. Blood is the only specimen taken during early infection.

   b. CSF and joint fluid may be needed as specimens in cases of later-stage infection.

   c. For primary infection, therapy is with doxycycline, amoxicillin, or cefuroxime.

   d. For carditis and meningitis, therapy is with ceftriaxone.

   e. For arthritis, treatment is with doxycycline or azithromycin.

2. **Prevention**

   a. **Endemic areas** for Lyme disease are Minnesota, Wisconsin, and the northeastern seaboard of the United States; however, it occurs worldwide.

b. The highest incidence of Lyme disease correlates with tick season (summer).

c. If a tick is visibly attached and embedded, it should be carefully removed without squeezing the body; remnants of its mouth parts should not be left in the skin.

IV. *Ehrlichia*

–is tick borne.

–is a rickettsia that causes human disease endemic to the United States.

–enters monocytes or granulocytes (depending on the species) by *Ehrlichia*-induced phagocytosis and replicates in phagosomes.

–causes fever, myalgia, headache, malaise, leukopenia, and thrombocytopenia but no rash. There have been some fatalities. (It appears similar to Rocky Mountain spotted fever but without the rash.)

–may appear as mulberry-like structures (morulae) in infected cells.

–infection is treated with tetracycline.

V. *Rickettsia rickettsii*

A. General characteristics—*Rickettsia rickettsii*

–is a weakly staining gram-negative **obligate intracellular bacterium** with a specific predilection for endothelial cells of capillaries.

–causes a **zoonotic** disease in which ticks are vectors of human disease. *R. rickettsii* has dogs and rodents as its primary reservoir.

–induces **variable clinical manifestations,** ranging from benign and self-limiting to highly fulminant, which is highly fatal.

B. Classification—*Rickettsia rickettsii*

–is related to less common organisms.

–is listed by disease and symptomatology in Table 3–9.

C. Attributes of pathogenicity—*Rickettsia rickettsii*

–takes up intracellular (cytoplasmic) residence within endothelial cells of the vascular system.

–has an endotoxin.

D. Clinical manifestations

1. **Multisystemic diseases** of endothelial cells occur, resulting in hyperplasia, thrombus formation, inhibited blood supply, angiitis, and peripheral vasculitis.

2. **General rickettsial manifestations** involve **abrupt onset** of high fever, chills, headache (severe, frontal, unremitting), and myalgias; a few days later, hemorrhagic rash, stupor, delirium, and shock develop.

3. **Rocky Mountain spotted fever** (*R. rickettsii,* carried by ticks) initially causes a rash on the extremities, which spreads to the trunk. The fatality rate varies from 20% to 30%.

E. Laboratory diagnosis

1. **Identification**

–depends heavily on clinical manifestations, especially rash and abrupt onset of fever, headache, and chills with recent exposure to ticks.

Table 3–9. Important Rickettsial Diseases

Group	Disease	Organism	Spread	Clinical Presentation
Typhus	Epidemic	*Rickettsia prowazeckii*	Lice	Trunk rash, progressing to extremities, gangrene, shock, renal, heart
	Epidemic	*Rickettsia typhi*	Rat fleas	Trunk rash, progressing to extremities (less severe than epidemic typhus)
Spotted fever	Rocky Mountain spotted fever	*Rickettsia rickettsii*	Ticks	Rash on extremities, progressing to trunk, fulminant vasculitis
	Rickettsialpox	*Rickettsia akari*	Mites	Rash similar to chickenpox (benign course), adenopathy, eschars
Q fever		*Coxiella burnetii*	Dust	Pneumonitis without rash; atypical pneumonia with hepatitis
Cat scratch fever		*Rochalimea henselae*	Cat scratches	Skin, eye rashes, temporary blindness

–may be determined by comparing acute and convalescent sera measurements, using agglutination reactions and cross-reacting *Proteus* antigens, immunofluorescence reactions, and complement fixation tests.

2. **Clinical specimens** for antibody detection are obtained from blood.

F. Control

1. **Treatment**

   a. **Doxycycline** is the drug of choice.

   b. **Chloramphenicol** should be used if there is no time to differentiate between Rocky Mountain spotted fever and infection with *N. meningitidis*.

   c. If Rocky Mountain spotted fever is suspected, treatment should be initiated immediately.

   d. The patient should continue the prescribed regimen of antibiotics. (After the rash disappears, patients tend to discontinue treatment.)

   e. Treatment failures are expected.

2. **Prevention**

   a. Vectors should be avoided.

   b. The **endemic area** in the United States for Rocky Mountain spotted fever is primarily in the Appalachian states.

VI. *Coxiella burnetii*

A. General characteristics—*Coxiella burnetii*

–is a genus of Rickettsiaceae and therefore a gram-negative, intracellular organism that replicates in the cytoplasm.

–grows to high titers in infected pregnant animals.

–is transmitted by aerosols to humans aiding animals giving birth. May be milk borne, or, because of a resistant form, may be dust borne.

B. Attributes of pathogenicity include:

–a desiccation-resistant form

–intracellular replication

–endotoxin

–phase variation in surface polysaccharide

C. Clinical manifestations include:

–fever, chills, headache, but no rash

–interstitial pneumonia that may be mild

–hepatosplenomegaly with abnormal liver enzymes

–complications of myocarditis, pericarditis, endocarditis, or encephalitis

D. Laboratory diagnosis is by establishing an increasing complement fixation titer or by IFA or ELISA.

E. Treatment is with tetracyclines.

VII. *Francisella tularensis* (see Table 3–8)

A. General characteristics—*Francisella tularensis*

–causes a **zoonotic** disease, seen mainly in rabbits and rodents, that can be transmitted to humans through ingestion or handling of infected animals or through the bites of ticks, deer flies, black flies, mosquitoes, mites, or lice.

–is the gram-negative bacterium causing **tularemia** (also called deer fly fever or rabbit fever).

B. Attributes of pathogenicity. *Francisella* takes up intracellular residence within fixed macrophages of the reticuloendothelial system and within mononuclear phagocytes.

C. Clinical manifestations

1. **Tularemia** is characterized by macrophage infiltration, granulomas, and necrosis of infected tissues. Regional lymph nodes become infected and suppurate. Spread to the lungs, liver, and spleen is common.

2. Initial manifestations include abrupt onset of fever, headache, and regional (painful) adenopathy; back pain, anorexia, chills, sweats, and prostration follow. The fatality rate is 1%.

3. Manifestations vary according to the site of organism entry.

   a. **Ulceroglandular tularemia** (the most common manifestation) is a skin infection.

   b. **Oculoglandular tularemia** involves an eye infection (granulomatous conjunctivitis).

      c. Glandular or **pneumonic tularemia** involves lung infection; it results from inhaling infected dust.

      d. Typhoidal tularemia causes gastrointestinal symptoms; it results from ingesting contaminated meat.

  D. Laboratory diagnosis

    1. Identification

      a. The organism is a gram-negative coccobacillus.

      b. The organism is difficult to culture in vitro.

      c. Agglutination reaction can detect a rise in antibody titers from acute to convalescent sera.

      d. A skin test is available.

    2. Clinical specimens

      a. The organism is contagious after in vitro growth.

      b. Routine laboratory culture should be avoided.

  E. Control

    1. Treatment

      –is with **streptomycin;** if the infection is in an early stage, a rapid cure is anticipated; more advanced infection is more difficult to cure.

      –may not prevent relapses, which are attributed to the intracellular residence of the organism.

    2. Prevention

      a. Meat should be cooked thoroughly (especially rabbit meat).

      b. A vaccine is recommended for high-risk groups, such as sheep handlers, trappers, and laboratory workers.

VIII. *Brucella* (see Table 3–8)

  A. General characteristics. *Brucella* causes zoonosis, with most human infections occurring in livestock farmers and meat processors.

  B. Classification. Three species of the genus cause human **brucellosis:**
    –*Brucella suis* (swine)
    –*Brucella melitensis* (goats)
    –*Brucella abortus* (cattle)

  C. Attributes of pathogenicity

    1. Intracellular multiplication occurs in macrophages of the reticuloendothelial system.

    2. Initial exposure leads to phagocytosis by neutrophils, which carry organisms to the lymph nodes, spleen, bone marrow, and liver, with ensuing infection of these tissues.

  D. Clinical manifestations

    1. Organisms localize and cause **granulomas** in the spleen, liver, bone marrow, and lymph nodes.

2. The patient has intermittent fever and nondescript findings, including profound muscle weakness, chills, sweats, anorexia, headache, backache, depression, and nervousness.

3. Two types of infection occur:

   a. Acute infection, with relapses and fever

   b. Chronic infection, with protracted weakness, depression, arthralgias, and myalgias lasting more than 12 months

E. Laboratory diagnosis

–is by identification of gram-negative coccobacilli (stain after in vitro culture).

–is based primarily on prolonged clinical manifestations and a serologic agglutination reaction.

F. Control

1. **Treatment**

   a. Tetracycline and **streptomycin** are given for 3 to 6 weeks (the infection is hard to eradicate because of its intracellular residence).

   b. Relapses occur in 30% of cases.

2. **Prevention**

   a. Most infections in the United States are attributed to **contaminated milk and cheese;** routine pasteurization of milk and cheese has greatly reduced the incidence of infection.

   b. An effective vaccine exists only for animals.

   c. Brucellosis poses a continued problem for farmers and meat processors.

IX. *Bacillus anthracis*

A. General characteristics—*Bacillus*

–causes anthrax (a zoonosis), which is especially prevalent in goats, sheep, and cattle.

–spores play an important role in transmission; they can survive in soil for 30 years.

B. Attributes of pathogenicity—*Bacillus anthracis*

–possesses a capsular polypeptide of D-glutamic acid (unique because bacterial capsules usually contain polysaccharide) that inhibits phagocytosis.

–produces a potent **exotoxin** that causes CNS distress with respiratory failure and anoxia; the exotoxin is composed of a protective antigen, a lethal factor, and an edema factor.

–spores are phagocytosed by macrophages that carry them to lymph nodes and induce infection.

C. Clinical manifestations. *Bacillus anthracis* causes a **profound toxemia** (on entry of a potent exotoxin into the circulation); death occurs within 2 to 5 days. Manifestations depend on the route of spore entry.

1. **Cutaneous manifestations,** seen in 95% of anthrax cases, result from

entry of spores into a cut or an abrasion (especially on the hands, forearms, or head).

    a. A **small pustule** develops into a large vesicle containing dark fluid (eschar) surrounded by a characteristic inflammatory ring at the base.

    b. The fatality rate is 10%.

2. Pulmonary manifestations (known as wool sorters' disease) occur in 5% of anthrax cases and result from entry of spores into the lungs.

    a. This disease form is characterized by abrupt onset of high fever, malaise, cough, myalgias, marked hemorrhagic necrosis of the lymph nodes, respiratory distress, and cyanosis.

    b. The fatality rate is 50%.

D. Laboratory diagnosis

1. Identification

    a. The organism is gram-positive with large rods; spores are absent in the clinical specimen.

    b. Blood agar is used to isolate colonies.

    c. Toxicity is demonstrated by injecting *Bacillus anthracis* into mice; death occurs in a few days, with large numbers of bacilli in the blood.

    d. Antibody tests should be performed on acute and convalescent sera.

2. Clinical specimens

    a. A blood sample should be obtained; if organisms are detected, the prognosis is poor.

    b. A vesicle fluid sample should be obtained.

E. Control

1. Treatment of anthrax

    a. **Early detection** is the key to diagnosing cutaneous anthrax; pulmonary and gastrointestinal anthrax are usually diagnosed on postmortem examination.

    b. **Penicillin** should be given intravenously to kill the organisms and stop elaboration of the exotoxin.

2. Prevention of anthrax

    a. Infected animals should be killed and buried deeply (to minimize spores); animals should not be incinerated because spores would be released into the air.

    b. In endemic areas (Louisiana, Texas, California, South Dakota, Nebraska), commercial wool, hair, and hides should be gas sterilized.

    c. An effective **vaccine** is routinely used in animals in areas where outbreaks have occurred.

    d. Farmers and animal processors are at risk (the disease has a very low incidence in the United States).

Table 3–10. Properties of Bacterial Pathogens

Bacterium	Distinguishing Characteristics	Diseases
Actinomyces	Anaerobe, branching rod "Sulfur" granular microcolonies Contiguous growth through anatomic barriers Cervicofacial, thoracic, and abdominal lesions	Actinomycosis
Bacillus anthracis	Potent exotoxin Capsular polypeptide inhibits phagocytosis Spore transmission	Cutaneous anthrax Pulmonary anthrax
Bacteroides fragilis	Non–spore-forming pleomorphic anaerobe Mixed infections Capsulated Possesses a beta-lactamase Wound débridement important	Brain abscess Gastrointestional (GI) abscess Cellulitis Pelvic inflammatory disease (PID)
Bordetella pertussis	Paroxysmal cough due to toxin Attaches via pili Component of DPT vaccine	Whooping cough
Borrelia burgdorferi	*Ixodes* transmission Corkscrew-shaped motile spirochete	Lyme disease
Campylobacter jejuni	Comma-shaped rod A frequent cause of diarrhea Enterotoxin Neutrophils and blood in stool	Gastroenteritis
Chlamydia pneumoniae	Obligate intracellular parasite Elementary and reticular body Divides by binary fission	Pneumonia
Chlamydia psittaci	Zoonotic (birds, parrots) Sudden onset	Respiratory disease
Chlamydia trachomatis	As for *C. pneumoniae* 15 Serotypes	Chronic keratoconjunctivitis (subtypes A–C) Sexually transmitted infection (D–K) Lymphogranuloma venereum (L subtype) Arthritis, PID

Table 3–10. (*continued*)

Bacterium	Distinguishing Characteristics	Diseases
Clostridium botulinum	Spore-forming anaerobe Exotoxin acting at myoneural junction Suppresses acetylcholine release by peripheral nerves Produces flaccid muscle paralysis Caused by ingestion of preformed toxin or by ingestion of spores by infants	Botulism
Clostridium difficile	Spore-forming anaerobe Part of normal gastrointestinal flora Activated by antibiotic disruption of other flora Secrete an enterotoxin and cytotoxin	Gastroenteritis Pseudomembranous colitis
Clostridium perfringens	Spore-forming anaerobe Spores introduced by severe trauma Possesses an alpha toxin (lecithinase)	Gas gangrene Food poisoning Soft tissue cellulitis
Corynebacterium diphtheriae	Phage-induced A/B exotoxin Lysogenic conversion Fragment A inhibits tRNA EF-2	Pharyngeal diphtheria Cutaneous diphtheria
Coxiella burnetii	Intracellular bacterium (rickettsia) Dust and tick transmitted Absence of rash	Q fever Pneumonitis
Ehrlichia	Tick-transmitted zoonosis Strict intracellular pathogen (WBC) Belong to family Rickettsiaceae	Ehrlichiosis
Enterococcus	Formerly group D streptococci Most are alpha- or gamma-hemolytic Antibiotic resistance is a problem Beta-lactamase Nosocomial opportunist	Urinary tract infection Endocarditis
Escherichia coli	Enterotoxigenic: heat-labile toxin stimulates adenylate cyclase similar to cholera toxin; heat-stable toxin activates guanylate cyclase Enteropathogenic: adherence to enterocytes→infantile diarrhea Enterohemorrhagic: Shiga-like verotoxin→bloody diarrhea (serotype 0157) Enteroinvasive: properties similar to shigellosis All strains possess endotoxin	Genitourinary tract infections Gastroenteritis Septic shock Neonatal meningitis

Table 3–10. (*continued*)

Bacterium	Distinguishing Characteristics	Diseases
Fusobacterium nucleatum	Polymorphic, slender filaments Oral anaerobe Synergizes with *Borrelia vincentii*	Vincent's angina Brain abscess Head, neck, chest infections
Haemophilus aegyptius	Antiphagocytic polysaccharide capsule	Conjunctivitis (pinkeye)
Haemophilus influenzae	Antiphagocytic polysaccharide capsule Pyrogenic IgAase Grow on chocolate agar or with X and V factors Epiglottis requires a tracheotomy	Genitourinary (GU) infections Meningitis (to 6 years old) Epiglottitis
Helicobacter pylori	Curved rod Produces a potent urease and cytotoxin Treat with bismuth salts, metronidazole, and antibiotic	Gastric and peptic ulcers Increases risk for gastric adenocarcinoma
Legionella pneumophila	Aquaphile–inhalation transmission Association with amoeba Possesses a cytotoxin and endotoxin Beta-lactamase Stains with Dieterle silver stain; no Gram stain Requires cysteine and iron for growth Intracellular parasite	Legionnaires' disease (pneumonia)
Listeria monocytogenes	Animal reservoir Infects monocytes (monocytosis) Hemolysin destroys vesicular membranes	Granulomas Abscesses Meningitis (newborns)
Mycobacterium avium-intracellulare	Group of acid-fast organisms Drug resistance Common infection in AIDS; noncontagious	Pulmonary disease
Mycobacterium tuberculosis	Peptidoglycan–arabinogalactam cell wall Mycolic acids require acid-fast stain Cord factor (trehalose mycolate) induces granuloma Purified protein derivative (PPD) skin test Becoming isoniazid and rifampin resistant Bacille Calmette Guérin (BCG) vaccine	Tuberculosis Granulomas
Mycoplasma pneumoniae	Lacks a cell wall Smallest extracellular bacterium; not an L form Mucosal tissue tropism Requires cholesterol	Primary atypical pneumonia

Table 3–10. (*continued*)

Bacterium	Distinguishing Characteristics	Diseases
Neisseria gonorrhoeae	Intracellular gram-negative diplococcus Produces an IgAase and a penicillinase plasmid Purulent exudate Requires chocolate agar (Thayer-Martin) Oxidase positive	Urethritis PID Conjunctivitis in newborns
Neisseria meningitidis	Antiphagocytic capsule Endotoxin (lipopolysaccharide) IgAase Vasculitic purpura Headache and stiff neck are common	Meningococcemia Waterhouse-Fridericksen syndrome
Nocardia	Aerobic soil bacterium Inhalation transmission	Pulmonary infections
Prevotella melaninogenica	Aerobic black colonies on agar Found in mouth, GI and GU tract Putrid sputum Débride and drain lesion Formerly in genus *Bacteroides*	Lung abscesses Female GU infections
Proteus mirabilis	Highly motile Produces urease	Pneumonia Nosocomial infections
Pseudomonas aeruginosa	Glycocalyx slime layer Pyocyanin–blue-green pigment Exotoxin similar in action to diphtheria Endotoxin (lipopolysaccharide)	Burn infections Cystic fibrosis infections Septic shock
Rickettsia rickettsii	Tick transmission Intracellular dwelling bacterium	Rocky Mountain spotted fever
Salmonella	Wide host range; except *S. typhosa* Many serotypes Intracellular multiplication Can invade bloodstream Endotoxin lipopolysaccharide Enterotoxin	Enterocolitis Septicemia Enteric fever (typhoid)
Shigella	No known animal reservoir Pathogenic in small numbers Perpetuation by small numbers Perpetuation by human carriers Possesses an endotoxin and an exotoxin Stools can contain mucus, pus, and blood Bloodstream invasion is rare Culture on differential and selective media Only *Shigella sonnei* ferments lactose	Shigellosis

Table 3-10. (*continued*)

Bacterium	Distinguishing Characteristics	Diseases
Staphylococcus aureus	Grape-like cluster morphology Antibiotic resistance Catalase and coagulase positive Enterotoxin Short incubation period (hours)	Local abscesses Impetigo Food poisoning
Staphylococcus epidermidis	Slime layer Instrument contamination Noninvasive nosocomial infections	Urinary tract infections Endocarditis
Staphylococcus saprophyticus	Noninvasive nosocomial infections	Urinary tract infections
Streptococcus agalactiae	Group B Can be part of normal vaginal and oral flora Capsule Inhibits complement	Neonatal sepsis (early and late onset) Meningitis
Streptococcus pneumoniae	Alpha-hemolytic Large antiphagocytic capsule Diplococcus Sensitive to bile and optochin Quellung reaction Vaccine contains 23 capsular serotypes Anticapsular antibody is protective Differentiates from *S. viridans*	Pneumonia Otitis media Septicemia
Streptococcus pyogenes	Group A M protein; (more than 80 types); antiphagocytic Beta-hemolytic Sensitive to bacitracin Erythrogenic exotoxins	Pharyngitis Scarlet fever Rheumatic fever Acute glomerulonephritis (GLN) Impetigo Cellulitis–erysipelas Endocarditis
Treponema pallidum	Spirochete Unable to be cultured Immunosuppressive Darkfield microscopy examination Serologic tests	Syphilis, 1°, 2°, 3°

Table 3–10. (*continued*)

Bacterium	Distinguishing Characteristics	Diseases
Vibrio cholerae	Comma-shaped morphology A/B enterotoxin overproduces cyclic AMP Vomiting and rice-water diarrhea Must replace copious fluid loss	Cholera
Viridans streptococci	Noninvasive opportunist in normal oral flora Alpha-hemolytic Differentiate from *S. pneumoniae* because the *S. viridans* are bile insoluble and not inhibited by optochin	Endocarditis Dental caries
Yersinia pestis	Zoonotic disease (rats and fleas) Intracellular multiplication Fever, conjunctivitis, regional buboes	Bubonic plague Pneumonic plague Yersiniosis

X. *Actinomyces*

A. General characteristics—*Actinomyces*

–is a non–acid-fast, gram-positive **bacterium.**

–is **anaerobic.**

–may branch in tissues and convert to rod forms.

–is found as a commensal organism in the gingival crevices and female genital tract.

–causes **chronic granulomatous infections,** mainly of the soft tissues (although it does invade bone), with swelling and a tendency to form **sinus tracts** to the surface; exudate from these sinus tracts contains hard microcolonies called **granules.**

B. Classification.
The organism is related to the mycobacteria and belongs to the Actinomycetes.

C. Attributes of pathogenicity.
The organism grows contiguously without respect for anatomic barriers.

D. Clinical disease

1. **Cervicofacial actinomycosis** (lumpy jaw) most commonly begins after dental work is performed.

2. **Thoracic actinomycosis** may involve the lungs and ribs.

3. **Abdominal actinomycosis** starts in the ileocecal region and frequently produces sinus tracts to the skin surface.

4. **Mycetoma** is an infection of the limb, with swelling, sinus tract formation, and granules.

E. Laboratory diagnosis
is by Gram stain of granules and anaerobic culture.

F. Control. Treatment commonly involves penicillin and surgical drainage of necrotic tissues.

XI. *Staphylococcus aureus* (see Skin and Soft Tissue Infections)

–is a catalase-positive, coagulase-positive, gram-positive coccus.

A. Clinical disease—toxic shock syndrome

1. TSST-1 circulates from the nidus of infection (e.g., tampon or surgical infection), acting as a superantigen, reducing liver clearance of endogenous endotoxin (from gram-negative organism in the body's normal flora), and triggering shock and other symptoms. (TSST-1–negative staphylococci and group A streptococci also cause toxic shock syndrome.)

2. Symptoms include high fever, diarrhea, collapse of peripheral circulation, hypotensive shock, scarlatiniform rash with desquamation of palms and soles.

3. Toxic shock syndrome may be associated with menstruating women using tampons, but it also occurs in other individuals, including patients with surgical packing.

B. Control

1. **Treatment** is with antibiotics and supportive care.

2. **Prevention,** in menstruating women, is by careful use of "super tampons."

XII. *Staphylococcus aureus* (see Skin and Soft Tissue Infections)—Clinical disease

–*S. aureus* is the major causative agent of hematogenously acquired osteomyelitis in adults and children.

–Disease is characterized by swelling, redness, pain, and fever.

XIII. Other

A. *Haemophilus influenzae* arthritis or osteomyelitis

–is generally caused by type B strains in children younger than 2 years old who have not been vaccinated.

B. *Yersinia enterocolitica*

–is a gram-negative Enterobacteriaceae (oxidase negative, catalase positive, fermentor of glucose, nonfermentor of lactose).

–may be zoonotic.

–may be transmitted in humans by the fecal–oral route or by blood transfusion.

–grows in the cold.

1. **Clinical disease**

   a. **Enterocolitis** occurs as fever, diarrhea, and abdominal pain, resembling appendicitis; symptoms include invasive infection-producing mesenteric lymphadenitis, terminal ileitis, septicemia and, generally in adults, arthritis.

   b. **Septicemia** is associated with blood transfusions. (Low numbers of bacteria replicate in the cold storage of the blood.)

2. **Control.** The disease is generally self-limiting.

Review Test

Directions: Each of the numbered items or incomplete statements in this section is followed by answers or by completions of the statement. Select the **one** lettered answer or completion that is **best** in each case.

1. A 22-year-old cystic fibrosis patient presents because of fever and increasing dyspnea. A gram-negative organism is found in unusually high numbers in the mucus. Which virulence factor is most important in colonization and maintenance of the organism in the lungs?

(A) Exotoxin A
(B) Pyocyanin (blue-green pigment)
(C) Polysaccharide slime
(D) Endotoxin

2. Exotoxin A mentioned in question 1 most closely resembles the cellular mechanism of which of the following?

(A) Heat-labile (LT) *Escherichia coli*
(B) Shiga toxin
(C) Diphtheria toxin
(D) *Vibrio cholerae* toxin
(E) Verotoxin

3. What is the most likely causative agent of gastroenteritis starting on day 5 of clindamycin treatment?

(A) *Clostridium perfringens*
(B) *Clostridium difficile*
(C) *Pseudomonas aeruginosa*
(D) *Shigella sonnei*

4. Which of the following statements about clinical manifestations of clostridial infections is correct?

(A) *Clostridium perfringens* does not infect nontraumatized tissues due to the high E_h of normal tissue.
(B) Infant botulism results from ingestion of preformed toxins in contaminated food.
(C) Tetanus causes death from cardiac dysfunction.
(D) The anaerobic cellulitis produced by *C. perfringens* spreads to surrounding healthy tissues.
(E) *Clostridium difficile* produces a mild gastroenteritis.

5. Which of the following statements about treatment of clostridial infections is true?

(A) Anaerobic cellulitis may require amputation or skin grafting.
(B) Clostridial food poisoning is severe, and patients infected with either *Clostridium perfringens* or *Clostridium botulinum* frequently require hospitalization.
(C) Infant botulism should be treated with antibiotics to eradicate the organism.
(D) Antitoxins must be administered as soon as clostridial infection is suspected.
(E) Patients with anaerobic cellulitis should be given antitoxin and antibiotics.

6. Which of the following is a characteristic of *Bacteroides fragilis?*

(A) Colonies have a distinctive black appearance.
(B) Organisms are susceptible to penicillin.
(C) Organisms possess a beta-lactamase.
(D) Organisms are rarely found in the gastrointestinal tract.

7. Which of the following conditions is necessary for effective diagnosis of anaerobic infections?

(A) Streaking on eosin–methylene blue (EMB) agar
(B) Rapid transport of culture to the laboratory
(C) Assay for superoxide dismutase
(D) Sputum sampling

8. Which one of the following statements concerning *Vibrio cholerae* infections is correct?

(A) Death occurs in 2 to 4 weeks from exhaustion and respiratory failure.
(B) The disease is marked by organism invasion and hemorrhagic necrosis of the small intestine.
(C) It is one of the most devastating diseases in humans.
(D) *V. cholerae* produces an acute febrile disease with meningitis.
(E) There is no need to hospitalize patients with *V. cholerae* infections. Organisms in stools are not contagious because the organism is sensitive to acid pH.

9. Which of the following statements about Lyme disease and its clinical manifestations is true?

(A) It is characterized by a rash throughout the trunk and extremities.
(B) The three stages of the disorder are distinctive and do not overlap.
(C) It is caused by *Borrelia burgdorferi*.
(D) Manifestations of stage 3 may appear within 4 weeks of the initial infection.

10. Which of the following statements about congenital syphilis is correct?

(A) Syphilis serology test should be performed in the first and third trimesters of pregnancy.
(B) Clinical manifestations are generally mild.
(C) Newborns are infected only when they pass through the infected birth canal.
(D) Specimens should be cultured on blood agar.

11. A patient has a gastric ulcer not induced by nonsteroidal anti-inflammatory agents. Which characteristic appears to play the most central role in the ability of the organism to colonize the stomach?

(A) Phospholipase C production
(B) Urease production
(C) Microaerophilic lifestyle
(D) O-antigens
(E) Motility

12. Which of the following statements about mycobacterial disease is correct?

(A) Nontuberculous disease is as contagious as tuberculosis.
(B) Tuberculosis is caused by *Mycobacterium tuberculosis*, and nontuberculous disease is caused by other mycobacteria, including *Mycobacterium bovis*, *Mycobacterium kansasii*, and *Mycobacterium avium-intracellulare*.
(C) Water is a source of exposure to nontuberculous mycobacteria.
(D) Only nontuberculous disease is seen with great frequency in patients with acquired immune deficiency syndrome (AIDS).
(E) *M. tuberculosis* is the only acid-fast mycobacteria.

13. Which of the following organisms grows contiguously in tissues with no respect to anatomic barriers?

(A) *Actinomyces israelii*
(B) *Mycobacterium leprae*
(C) *Mycobacterium kansasii*
(D) *Mycobacterium tuberculosis*

14. The Ghon complex, a lesion in the lung and regional lymph nodes, is found in

(A) actinomycotic mycetoma.
(B) tuberculoid leprosy.
(C) primary tuberculosis.
(D) cervical facial actinomycosis.
(E) soft tissue infections caused by *Mycobacterium marinum*.

15. Which of the following statements is true about the two major forms of leprosy (tuberculoid and lepromatous)?

(A) Tuberculoid leprosy is the hardest to treat due to poor cell-mediated immunity.
(B) In either extreme form of leprosy, the lepromin test will be positive.
(C) Diagnostic workup on the patient should include a physical examination, skin test, and cultures.
(D) Biopsy sample of lesions from a lepromatous leprosy patient is generally loaded with *Mycobacterium leprae*.
(E) Lepromatous leprosy patients usually have few lesions.

16. Which one of the following statements about *Francisella tularensis* infections and their treatment is correct?

(A) Culture of the suspected infection by the hospital laboratory is important.
(B) An effective vaccine is available but only for use in high-risk groups.
(C) *F. tularensis* causes a noninvasive focal skin infection.
(D) Relapses do not occur after treatment.
(E) The hallmark of *F. tularensis* infection is regional buboes.

17. Which of the following statements about *Brucella* infections is true?

(A) *Brucella suis* is the human pathogen; *Brucella melitensis* and *Brucella abortus* cause infections in animals only.
(B) *Brucella* infection produces profound muscle weakness along with other relatively nondescript manifestations.
(C) *Brucella* infection is a zoonotic disease spread to humans primarily by rat fleas.
(D) Untreated infections are self-limiting and resolve in 2 weeks.
(E) *Brucella* is an extracellular parasite.

18. Which of the following statements about anthrax infections is correct?

(A) The early cutaneous form may mimic a staphylococcal furuncle or insect bite.
(B) Pulmonary and gastrointestinal anthrax tend to be chronic, with frequent treatment failure.
(C) Spores are routinely observed in lesion aspirates.
(D) The capsule is a long-chain polysaccharide.
(E) Primary animal reservoirs are rabbits and other rodents.

19. Which of the following is a virulence factor for *Streptococcus pneumoniae*?

(A) C-reactive protein
(B) Bacitracin
(C) Endotoxic lipopolysaccharide
(D) Capsular polysaccharide

20. Which one of the following statements about laboratory diagnosis of diphtheria is correct?

(A) Organisms are delicate and survive poorly outside the host.
(B) It is sufficient to identify *Corynebacterium diphtheriae* in the isolate.
(C) Organisms are impossible to identify by Gram stain because of their small size.
(D) Culture on Löffler's medium or tellurite medium should reveal characteristic Chinese letter formation.
(E) Organisms are coagulase-positive.

21. Which of the following statements about laboratory diagnosis of whooping cough is correct?

(A) Lymphocyte numbers are greatly decreased.
(B) Cough plate is the method of choice to isolate organisms from the patient.
(C) The clinical specimen should be plated on Bordet-Gengou agar.
(D) The best chance to isolate the organism is during the paroxysmal stage.
(E) The causative organism is a gram-positive rod.

22. A 54-year-old man develops a pyogenic infection along the suture line following knee surgery. The laboratory gives a preliminary report of a β-hemolytic, catalase-positive, coagulase-positive, gram-positive coccus. The most likely causative agent is

(A) *Moraxella catarrhalis*
(B) *Staphylococcus aureus*
(C) *Staphylococcus epidermidis*
(D) *Streptococcus agalactiae*
(E) *Streptococcus pyogenes*

23. Which of the following statements about treatment and prevention of *Haemophilus* is correct?

(A) Give rifampin to index case of *Haemophilus influenzae* meningitis and to family members to eradicate the carrier state.
(B) Bacterial pinkeye is treated with intravenous ampicillin.
(C) Soft chancre is poorly contagious, and asymptomatic sexual partners need not be treated.
(D) Haemophilus capsular vaccine is highly effective in target population of children age 3 months to 6 years.
(E) Meningitis patients should be treated for 14 days with oral antibiotics.

24. Which one of the following statements about laboratory diagnosis of *Neisseria gonorrhoeae* is correct?

(A) Purulent discharge contains primarily neutrophils and intracellular diplococci.
(B) Asymptomatic patients are identified by culturing organisms from a clinical specimen with a lubricated swab.
(C) Purulent discharge contains only intracellular diplococci.
(D) Clinical specimens should be plated onto blood agar to determine type of hemolysis.
(E) In disseminated infections, organisms can be routinely isolated from skin lesions.

Directions: Each of the numbered items or incomplete statements in this section is negatively phrased, as indicated by a capitalized word such as NOT, LEAST, or EXCEPT. Select the **one** lettered answer or completion that is **best** in each case.

25. All of the following statements about clinical manifestations of *Haemophilus influenzae* are correct EXCEPT

(A) acute bacterial epiglottitis is a mild disease in children.
(B) severe CNS deficits occur in one-third of recovered meningitis patients.
(C) pus production is typical.
(D) during viral influenza outbreaks, incidence of *H. influenzae* increases.
(E) pneumonia is a complication usually seen in children or the aged.

26. Which of the following is NOT characteristic of plague infections?

(A) They are marked by intravascular coagulation and purpuric skin lesions.
(B) They are transmitted between humans via respiratory droplets.
(C) They cause septicemia, primarily in debilitated patients.
(D) They are termed yersiniosis if caused by *Yersinia enterocolitica*.
(E) They are spread by fleas.

27. All of the following statements about *Mycoplasma pneumoniae* infections are true EXCEPT

(A) Eaton agent causes primary atypical pneumonia.
(B) *M. pneumoniae* produces surface mucous membrane infections that do not disseminate to other tissues.
(C) *M. pneumoniae* is a slow-growing organism that requires 1 to 3 weeks to culture in the laboratory.
(D) serologic tests for *M. pneumoniae* involve complement fixation or cold agglutination.
(E) incidence of *M. pneumoniae* is highest in elderly persons.

28. All of the following are characteristics of *Legionella* EXCEPT

(A) it is associated with water.
(B) it causes granulomatous lung infection.
(C) it is weakly gram-negative.
(D) it is a facultative, intracellular parasite.
(E) it is catalase-positive.

29. All of the following statements about non–spore-forming anaerobes are correct EXCEPT

(A) they are pleomorphic and can be either gram-negative or gram-positive.
(B) they are a common cause of intra-abdominal infections.
(C) they usually are found in mixed infections.
(D) they represent a minority of the total fecal flora.
(E) they include the *Fusobacterium* genus found in the oral cavity.

30. All of the following statements about *Campylobacter* infections are correct EXCEPT

(A) sepsis is a problem in debilitated patients with *Campylobacter fetus* species infection.
(B) human infections with *Campylobacter jejuni* are rare relative to *Salmonella* and *Shigella* infections.
(C) *C. jejuni* infection is usually self-limiting.
(D) *C. jejuni* clinical specimens should be incubated at 42°C.

31. All of the following are characteristics of Enterobacteriaceae EXCEPT they

(A) commonly cause hospital-acquired infections.
(B) are usually noninvasive and are part of the normal intestinal flora.
(C) can produce both endotoxins and exotoxins.
(D) have a short incubation period (several hours), leading to gastrointestinal disturbances.
(E) ferment glucose.

32. All of the following statements about the incidence of bacterial shock are correct EXCEPT

(A) it is usually a hospital-induced syndrome.
(B) it can occur after catheterization.
(C) it is reversible by penicillin.
(D) mortality is dependent on admission prognosis.
(E) it is usually preceded by a fever spike.

33. All of the following are characteristics of *Salmonella typhimurium* EXCEPT it

(A) has a multianimal reservoir.
(B) is one of the most common causes of enterocolitis.
(C) ferments lactose.
(D) is a common contaminant of poultry.
(E) is a gram-negative, motile, endotoxin-bearing rod.

34. All of the following statements about *Listeria monocytogenes* infection are correct EXCEPT

(A) abscesses and granulomas occur in many different tissues.
(B) laboratory isolation involves cold enrichment technique.
(C) neonatal infections have poor prognosis.
(D) bacteria parasitize neutrophils and monocytes.
(E) neonatal infections occur only during passage through the infected birth canal.

35. All of the following statements about *Yersinia pestis* infections are true EXCEPT

(A) wild rodents and their infected fleas are the primary reservoir.
(B) a key early manifestation is a slowly progressing malaise.
(C) the pneumonic form is far more contagious than the bubonic form.
(D) the bubonic form may progress to the pneumonic form.

36. All of the following statements are true of staphylococcal and *Neisseria* infections EXCEPT

(A) pus production is a helpful diagnostic aid.
(B) localized infections may disseminate and cause severe clinical problems.
(C) both types of organisms cause urinary tract infections.
(D) Gram stain of clinical specimens is an important diagnostic aid.
(E) they both produce an enzyme that degrades IgA (IgAase).

37. All of the following are characteristics of group A streptococci EXCEPT they

(A) are part of the normal intestinal flora.
(B) attach to epithelial cells via fimbriae containing lipotechoic acid.
(C) are rarely resistant to penicillin.
(D) produce β-hemolysis with streptolysin S.

38. All of the following are characteristic of group B streptococci EXCEPT

(A) an effective vaccine incorporates proteinaceous capsular antigens.
(B) they are part of the normal vaginal flora.
(C) they are bacitracin-resistant.
(D) they precipitate with *Streptococcus agalactiae* antiserum.
(E) they cause neonatal sepsis and meningitis.

Directions: Each group of items in this section consists of lettered options followed by a set of numbered items. For each item, select the **one** lettered option that is most closely associated with it. Each lettered option may be selected once, more than once, or not at all.

Questions 39–45

Match each of the following organisms with the appropriate characteristic.

(A) *Rickettsia akari*
(B) *Rickettsia typhi*
(C) *Rickettsia rickettsii*
(D) *Coxiella burnetii*
(E) All of the above

39. Spread through inhalation of infected dust

40. Characterized by abrupt onset of fever, chills, and unremitting headache

41. Rash initially on extremities, spreading to trunk

42. Zoonosis spread to humans by arthropod vectors

43. Obligate intracellular bacteria with predilection for multiplication within capillary endothelial cells

44. Pneumonitis resembling atypical pneumonia

45. Mite-borne agent causing a rash that may be confused with chickenpox

Questions 46–49

Match each of the following organisms with the appropriate characteristic.

(A) *Vibrio cholerae*
(B) *Vibrio parahaemolyticus*
(C) *Salmonella typhi*
(D) *Shigella sonnei*

46. Causes a relatively mild form of gastroenteritis

47. Causes septicemic disease

48. Has diverse animal reservoir

49. Invades mucosal epithelial cells

Questions 50–54

Match each of the following characteristics with the appropriate organism.

(A) Secretes an enterotoxin
(B) Contains an endotoxin
(C) Possesses both an enterotoxin and endotoxin
(D) Possesses neither an enterotoxin nor an endotoxin

50. *Streptococcus pneumoniae*

51. *Pseudomonas aeruginosa*

52. *Shigella dysenteriae*

53. *Salmonella typhimurium*

54. *Vibrio cholerae*

Questions 55–57

Match each of the following infectious diseases with the causative spirochete.

(A) *Treponema*
(B) *Borrelia*
(C) *Leptospira*

55. Relapsing fever transmitted by lice or ticks

56. Acute icteric disease with protean manifestations

57. Zoonotic disease transmitted to humans primarily by contact with animal urine

Questions 58–61

Match each of the following characteristics with the appropriate actinomycete.

(A) *Nocardia*
(B) *Actinomyces*
(C) Mycobacteria

58. Anaerobic

59. Partially acid-fast and filamentous

60. Generally rod-shaped and acid-fast

61. Very slow growers

Questions 62–65

Match the characteristics with the following corresponding components of *Mycobacterium tuberculosis*.

(A) Cord factor
(B) Mycolic acid
(C) Purified protein derivative (PPD)
(D) Sulfatides
(E) Wax D

62. Promotes intracellular survival by inhibiting phagosome–lysosome fusion

63. Used for skin testing

64. Responsible for the acid-fast property of the organism

65. Interrupts mitochondrial function

Questions 66–68

Match the following clinical manifestations with the associated staphylococcal organism.

(A) *Staphylococcus aureus*
(B) *Staphylococcus epidermidis*
(C) *Staphylococcus haemolyticus*
(D) *Staphylococcus saprophyticus*

66. Subacute bacterial endocarditis occurring 2 months or more after heart surgery

67. Acute bacterial endocarditis occurring within 2 months after heart surgery

68. Urinary tract infections, primarily in the adolescent female

Questions 69–71
Match the following characteristics to the corresponding group A streptococcal disease.

(A) Impetigo
(B) Scarlet fever
(C) Rheumatic fever
(D) Cellulitis

69. Highly communicable in infants

70. Characterized by rash due to erythrogenic toxins

71. Skin infection capable of giving rise to a septicemia

Questions 72–74

Match the following organisms with the corresponding characteristic.

(A) Enterococcus faecalis
(B) *Streptococcus pneumoniae*
(C) Group B streptococci
(D) *Viridans* streptococci

72. Grows in 40% bile

73. Causes neonatal sepsis

74. Most frequent cause of bacterial endocarditis

Answers and Explanations

1–C. *Staphylococcus aureus* and *Pseudomonas aeruginosa* are two primary pulmonary colonizers that cause pneumonia in patients with cystic fibrosis. Of the two, *Pseudomonas* is gram-negative. Its slime material (alginate) produces the resistance to phagocytic killing and poor penetration of antibiotics to the site, which, in conjunction with the antibiotic resistance of *Pseudomonas*, make these serious infections.

2–C. Both *Pseudomonas* exotoxin A and *Corynebacterium diphtheriae* toxin inhibit protein synthesis through the inhibition of transfer RNA elongating factor (EF-2). Shiga toxin is a cytotoxin, enterotoxin, and neurotoxin. *V. cholerae* enterotoxin and *E. coli* labile toxin (LT) both result in increased cyclic adenosine monophosphate (cyclic AMP).

3–B. *Clostridium difficile* has been shown to be the major causative agent of pseudomembranous colitis, which causes diarrhea most commonly starting after 3–4 days of antibiotic administration.

4–A. *C. perfringens* requires a low oxidation-reduction potential (E_h) to reproduce and does not infect nontraumatized tissues with a high E_h. Infant botulism results from ingesting spores in food.

Death from tetanus occurs as a result of exhaustion and respiratory failure. Anaerobic cellulitis does not spread to healthy tissues. Gastroenteritis caused by *C. difficile* is severe.

5–D. Antitoxin should be administered as soon as clostridial infection is suspected, because once the toxin is bound, the antitoxin is ineffective. Myonecrosis caused by *C. perfringens*, but not anaerobic cellulitis, may require amputation or skin grafting; treatment of anaerobic cellulitis involves only removal of necrotic tissue. Food poisoning due to *C. perfringens* is self-limiting and does not require treatment. Antibiotic therapy should not be used to treat infant botulism, because the antibiotics rapidly kill the organisms, thereby releasing the toxin and increasing the severity of disease. Patients with cellulitis should be given antibiotics.

6–C. Most of the *Bacteroides* are resistant to tetracyclines, penicillin, and cephalosporins, possessing a beta-lactamase. This organism is found mainly in the gut and the female genital tract. *Prevotella melaninogenicus* is the species possessing a black colonial pigment.

7–B. The culture should be transported to the laboratory immediately in an anaerobic transport tube, because oxygen is lethal to these organisms. These organisms do not grow on eosin–methylene blue (EMB) agar and do not contain superoxide dismutase. Sputum sampling is ineffective because normal flora interferes with interpretation.

8–C. The disease is rapidly progressive and may be fatal in 2 days because of bacterial multiplication and shock. Organisms do not invade. Although *V. cholerae* are sensitive to acid pH, the "rice water" stools are highly contagious.

9–C. The causative agent in Lyme disease is *Borrelia burgdorferi*. The three stages frequently overlap. Stage 3 manifestations are slow to develop and may not emerge until several months or years after the initial infection. The hallmark rash is circular, spreading out from the site of the tick bite.

10–A. Serology should be evaluated in the first and third trimesters of pregnancy. The clinical manifestations of congenital syphilis are generally severe and may include abortion, stillbirth, or birth defects. *Treponema pallidum* readily penetrates the maternal–fetal barrier and can infect in utero. *T. pallidum* cannot be grown in vitro.

11–B. The major virulence factor of *Helicobacter pylori* appears to be the neutralizing ability of the urease.

12–C. The nontuberculous mycobacteria are not considered contagious; they are picked up from the environment, for example, from surface water of lakes and some water supplies. Tuberculosis is caused by both *M. tuberculosis* and *M. bovis*. Both tuberculous and nontuberculous mycobacterial infections are seen in AIDS patients, and all *Mycobacteria* are acid-fast.

13–A. *A. israelii* grows contiguously in tissues, crossing anatomic barriers; thus, it often invades bone. *M. tuberculosis* may be hematogenously spread to any tissue.

14–C. The Ghon complex is the combination of the initial Ghon lesion at the site of *Mycobacterium tuberculosis* infection in the lung and involvement of the adjoining lymph node. This lesion heals after primary tuberculosis.

15–D. Numerous *M. leprae* organisms are found in the skin in lepromatous leprosy, and the patient has many skin lesions from failure of cell-mediated immunity to restrict infection. Lepromatous leprosy patients usually have a poor response to the lepromin skin test. Leprosy is diagnosed by cytologic findings and a lepromin skin test, not by culture, because the organism cannot be cultured in vitro.

16–B. A vaccine is recommended for high-risk groups, such as sheep handlers, fur trappers, and laboratory workers. This organism is highly contagious after in vitro growth and only specially equipped laboratories (not hospitals) should attempt to culture it. When *F. tularenis* is implanted into skin, it is carried to lymph nodes where it also replicates causing ulceroglandular tularemia. These bacteria parasitize fixed macrophages and mononuclear phagocytes, and relapses may occur because of failure to eradicate intracellular organisms.

17–B. Typically, the patient with *Brucella* infection has intermittent fever and nondescript findings, including profound muscle weakness. The infection is hard to eradicate; acute infections are marked by relapses. Chronic infection may last more than 12 months. All three species of *Brucella* are human pathogens. *Brucella* is spread to humans primarily by the handling of infected meat. The organism is an intracellular parasite of macrophages.

18–A. The early cutaneous form of anthrax infection may mimic a staphylococcal furuncle (or boil) or insect bite. Pulmonary and gastrointestinal infections are rapidly fatal. Spores are never observed within lesions. The capsule of *Bacillus anthracis* is unique for bacteria in that it is a polypeptide of glutamic acid. Sheep and cattle are the usual sources of infection.

19–D. Capsular polysaccharide is the virulence determinant. This organism does not have an endotoxin. C-reactive protein is an endogenous host factor in response to *S. pneumoniae*. Bacitracin is an antibiotic.

20–D. Organisms are fairly resistant to environmental influences and can survive for weeks in dried pseudomembranes. Organisms can be routinely Gram stained but cannot be distinguished from normal oral flora diphtheoids. Therefore, it is important to demonstrate toxin production by the isolate. Only *S. aureus* and *Yersinia pestis* are coagulase positive.

21–C. Lymphocytosis is prevalent. The nasopharyngeal swab is used to isolate organisms, which are plated on Bordet-Gengou agar. The organism is a gram-negative coccobacillus, most readily isolated during the catarrhal stage.

22–B. In this list, only the streptococci and staphylococci are gram-positive. The streptococci are catalase negative and staphylococci are catalase positive. Of the two staphylococci, *Staphylococcus aureus* is the β-hemolytic, coagulase-positive one and thus the correct answer.

23–A. Meningitis is treated with intravenous antibiotics, but rifampin is still necessary to eliminate carriage. Bacterial pinkeye is relatively mild and can be treated with topical sulfonamides. Soft chancre is highly contagious and partners have to be treated. *Haemophilus* capsular vaccine is poorly immunogenic in the target population, especially in children 3 months to 2 years old.

24–A. Culturing organisms from a clinical specimen is the only method to diagnose gonorrhea in asymptomatic patients. Organisms should be cultured on Thayer-Martin agar in a candle jar. However, organisms are labile and will be killed by lubricants.

25–A. Epiglottitis is a medical emergency requiring hospitalization. It can be fatal in 24 hours. Severe CNS defects occur in one-third of meningitis patients. Pus production is diagnostic. Pneumonia occurs primarily in adults older than age 50 years or in young children.

26–D. In debilitated patients, septicemia with abscesses may occur. Yersiniosis is marked by lesions in the wall of the small intestine and mesenteric lymphadenitis. "Black death" applies only to plague, which is caused by infection with *Y. pestis*, and is not considered a yersiniosis. Yersiniosis includes *Yersinia enterocolitica* and *Yersinia pseudotuberculosis* infections, which are spread through infected food and water. Plague is transmitted by droplet infection and spread by fleas.

27–E. The incidence of *M. pneumoniae* is highest in the young (5–15 years of age), not in the elderly.

28–B. *Legionella* causes a fibrinopurulent pneumonia, not a granulomatous pulmonary infection. It is a weakly gram-negative, facultative, intracellular parasite found in streams and air-conditioning cooling tanks and is both catalase- and oxidase-positive.

29–D. The non–spore-forming anaerobes are present to the extent of 10^{11} organisms/g of stool, comprising approximately 99% of the normal fecal flora.

30–B. *C. jejuni* infections are at least as common as *Salmonella* and *Shigella* infections.

31–D. One of the differentiating characteristics between gastrointestinal upsets caused by *Staphylococcus* or the Enterobacteriaceae is the shorter incubation period following infection by the staphylococci (approximately 6 hours versus 1–2 days for the enterics).

32–C. Although penicillin may lower the number of bacteria, the endotoxin component responsible for shock is liberated and is unaffected by antibiotics.

33–C. *Salmonella* species do not ferment lactose, although some species produce acid, gas, and hydrogen sulfide from glucose.

34–E. Neonatal infections can arise either from infection during delivery or from an in utero infection. In either case, the prognosis is poor.

35–B. Key early manifestations of *Y. pestis* infection are a sudden onset of fever, conjunctivitis, and regional bubo formation. No exotoxin has been described.

36–E. Only *Neisseria* possesses the ability to degrade the IgA antibody, which protects against invasion of the mucosal surfaces.

37–A. Group A streptococci are not part of the normal oral or intestinal flora. When present, antibiotic treatment should be begun.

38–A. Group B streptococci have polysaccharide capsules, which are poorly antigenic in neonates and children.

39–D. *C. burnetii* is the only rickettsial disease that can be spread via dust particles. All other rickettsia rapidly die in the environment.

40–E. Rickettsial diseases in general exhibit these three manifestations.

41–C. Rocky Mountain spotted fever rash characteristically appears initially on hands and feet.

42–E. All of these organisms are associated with zoonosis spread to humans by arthropod vectors. *C. burnetii* is usually transmitted by dust particles but can be transmitted by ticks.

43–E. All of these organisms are obligate intracellular bacteria with a predilection for multiplication within capillary endothelial cells.

44–D. *C. burnetii;* only *Coxiella* causes a pneumonia.

45–A. *R. akari* results in a vesicular rash typical of chickenpox, with the greatest concentration on the trunk. There is generally a smaller eschar at the site of the mite bite.

46–B. *V. cholerae* causes classic cholera; *V. parahaemolyticus*, in contrast, causes a relatively mild gastroenteritis.

47–C. Septicemia due to *Salmonella* is a fulminant, sometimes fatal, extraintestinal disease; bloodstream invasion by *Shigella* is rare.

48–C. *Salmonella* is associated with intestinal tracts of humans, other animals, reptiles, amphibians, fish, and birds.

49–D. *Shigella* invades the intestinal epithelium, resulting in liquid stools containing mucus, pus, and occasionally blood.

50–D. The gram-positive organism *S. pneumoniae* contains neither an endotoxin nor an exotoxin; rather, it expresses its toxicity through sheer numbers.

51–C. Many if not all gram-negative bacteria contain an endotoxin. In addition, many such as *Pseudomonas*, *Shigella*, *Salmonella*, and *Vibrio* also secrete an exotoxin.

52–C. *S. dysenteriae* possesses an endotoxin and an enterotoxin.

53–C. *S. typhimurium* possesses an endotoxin and an enterotoxin.

54–C. *V. cholerae* possesses both an enterotoxin and an endotoxin.

55–B. *Borrelia recurrentis* causes epidemic relapsing fever, which is transmitted by lice; other species cause tick-borne relapsing fever.

56–C. The acute icteric disease caused by *Leptospira* is characterized by abrupt onset of fever, chills, headache, myalgia, gastrointestinal upset, conjunctival suffusion, and aseptic meningitis.

57–C. Leptospirosis infects humans through contact with the urine of wild rodents and domestic animals.

58–B. Only *Actinomyces* is anaerobic; the rest are aerobic.

59–A. *Nocardia* is a gram-positive filamentous bacteria that is partially acid-fast.

60–C. Mycobacteria are slender rods and are acid-fast.

61–C. The mycobacteria are mostly very slow growers; *Mycobacterium leprae* cannot be cultured in vitro.

62–D. Sulfatides decrease the ability of phagocytes to kill *M. tuberculosis* by inhibiting phagosome–lysosome fusion.

63–C. PPD is used in skin testing for infection.

64–B. The long-chain fatty acids, or mycolic acids, confer acid-fastness to the organism.

65–A. Cord factor disrupts the mitochondrial membrane, ultimately interrupting mitochondrial function.

66–B. *S. epidermidis* is ubiquitous as part of the normal flora. Organisms are introduced into the host during invasive procedures.

67–A. The anterior nares of hospital personnel and patients are a major habitat of *S. aureus*. From this "vantage point," organisms can be passed to postsurgical patients.

68–D. *S. saprophyticus* is the etiologic agent in 10% to 20% of primary urinary tract infections in young women.

69–A. Impetigo causes local infection of superficial skin layers and is highly communicable in infants.

70–B. Scarlet fever is marked by a rash due to erythrogenic toxins.

71–D. Group A streptococci infection of the skin can invade and quickly traverse the lymphatics to the bloodstream, giving rise to a potentially lethal septicemia.

72–A. Enterococci can be differentiated by their reactivity with group D antiserum, bacitracin resistance, and growth in 40% bile or pH 9.6.

73–C. Group B streptococci cause neonatal sepsis in two forms: an early-onset form, occurring in infants from birth to 4 days old, and a late-onset form, occurring in infants from age 7 days to 4 months old.

74–D. The *Viridans* streptococci are the most frequent cause of bacterial endocarditis.

4

Virology

I. Nature of Animal Viruses

A. Virus particles

–are called **virions.**

–are composed of either RNA or DNA that is encased in a protein coat called a **capsid.**

–are either naked or enveloped, depending on whether the capsid is surrounded by a lipoprotein **envelope.**

–replicate only in living cells and therefore are **obligate intracellular parasites.**

–cannot be observed with a light microscope.

1. The viral genome

–may be single-stranded or double-stranded, linear or circular, and segmented or nonsegmented.

–is used as one criterion for viral classification.

–is associated with viral-specific enzymes, other proteins within the virion, or both.

2. The viral capsid

–is composed of structural units called **capsomers,** which are aggregates of **viral-specific polypeptides.**

–has a symmetry that is classified as **helical, icosahedral** (a 20-sided polygon), or **complex.**

–is used as a criterion for viral classification.

–serves four functions:

a. As protection of the viral genome

b. As the site of receptors necessary for naked viruses to initiate infection

c. As the stimulus for antibody production

d. As the site of antigenic determinants important in some serologic tests

3. The viral nucleocapsid

–refers to the capsid and enclosed viral genome.

–is identical to the virion in naked viruses.

4. The viral envelope

–surrounds the nucleocapsid of enveloped viruses.

–is composed of **viral-specific glycoproteins** and **host-cell–derived lipids and lipoproteins.**

–contains molecules that are necessary for enveloped viruses to initiate infection, act as a stimulus for antibody production, and serve as antigens in serologic tests.

–is the basis of ether sensitivity of a virus.

B. Viral classification

–is based on chemical and physical properties of virions.

–has resulted in the classification of viruses into **major families,** which are further subdivided by physiochemical and serologic characteristics into **genera.**

C. DNA viruses (Table 4–1)

–contain double-stranded DNA (except for parvovirus).

–are naked viruses (except for herpesviruses, poxviruses, and hepadnaviruses).

–have icosahedral capsids and replicate in the nucleus (except for poxviruses).

D. RNA viruses (Tables 4–2 through 4–4)

–contain single-stranded RNA (except for reoviruses).

–are enveloped (except for caliciviruses, picornaviruses, and reoviruses).

–have helical capsids (except for picornaviruses, reoviruses, and togaviruses).

–are classified positive, negative, or ambisense depending on the ability of virion RNA to act as messenger RNA (see II C 1).

Table 4–1. Virion and Nucleic Acid Structure of DNA Viruses

Virus Family	Prominent Examples	Virion Structure	Virion Polymerase	Capsid Symmetry	DNA Structure
Adenoviridae	Adenoviruses	Naked	No	Icosahedral	Linear, double-stranded
Herpesviridae	Herpes simplex virus Varicella-zoster virus Epstein-Barr virus Cytomegalovirus	Enveloped	No	Icosahedral	Linear, double-stranded
Poxviridae	Smallpox virus Vaccinia virus Molluscum contagiosum virus	Brick-shaped, enveloped	Yes	Complex	
Papovaviridae	Papillomaviruses Polyomaviruses	Naked	No	Icosahedral	Circular, double-stranded
Hepadnaviridae	Hepatitis B virus	Enveloped	Yes	Icosahedral	Circular, double-stranded
Parvoviridae	B19 virus	Naked	No	Icosahedral	Linear, single-stranded

Table 4–2. Virion and Nucleic Acid Structure of Positive-Sense RNA Viruses

Virus Family	Prominent Examples	Virion Structure	Virion Polymerase	Capsid Symmetry	RNA Structure
Caliciviridae	Norwalk agent	Naked	No	Icosahedral	Linear, single-stranded, nonsegmented
Picornaviridae	Coxsackieviruses Echoviruses Enteroviruses Hepatitis A virus Polioviruses Rhinoviruses	Naked	No	Icosahedral	Linear, single-stranded, nonsegmented
Flaviviridae	Dengue virus Hepatitis C virus St. Louis encephalitis virus Yellow fever virus	Enveloped	No	Icosahedral	Linear, single-stranded, nonsegmented
Togaviridae	Eastern, Western, and Venezuelan equine encephalitis viruses Rubella virus	Enveloped	No	Icosahedral	Linear, single-stranded, nonsegmented
Retroviridae	Human immunodeficiency virus Leukemia viruses Sarcoma viruses	Enveloped	No*	Helical	Linear, single-stranded, nonsegmented*
Coronaviridae	Coronaviruses	Enveloped	No	Helical	Linear, single-stranded, nonsegmented

* Retroviruses are diploid and have a reverse transcriptase.

—replicate in the cytoplasm (except for orthomyxoviruses and retroviruses, which have both a cytoplasmic and a nuclear phase).

II. Viral Replication and Genetics

A. Viral replication

—occurs only in living cells.

—involves many host-cell enzymes and functions.

—may be incomplete in some cells (**abortive infection**) and yield **defective particles** (lack a functional replication gene) in some cells.

—may lead to the death of the host cell (**virulent viruses**) or may occur without apparent damage to the host cell (**moderate viruses**).

—is similar for all viruses in a specific family.

Table 4–3. Virion and Nucleic Acid Structure of Negative-Sense RNA Viruses

Virus Family	Prominent Examples	Virion Structure	Virion Polymerase	Capsid Symmetry	RNA Structure
Paramyxoviridae	Mumps virus Measles virus Parainfluenza virus Respiratory syncytial virus	Enveloped	Yes	Helical	Linear, single-stranded, nonsegmented
Rhabdoviridae	Rabies virus Vesicular stomatitis virus	Enveloped	Yes	Helical	Linear, single-stranded, nonsegmented
Filoviridae	Ebola virus Marburg virus	Enveloped	Yes	Helical	Linear, single-stranded, nonsegmented
Orthomyxoviridae	Influenza viruses	Enveloped	Yes	Helical	Linear, single-stranded, eight segments
Bunyaviridae	California encephalitis virus Hantavirus	Enveloped	Yes	Helical	Circular, single-stranded, three segments

Table 4–4. Virion and Nucleic Acid Structure of Other RNA Viruses

Virus Family	Prominent Examples	Virion Structure	Virion Polymerase	Capsid Symmetry	RNA Structure
Arenaviridae	Lassa fever virus Lymphocytic choriomeningitis virus	Enveloped	Yes	Helical	Circular, single-stranded, two segments (one negative sense and one ambisense)
Reoviridae	Colorado tick fever virus Reoviruses Rotaviruses	Naked	Yes	Icosahedral	Linear, double-stranded, 10–11 segments

1. **Replication process**

   –has a sequential pattern that includes the following steps:

   a. Attachment

   b. Penetration

   c. Uncoating of the viral genome

   d. Synthesis of early proteins involved in genome replication

   e. Synthesis of late proteins (structural components of the virion)

   f. Assembly

   g. Release

2. Plaques and pocks

–are focal areas of viral-induced cytopathology observed in tissue culture cells, monolayers, and membranes of embryonated eggs.

–are counted after application of serial dilutions of a virus suspension to susceptible cells to quantitate the infectious virions present.

3. One-step multiplication curves

–are plots of time after infection versus the number of viral plaques or pocks.

–show that viruses have an **eclipse period** (the time from the start of infection to the first appearance of intracellular infectious virus) and a **latent period** (the time from the start of infection to the first appearance of extracellular virus).

–indicate that viruses take a much longer time (hours or days) to replicate than phage.

4. Attachment

–involves the interaction of viral receptors and specific host-cell receptor sites.

–plays an important role in viral pathogenesis, determining **viral cell trophism.**

–may be inhibited by antibodies (neutralizing antibodies) against viral receptors or cellular receptor sites.

5. Penetration

–can occur by a cellular mechanism called **receptor-mediated endocytosis,** which is referred to as **viropexis** when viruses are involved.

–can involve the fusion of the virus envelope with the plasma membrane of the host cell.

6. Uncoating

–refers to the separation of the capsid from the viral genome.

–results in the loss of virion infectivity.

7. Budding

–is the process by which enveloped viruses obtain their envelope.

–is preceded by the insertion of virus-specific glycoproteins into the membranes of a host cell.

–occurs most frequently at the plasma membrane, but also occurs at other membranes.

–confers infectivity to enveloped viruses.

B. DNA viruses (see Table 4–1)

1. Transcription

–occurs by host-cell DNA-dependent RNA polymerases (except for virion-associated RNA polymerase of poxviruses).

–results in transcripts that must have a poly A tail and methylated cap added before translation.

–occurs in a specific temporal pattern, such as immediate early, delayed early, and late messenger RNA (mRNA) transcription.

–may be followed by **post-transcriptional processing** of primary mRNA transcripts (late adenovirus transcripts).

–occurs in the nucleus (except for poxviruses).

2. Translation

–occurs on cytoplasmic polysomes.

–is followed by transport of newly synthesized proteins to the nucleus (except for poxviruses).

3. Genome replication

–is **semiconservative.**

–is performed by a DNA-dependent DNA polymerase, which may be supplied by the host cell (adenoviruses) or may be virus-specific (herpesviruses).

–occurs after the synthesis of the early proteins.

4. Assembly

–occurs in the nucleus (except for poxviruses).

–is frequently an inefficient process that leads to accumulation of viral proteins that may participate in the formation of **inclusion bodies.**

C. RNA viruses (see Tables 4-2 through 4-4)

1. The viral genome

–may be single-stranded or double-stranded, segmented or nonsegmented.

–may have **messenger (positive-sense) polarity** if it is single-stranded and able to act as mRNA (picornaviruses and retroviruses).

–may have **antimessenger (negative-sense) polarity** if it is single-stranded and complementary to mRNA (orthomyxoviruses and paramyxoviruses).

–is **ambisense** if it is single-stranded with segments of messenger polarity and segments of antimessenger polarity.

2. Transcription

–involves an RNA-dependent RNA polymerase for all viruses, except retroviruses, which use a host-cell DNA-dependent RNA polymerase.

–involves a virion-associated enzyme (transcriptase) with negative-sense viruses.

3. Translation

–occurs on cytoplasmic polysomes.

–may result in the synthesis of a large polyprotein that is subsequently cleaved (in **post-translational processing**) into individual viral polypeptides (picornaviruses and retroviruses).

4. Genome replication

–occurs in the cytoplasm (except for orthomyxoviruses and retroviruses).

–is performed by a viral-specific **replicase enzyme** (except for retroviruses).

–involves a replicative intermediate RNA structure for all single-stranded RNA genomes.

–is asymmetric and conservative for double-stranded RNA genomes.

D. Genetics

1. **Phenotypic mixing**

   –occurs when pairs of related viruses with similar but distinct surface antigens infect the same cell.

   –results when surface antigens from two related viruses enclose the genome of one of the viruses.

2. **Phenotypic masking (transcapsidation)**

   –occurs when pairs or related viruses infect the same cell.

   –results when the genome of one virus is surrounded by the capsid or capsid and envelope of the other virus.

3. **Complementation**

   –can occur when two mutants of the same virus or, less frequently, two mutants of different large DNA viruses, infect the same cell.

   –results when one mutant virus supplies an enzyme or factor that the other mutant lacks.

4. **Genetic reassortment**

   –can occur when two strains of mutants of a segmented RNA virus infect a cell.

   –results in a stable change in the viral genome.

5. **Viral vectors**

   –can be constructed with recombinant DNA technology and allow gene transfer into cells.

   –are usually defective viruses that cannot replicate but can infect cells.

   –have been used for the production of some vaccines (e.g., hepatitis B vaccine).

III. Viral Pathogenesis

A. General characteristics—viral pathogenesis

–is the process of disease production following infection.

–may lead to **clinical** or **subclinical** (asymptomatic) disease.

–is the result of several viral and host factors.

1. **Viral entry into a host**

   –occurs most often through the mucosa of the respiratory tract.

   –may occur through the mucosa of the gastrointestinal or genitourinary tract.

   –can be accomplished by direct virus injection into the bloodstream via a needle or an insect bite.

2. **Asymptomatic viral disease**

   –may also be called **subclinical infection** because no clinical symptoms are evident.

   –occurs with most viral infections.

   –can stimulate humoral and cellular immunity.

3. **Clinical viral disease**

   –frequently depends on the size of the viral inoculum.

   –does not always follow infection and therefore is not an accurate index of viral infection.

—results from direct or indirect viral effects (e.g., viral-induced cytolysis, immunologic attack on infected cells, etc.), which lead to physiologic changes in infected tissues.

—is much less common than inapparent infection.

—is associated with a particular **target organ** for a specific virus.

B. Viral aspects of pathogenesis

1. Viral surface receptors

—interact with cellular receptor sites to initiate infection.

—may react with specific antibodies (neutralizing antibodies) and become incapable of interaction with cellular receptor sites.

—can be inactivated by pH, enzymes, and other host biochemical factors.

2. Viral virulence

—refers to the ability of a particular viral strain to cause disease.

—is genetically determined.

—is a composite of all the factors that allow a virus to overcome host defense mechanisms and damage its target organ.

—is decreased with **attenuated strains** of virus.

C. Cellular aspects of pathogenesis

1. Cellular receptor sites

—interact with virion receptors to initiate infection.

—help determine **cell trophism** of viruses.

—may be determined by the differentiation stage of a cell.

2. Cell trophism

—refers to the propensity of a virus to infect and replicate in a cell.

—is largely determined by the interaction of virus receptors and cellular receptor sites and the ability of the cell to provide other components (e.g., substrates and enzymes) essential for viral replication.

3. Target organ

—refers to that organ responsible for the major clinical signs of a viral infection.

—is largely determined by viral virulence and cell trophism.

4. Cellular responses to viral infection

—result in clinical disease.

— may be inapparent or may include:

a. Cytopathic effects

b. Cytolysis

c. Inclusion body formation

d. Chromosomal aberrations

e. Transformation

f. Interferon synthesis

5. Cytopathogenic effects

–include inhibition of host-cell macromolecular biosynthesis, alterations of the plasma membrane and lysosomes, and development of **inclusion bodies** (focal accumulation of virion or viral gene products).

–may occur without the production of infectious virus progeny.

–may aid in identification of certain viruses (e.g., polykaryocyte formation by measles virus).

D. Types of infections

1. Inapparent infections

–occur when too few cells are infected to cause clinical symptoms.

–are synonymous with **subclinical disease.**

–can result in sufficient antibody stimulation to cause immunity from further infections.

–occur frequently when the virus inoculum is small.

–occur when the virus does not reach its target organ.

2. Acute infections

–occur when clinical manifestations of disease are observed for a short time (days to weeks) after a short incubation period.

–have recoveries associated with elimination of the virus from the body.

–are classified as **localized** or **disseminated,** depending on whether the virus has traveled from its site of implantation to its target organ.

–may lead to **persistent** or **latent** infections.

3. Persistent infections

–are associated with the continuing presence of the infectious virus in the body for an extended, perhaps lifelong, period.

–may or may not involve clinical symptoms.

–may involve infected individuals known as **carriers.**

–provide constant viral antigenic stimulation that leads to high antibody titers for some antigens.

4. Latent infections

–occur when the infecting virus persists in the body in a noninfectious form that can periodically reactivate to an infectious virus and produce clinical disease.

–are synonymous with **recurrent disease.**

–produce antibody stimulus only during the initial (**primary**) infection and during recurrent episodes.

–can have subclinical reactivations.

–are difficult to detect in cells because viral antigen production is not detected and cytopathology is not observed during "silent" periods.

5. Slow infections

–have a **prolonged incubation** period lasting months or years.

–do not cause clinical symptoms during incubation.

–produce some infectious viruses during incubation.

–are most often associated with **chronic, progressive, fatal viral diseases** of the **central nervous system (CNS),** such as kuru and Creutzfeldt-Jakob disease.

E. Patterns of acute disease

1. **Localized disease**

   –occurs when viral multiplication and cell damage remain localized to the site of viral entry into the body.

   –has a short incubation time.

   –may have systemic clinical features (e.g., fever).

   –is not associated with pronounced viremia (virions in the blood).

   –occurs in the **respiratory tract** (influenza, rhinovirus), **alimentary tract** (picornaviruses, rotaviruses), **genitourinary tract** (papillomavirus), and the **eye** (adenovirus).

   –can spread over the surface of the body to other areas where it causes another localized infection (picornavirus-induced conjunctivitis).

   –induces a much weaker immune response than disseminated infections.

2. **Disseminated infections**

   a. **General characteristics—disseminated infections**

      –involve the spread of virus from its entry site to a target organ.

      –involve a **primary viremia** and perhaps a **secondary viremia.**

      –involve moderate incubation times (e.g., weeks).

      –have their main clinical symptoms associated with infection of one target organ, although infection of other organs is involved.

      –generate a substantial immune response that frequently confers lifelong immunity to the host.

      –allow more time for the host's immune system to eliminate the virus infection.

   b. **Viral dissemination**

      –is a major feature of disseminated infections.

      –may involve virus travel in other cells (red blood cells and mononuclear peripheral white blood cells), the plasma, extracellular spaces, and nerve fibers.

      –is prevented by viral-specific cytotoxic cells and neutralizing antibodies.

3. **Congenital infections**

   –are viral infections of a fetus.

   –result from maternal viremia.

   –lead to **maldeveloped organs.**

   –are serious because of the immaturity of the fetal immune system, the placental barrier to maternal immunity, and the undifferentiated state and rapid multiplication of fetal cells.

IV. Host Defenses to Viruses

A. Host defense mechanisms

–are responsible for the self-limiting nature of most viral infections.

–have immune and nonimmune aspects.

–operate during all stages of a virus infection.

–may contribute to the clinical pattern of disease (immunopathology).

B. Nonimmune defenses

1. Innate immunity

–includes **anatomic barriers** (dead cells of the epidermis) and **chemical barriers** (mucous layers) that limit contact of the virus with susceptible cells.

–includes the complex parameters associated with the **age and physiologic status** of the host.

2. Cellular resistance

–involves **nonpermissive cells,** which lack factors necessary for virus replication.

–involves **lack of receptor sites** for virus on cells.

3. Inflammation

–limits the spread of virus from an infection site.

–results in unfavorable environmental conditions for viral replication (e.g., antiviral substances, low pH, elevated temperatures).

4. Interferon

–is a host-specific, viral-induced glycoprotein that inhibits viral replication (see Chapter 7, VII B 3, Table 7–2).

–is not viral-specific but is fairly species-specific.

–is the **first viral-induced defense mechanism** at the primary site of infection.

C. Humoral immunity

–involves the production of antibodies against viral-specific antigen by **B lymphocytes.**

–is the defense mechanism most important to cytolytic viral infections accompanied by viremia and viral infections of epithelial surfaces.

–involves both **virus-neutralizing antibodies** and **nonneutralizing antibodies.**

1. Neutralizing antibodies

–inhibit the ability of a virus to replicate.

–can inhibit viral attachment, penetration, or uncoating or all three processes.

–can induce lesions in the viral envelope, with the aid of complement.

–are most protective if they are present at the time of infection or during viremia.

2. Nonneutralizing antibodies

–enhance viral degradation.

–act as opsonins to enhance phagocytosis of virions.

D. Cell-mediated immunity

–involves cytotoxic **T lymphocytes,** antibody-dependent–cell-mediated cytotoxicity, natural killer cells, and activated macrophages.

–involves soluble factors from T lymphocytes (**lymphokines**) and macrophages (**monokines**) that regulate cellular immune responses.

–is the defense mechanism most important to noncytolytic infection in which the membrane of the virus-infected cell is antigenically altered by the virus.

E. Viral-induced immunopathology

–can contribute to the disease process.

–can result from various immunologic interactions, including immediate hypersensitivity, antibody–antigen complexes (as in hepatitis B virus, or HBV), and tissue damage due to cytotoxic cells or antibody and complement.

–is frequently observed in **persistent viral infections.**

F. Viral-induced immunosuppression

–results when infecting viruses alter the immune responsiveness or decrease the numbers of lymphocytes.

–can occur during cytolytic or noncytolytic infection.

–is frequently observed as a **transient consequence** of disseminated viral infections that involve lymphocyte infection by the virus.

V. Immunotherapy, Antivirals, and Interferon

A. Immunotherapy

1. Virus vaccines (Table 4–5)

–lead to **active immunization.**

–are effective in preventing infections caused by viruses with few antigenic types.

–may use **live virus, killed virus, virion subunits, viral polypeptides, or viral DNA.**

a. Live virus vaccines

–use **attenuated virus strains** that are relatively avirulent.

–have advantages of administration in a single dose by the natural route of infection and the ability to induce a wide spectrum of antibodies and cytotoxic cells.

–have the disadvantages of a limited shelf life, possible reversion to virulence, and possible production of persistent infection.

–include vaccines for **measles, mumps, rubella, chickenpox, polio (Sabin vaccine), yellow fever,** and some **adenovirus strains.**

b. Killed virus vaccines

–are prepared from whole virions by **heat** or **chemical inactivation** of infectivity.

–are injected into the body and stimulate antibodies only to surface antigens of the virus.

–have the advantage of easy combination into **polyvalent vaccines** (vaccines containing virions from several virus strains).

Table 4-5. Viral Immunotherapy

Virus	Passive Immunization*	Active Immunization (Vaccines)		
		Live Strain	Killed	Subunit
Adenovirus	No	Yes (military use)	No	No
Hepatitis A virus	Yes	No	Havrix	No
Hepatitis B virus	Yes	No	No	Engerix-B or Recombivax HB
Influenza virus	No	No	Yes	No
Measles virus	Yes	Moraten	No	No
Mumps virus	No	Jeryl Lynn	No	No
Poliovirus	No	Sabin	Salk	No
Rabies virus	Yes	No	Yes (Human diploid cell)	No
Rubella	No	RA 27/3 or Cendehill	No	No
Smallpox (variola) virus	No	Vaccinia	No	No
Varicella-zoster virus	Yes	Oka	No	No
Yellow fever virus	No	17D	No	No

* Commercial preparations available

  –have the disadvantages of lack of development of secretory IgA, need for boosters, poor cell-mediated response, and possible hypersensitivity reactions.

  –include vaccines for **poliovirus (Salk vaccine), rabies, influenza, and hepatitis A virus.**

c. **Virion subunit vaccines**

  –are purified proteins (viral receptors) obtained from virions.

  –have the same advantages and disadvantages as killed vaccines.

  –are available for **adenovirus.**

d. Viral polypeptides

    –are **polypeptide sequences of virion receptors** that have been synthesized or result from the purification of proteins made from cloned genes.

    –have the same advantages and disadvantages as killed vaccines.

    –are used in a vaccine for **HBV.**

e. DNA vaccines

    –are plasmid DNA expression vectors containing **specific viral genes** (usually envelope genes).

    –elicit both humoral and cell-mediated immune responses.

    –are being evaluated for human use to protect against **human immunodeficiency virus (HIV)** and **influenza viruses.**

2. Passive immunization (see Table 4–5)

    –is acquired by injection of pooled human plasma or gamma globulin fractions from immune individuals into high-risk individuals.

    –is valuable in prevention of some viral diseases but has little value after disease onset.

    –is used to prevent **rubella, measles, mumps, hepatitis A and B viruses, rabies,** and **varicella-zoster virus (VZV) infections.**

B. Antiviral agents (Table 4–6)

1. General characteristics—antiviral agents

    –must selectively inhibit viral replication without affecting the viability or functioning of the host cell (**selective toxicity**).

    –are of limited use.

    –include the licensed compounds acyclovir, amantadine, didanosine, famciclovir, foscarnet, ganciclovir, interferon-α (IFN-α), ribavirin, trifluridine, vidarabine, zalcitabine, and zidovudine.

2. Nucleoside analogues

    –constitute the majority of antiviral agents.

    –are effective against herpesviruses.

    –inhibit viral replication by inhibiting an enzyme involved in purine, pyrimidine, or DNA synthesis, or are incorporated into DNA and inhibit its synthesis or function.

    –are effective only against replicating virus, not latent virus.

a. Acyclovir (Zovirax)

    –is an analogue of guanosine.

    –is phosphorylated by herpesvirus thymidine kinase.

    –inhibits herpes viral DNA polymerase.

    –helps control serious **primary herpes simplex virus (HSV)** and **VZV** infections and genital herpes reactivity.

    –suppresses reactivation of latent herpesvirus infections including **cytomegalovirus (CMV)** in immunosuppressed and transplant patients.

b. Cytosine arabinoside (ara-C)

    –is a pyrimidine analogue.

Table 4–6. Licensed Antiviral Drugs in Current Use

Drug	Administration Route	Mechanism of Action	Indications
Acyclovir	Topical or systemic	Inhibits herpesviruses DNA polymerase	Primary genital herpes (HSV) encephalitis and keratitis Primary varicella infections Localized or ophthalmic zoster HSV, VZV, and CMV in immunocompromised or transplant patients
Amantadine	Systemic	Inhibits virus penetration or uncoating	Prophylaxis for influenza A virus
Didanosine	Systemic	Inhibits HIV reverse transcriptase	Acquired immune deficiency syndrome (AIDS)
Famciclovir	Systemic	Inhibits herpesvirus DNA polymerase	Zoster
Foscarnet	Systemic	Inhibits herpesviruses DNA polymerase	Acyclovir-resistant HSV and VZV infections Ganciclovir-resistant CMV retinitis
Ganciclovir	Systemic	Inhibits herpesviruses DNA polymerase	CMV retinitis Disseminated CMV infection of immunocompromised or AIDS patients Prophylaxis for disseminated CMV infections in transplant patients
Interferon-α	Systemic	Induces antiviral proteins	Chronic hepatitis B and hepatitis C virus infections
Ribavirin	Systemic	Inhibits nucleic acid polymerases	Severe RSV infection Lassa fever
Trifluridine	Topical	Inhibits herpesviruses DNA polymerase	HSV keratoconjunctivitis
Vidarabine	Topical and systemic	Inhibits herpesviruses DNA polymerase	HSV keratitis and encephalitis (acyclovir is the drug of choice)
Zalcitabine	Systemic	Inhibits HIV reverse transcriptase	In combination with zidovudine for advanced AIDS
Zidovudine	Systemic	Inhibits HIV reverse transcriptase	AIDS

CMV = cytomegalovirus; HSV = herpes simplex virus; RSV = respiratory syncytial virus; VZV = varicella-zoster virus.

–inhibits viral and cellular DNA polymerase.

–is immunosuppressive and cytotoxic.

c. Didanosine (Dideoxyinosine, or ddI)

–is an inosine analogue.

–inhibits HIV reverse transcriptase.

–is used for patients with advanced **acquired immune deficiency syndrome (AIDS)** who are not responding to zidovudine.

d. Famciclovir (Famvir)

–is an analogue of guanosine.

–has a similar mode of action and clinical spectrum as acyclovir.

–requires fewer doses per day than acyclovir.

e. Ganciclovir (DHPG; Cytovene)

–is an analogue of guanosine.

–inhibits CMV DNA polymerase.

–is used for treatment of **disseminated CMV infections** and **CMV retinitis** and for **prophylaxis in transplant patients.**

f. Idoxuridine

–is a halogenated pyrimidine.

–inhibits both **herpesvirus** and **cellular thymidine kinase.**

–can be toxic to humans.

g. Ribavirin (Virazole)

–is a nucleoside related structurally to guanosine.

–is active against **DNA and RNA viruses** in vitro.

–affects the synthesis of functional viral mRNA.

–is used for treatment of **respiratory syncytial virus** infections.

h. Trifluridine (Viroptic)

–is a fluorinated thymidine molecule.

–is used in the treatment of **herpes keratitis.**

i. Vidarabine (adenosine arabinoside, or vira A)

–is a purine analogue.

–blocks viral DNA polymerase.

–inhibits both **herpesvirus** and **poxvirus** replication.

–is relatively nontoxic but may cause nausea.

–is used in the treatment of **herpes encephalitis.**

j. Zalcitabine (dideoxycytidine, or ddC)

–is a cytodine analogue.

–inhibits HIV reverse transcriptase.

–is used in combination with zidovudine to treat patients with **advanced AIDS.**

k. Zidovudine (azidothymidine, or AZT; Retrovir)

–is a thymidine analogue.

–is converted to triphosphate form by cellular enzymes.

–inhibits HIV reverse transcriptase.

–is the current drug of choice for patients with AIDS.

3. Other types of antiviral agents

–affect viral penetration, uncoating, or assembly.

–inhibit viral-specific enzymes.

a. Amantadine (Symmetrel)

–blocks penetration and uncoating of **influenza A virus.**

–may be chemically modified to rimantadine **(Flumadine),** which has fewer side effects.

–is used for prophylaxis and treatment of **influenza A virus** infections.

b. Arildone (Win 51711 or Win 52084)

–stabilizes picornavirus virions and prevents uncoating.

–inhibits picornavirus replication in tissue culture and animal models of human **enterovirus disease.**

c. Foscarnet (phosphonoformic acid; Foscavir)

–inhibits herpesvirus DNA polymerase.

–is used in the treatment of **acyclovir-resistant HSV and VZV** and **ganciclovir-resistant CMV infections.**

–has been demonstrated to accumulate in bone.

d. Methisazone (Marboran)

–blocks a late stage in the replication of poxviruses.

–causes formation of noninfectious virions.

–was used to treat smallpox infections.

C. Interferons

–are host-coded proteins, or **glycoproteins,** produced in response to viruses, synthetic nucleotides, and foreign cells.

–are **host specific** but not viral specific.

–are divided into three groups or families: **IFN-α, IFN-β,** and **IFN-γ; IFN-α (Intron-A)** is licensed for treatment of chronic hepatitis B and C virus infections and can produce adverse effects at high doses or with chronic therapy.

–are produced in and secreted from virus-infected cells.

–bind to cell–surface receptors and **induce antiviral proteins,** including a **protein kinase and 2,5 A synthetase** (which synthesizes an oligoadenylic acid), leading to the destruction of viral mRNA.

–have toxic side effects, including bone marrow suppression.

VI. Diagnostic Virology

A. Laboratory viral diagnosis

–involves one of three basic approaches: **virus isolation; direct demonstration** of virus, viral nucleic acid, or antigens in clinical specimens; or **serologic testing** of viral-specific antibodies.

–is frequently not necessary because the clinical symptoms of a virus are often distinctive.

–begins with identification of the most likely viruses based on clinical symptoms and the patient's history.

–is often not possible during the first few days after infection.

B. Virus isolation

1. General characteristics—virus isolation

–depends on virus replication in susceptible cells.

–may involve tissue culture cells, embryonated eggs, or animal hosts.

–requires proper collection and preservation of specimens.

–is best accomplished during the onset and acute phase of disease.

2. Viral replication

–may be detected in live infected tissue culture cells by observing a characteristic **cytopathogenic effect** (CPE), such as polykaryocyte formation or hemadsorption (adhesion of red blood cells to infected cells).

–may be observed in fixed infected tissue culture cells by observing characteristic **inclusion bodies** (Table 4–7) or performing immunohistochemical staining of **viral antigens.**

–is detected in embryonated egg by pock formation and in animals by the development of clinical symptoms.

C. Direct examination of clinical specimens

–may be done on sections of tissue biopsies, tissue imprints or smears, blood, cerebrospinal fluid, urine, throat swabs, feces, or saliva.

–should be performed only on those specimens likely to contain the virus (e.g., throat swabs for respiratory tract infection).

–involves one of the following **assays** for virus detection: **viral-induced CPE, immunohistochemical staining, nucleic acid hybridization,** or **solid-phase immunoassay.**

Table 4–7. Viral Inclusion Bodies

Virus	Inclusion Site	Staining Properties	Inclusion Name
Adenovirus	Nucleus	B	. . .
Cytomegalovirus	Nucleus	B	Owl's eye
Herpes simplex virus	Nucleus	A	Cowdry type A
Poxvirus	Cytoplasm	A	Guarnieri bodies (smallpox) Molluscum bodies (molluscum contagiosum)
Rabies virus	Cytoplasm	A	Negri body
Reovirus	Cytoplasm	A	. . .
Rubella virus	Cytoplasm	A	. . .
Measles virus	Both	A	. . .

A = acidophilic; B = basophilic.

1. **Immunohistochemical staining**

    –uses fixed or fresh specimens and **chemically labeled (fluorescein)** or **enzymatically labeled (peroxidase) antibodies** to detect viral antigens.

    –may use impression slides made from specific tissues.

    –may involve either a **direct or an indirect staining method.**

2. **Nucleic acid hybridization**

    –involves the **detection of viral DNA or RNA sequences** in nucleic acid extracted from specimens.

    –may use **polymerase chain reaction** (PCR) techniques to amplify viral genes.

    –may involve **dot blot** hybridization techniques that usually use single-stranded, complementary **nucleic acid probes.**

    –is highly sensitive and specific.

    –is a popular technique for identifying adenovirus in nasopharyngeal washings, CMV in urine, and HIV in the blood of seronegative individuals.

3. **Solid-phase immunoassays**

    –are highly sensitive, specific assays used to detect **viral antigens.**

    –use specific viral antibodies and radioimmunoassay **(RIA)** or enzyme-linked immunosorbent assay **(ELISA)** techniques.

    –are popular for the detection of rotavirus and hepatitis A virus in feces.

D. **Serologic tests**

    –are used to determine the titer of specific antiviral antibodies.

    –are helpful in diagnostic virology if paired blood samples are taken (one sample at the onset and one sample during the recovery phase of the illness).

    –must show at least a fourfold increase in titer between the samples to indicate a current infection.

    –may be diagnostic without the use of paired samples if significant levels of IgM antiviral antibodies are obtained.

    –include virus neutralization, complement fixation, and hemagglutination inhibition tests and solid-phase immunoassays.

1. **Virus neutralization tests**

    –are based on the principle that certain antiviral antibodies will neutralize the CPE of the virus.

    –involve incubations of constant amounts of virus with decreasing amounts of serum added to susceptible cells.

    –are expensive to perform and must be standardized for each virus.

2. **Hemagglutination inhibition tests**

    –are based on the principle that antihemagglutinin antibodies in serum will inhibit viral agglutination of erythrocytes.

    –can be performed only on viruses with hemagglutinins on their surface (influenza, measles).

    –involve careful standardization of erythrocytes and viral hemagglutinin preparations.

3. **Solid-phase immunoassays**

   –are highly sensitive and specific assays used to detect **specific viral antibodies.**

   –use viral antigens in RIA and ELISA protocols.

   –are several hundred times more sensitive than other serologic tests.

VII. DNA Viruses (Table 4–8)

A. Human adenoviruses

–are naked viruses with an icosahedral nucleocapsid composed of **hexons, pentons,** and **fibers.**

–have **toxic activity** associated with pentons and **hemagglutinating activity** associated with pentons and fibers.

–contain **double-stranded DNA** that **replicates asymmetrically.**

–replicate in the nucleus of epithelial cells.

–cause localized infections of the eye, respiratory tract, gastrointestinal tract, and urinary bladder.

–frequently cause subclinical infections.

–can cause tumors in other animals because **EIA and EIB gene products bind to cellular tumor suppressor proteins p110^{Rb} and p53.**

1. **Classification—human adenoviruses**

   –are classified into seven groups (A through G), based on DNA homology.

   a. **Group A adenoviruses**

      –do not cause a specific clinical disease in humans.

      –induce **tumors** in newborn hamsters.

   b. **Group B adenoviruses**

      –cause acute respiratory disease, pharyngoconjunctival fever, and hemorrhagic cystitis.

      –can cause epidemics in military recruits (adenovirus type 7).

   c. **Group C adenoviruses**

      –cause approximately 5% of acute respiratory diseases in young children.

      –cause latent infections in the tonsils, adenoids, and other lymphatic tissue.

   d. **Group D adenoviruses**

      –are associated with sporadic and epidemic keratoconjunctivitis.

      –cause **pinkeye** (adenovirus type 8).

   e. **Group E adenoviruses**

      –are associated with acute respiratory disease accompanied by fever and with epidemic keratoconjunctivitis in military recruits.

   f. **Groups F and G adenoviruses**

      –cause gastroenteritis.

2. **Adenovirus vaccines**

   –are used by the military for protection against type 4 (group E) and type 7 (group B) adenoviruses.

   –may be of the **subunit (hexons and fibers) type** or the **live virus type.**

3. Diagnosis of adenovirus infections

– may be made by observing an increase in neutralizing antibody titer.

–may be made by virus isolation from the eyes, throat, or urine.

–may involve ELISA procedures on fecal specimens from patients with gastrointestinal infections.

B. Hepadnaviruses

–have a complex virion structure that includes an envelope.

–have **circular, double-stranded DNA** containing **single-strand breaks,** a primer protein, and a viral-specific DNA polymerase associated with the DNA.

–need a viral-coded reverse transcriptase to replicate because the virion DNA is synthesized from an RNA template.

–have their **DNA integrated into cellular DNA** during replication.

–cause liver disease as indicated by their names: human HBV, woodchuck hepatitis virus, and duck hepatitis virus.

1. Hepatitis B virus (HBV)

–causes **serum hepatitis** and frequently causes subclinical infections.

–has a special name given to its virion–the **Dane particle.**

–is associated with specific antigens: a surface antigen (**HBsAg or Australian antigen**) and core-associated antigens (**HBcAg** and **HBeAg**).

–has a viral-encoded reverse transcriptase involved in viral DNA replication.

–has been implicated in **hepatocellular carcinoma.**

2. Serum hepatitis

–has a long incubation period (50 to 180 days).

–involves antigen–antibody complexes.

–is usually contracted through a parenteral route.

–can progress to a **chronic carrier state** with or without clinical symptoms.

–is a potential high risk for the staff of hemodialysis units and health-care workers exposed to fresh blood.

–may be acute or chronic depending on the amount of HBeAg and HBsAg and of anti-HBs and anti-HBc, as determined by ELISA tests.

–may be treated prophylactically by **passive immunization** with hepatitis B immune globulin (HBIG) or HBsAg vaccine produced from particles in healthy carriers or from recombinant DNA techniques.

–may use IFN-α to treat chronic cases.

C. Herpesviruses

–are enveloped viruses with an **icosahedral nucleocapsid** containing **double-stranded DNA.**

–have linear DNA that consists of a short (18%) component and a long (82%) component, which are covalently linked and contain unique sequences flanked by inverted repeats.

–have a **tegument,** or fibrous material, between the nucleocapsid and envelope.

–replicate in the nucleus of the host cell.

–have **oncogenic potential.**

–can cause **latent infections** as well as **acute infections.**

Table 4–8. Properties of DNA Viruses

Virus Family	Virus Name	Unique Genes or Gene Products	Associated Acute Diseases	Associated Chronic or Persistent Diseases	Diagnostic Methods
Adenoviridae	Groups A–F adenoviruses	E1A E1B genes, hexons, pentons, fibers	Acute respiratory infection Keratoconjunctivitis Gastroenteritis (infants)	Lymphoid tissue	Virus isolation Serology
Hepadnaviridae	Hepatitis B virus	HB$_s$Ag (Australian ag) HB$_c$Ag (core ags) HB$_e$Ag Reverse transcriptase	Serum hepatitis	Hepatitis	ELISA test for antibodies and antigen
Herpesviridae	Herpes simplex virus type 1	...	Gingivostomatitis Cold sores Keratoconjunctivitis Encephalitis	Cold sores	Tzanck smear Cowdry type A inclusion Virus isolation
	Herpes simplex virus type 2	...	Genital herpes	Genital herpes	Tzanck smear Cowdry type A inclusion Virus isolation
	Varicella-zoster virus	...	Chickenpox Reye's syndrome	Shingles	Tzanck smear
	Cytomegalovirus	...	Congenital CID Heterophile-negative mononucleosis	Retinitis or pneumonia in immunocompromised patients	Owl's eye inclusion Virus isolation

Epstein-Barr virus	Early antigen	Infectious mononucleosis	...	Atypical lymphocytes (Downey cells) mononucleosis spot test
	Epstein-Barr nuclear antigen	Chronic fatigue syndrome		
	Viral capsid antigen			
	Lymphocyte-determined membrane antigen			
Human herpes virus type 6	...	Exanthem subitum (roseola)	...	...
Papovaviridae				
Human papilloma virus	E6 and E7	Warts	...	Keilocytotic cells FA or IP staining
		Laryngeal papillomas		
Polyomaviruses (BK, JC, and SV40)	Tumor antigens (7)	...	PML (JC virus) Urethral stenosis, hemorrhagic cystitis in immunocompromised patients (BK virus)	Pap smear or urinary sediment for viral inclusions FA or IP staining
Parvoviridae				
B19 virus	...	Erythema infectiosum (fifth disease)	...	ELISA test for IgM antibody
Poxviridae				
Variola virus	...	Smallpox (extinct)	...	...
Orf virus	...	Orf	...	...
Cowpox virus	...	Cowpox	...	...
Molluscum contagiosum virus	...	Molluscum contagiosum	...	Molluscum inclusion bodies

CID = cytomegalic inclusion disease; ELISA = enzyme-linked immunosorbent assay; FA = fluorescent antibody; HB_cAg = hepatitis B core antigen; HB_eAg = hepatitis B e antigen; HB_sAg = hepatitis B surface (Australia) antigen; IP = immunoperoxidase; PML = progressive multifocal leukoencephalopathy; SV40 = simian virus 40; Pap = Papanicolaou.

–are classified into subfamilies: **alphaherpesviruses** (e.g., HSV types 1 and 2 and VZV), **betaherpesviruses** (e.g., CMV), and **gammaherpesviruses** (e.g., Epstein-Barr virus [EBV]).

1. HSV types 1 and 2

–have approximately 50% DNA sequence homology.

–produce both **common antigens** and **type-specific antigens.**

–replicate by the regulated temporal synthesis of classes of proteins (alpha, beta, and gamma).

–produce a virus-specific DNA polymerase and thymidine kinase, which are necessary for replication.

–can cause transformation of hamster cells.

–are frequently **latent in neurons.**

–produce **defective virions** during serial passage.

–can produce distinctive cytopathology (cell rounding and **polykaryocyte formation**) or inclusion bodies (**Cowdry type A inclusions**) in infected cells.

–are treated clinically by acyclovir, famciclovir, trifluridine, and vidarabine.

a. HSV-1 disease

–may involve a primary infection (e.g., gingivostomatitis) or a recurrent infection (e.g., cold sores).

–is usually clinically inapparent as a primary disease.

–usually presents as a **lip, skin, or eye lesion.**

–can progress to a severe, fatal encephalitis.

–may be diagnosed by **Tzanck smear** for rapid identification when skin lesions are involved.

–may be diagnosed by virus isolation or serologic testing involving neutralization or complement fixation tests or ELISA procedures.

–cannot be treated prophylactically by vaccine.

b. HSV-2 disease

–may involve a primary or recurrent infection.

–affects the **genital or lip area.**

–is most frequently transmitted sexually.

–includes **neonatal herpes,** a severe generalized disease of the newborn caused by virus infection during passage through an infected birth canal.

–may be diagnosed and treated as described for HSV-1.

–may include cervical and vulvar carcinoma (viral nonstructural antigens have been found in biopsy specimens).

2. Varicella-zoster virus (VZV)

–causes an acute primary disease (chickenpox) and a recurrent disease (zoster).

–is **latent in neurons.**

a. Varicella (chickenpox)

–is a mild, highly infectious, generalized disease usually affecting children.

–is characterized clinically by vesicles on the skin and mucous membranes.

–may be diagnosed by **Tzanck smear** or **fluorescent antibody staining** of viral antigens in scrapings; **virus isolation** also is possible.

–may be prevented by a live, attenuated vaccine containing the Oka virus strain.

–may be treated prophylactically in immunocompromised children by giving varicella-zoster immune globulin.

b. Zoster

–is a reactivated virus infection in adults.

–is characterized by severe pain and the presence of vesicles in a specific area of the skin or mucosa supplied with nerves from one ganglia.

–can disseminate in immunocompromised individuals.

–is also called **shingles.**

–may be treated with famciclovir.

3. Cytomegalovirus (CMV)

–replicates more slowly and is more cell-associated than HSV.

–replicates only in human fibroblasts.

–can transform hamster and human cells in vitro.

–causes an acute primary infection and a latent infection that is reactivated to clinical disease only during immunosuppression.

–may be treated with ganciclovir.

a. Clinical manifestations

(1) CMV most commonly causes **inapparent disease** in children and adults, but can cause an **infectious mononucleosis-like disease.**

(2) **Retinitis** and **pulmonary disease** may occur in immunosuppressed individuals.

(3) **Cytomegalic inclusion disease**

–is a **generalized infection of infants,** with a distinct clinical syndrome that includes jaundice with hepatosplenomegaly, thrombocytopenic purpura, pneumonitis, and CNS damage.

–is caused by intrauterine (congenital) or early postnatal infection.

–may cause fetal death.

b. Diagnosis

(1) CMV forms owl's eye inclusions in cells found in urinary sediments of infected individuals.

(2) CMV can be isolated from the saliva and urine.

(3) Cytomegalic inclusion disease can be diagnosed by virus isolation from urine or peripheral blood leukocytes, serologic tests, and new **DNA hybridization tests** involving extraction of viral DNA from urine specimens.

4. Epstein-Barr virus (EBV)

–infects and can transform human B lymphocytes.

–produces several distinct antigens, including latent membrane proteins

(LMPs), nuclear antigens (EBNAs), early antigens (EAs), a membrane antigen (MA), and a viral capsid antigen (VCA).

–usually causes clinically inapparent infections, but may cause **infectious mononucleosis** and is associated with **Burkitt's lymphoma** and **nasopharyngeal carcinoma.**

a. Infectious mononucleosis

–is a disease of children and young adults (sometimes called **kissing disease**), characterized by fever and enlarged lymph nodes and spleen.

–is associated with the production of **atypical lymphocytes** and IgM **heterophile antibodies** identified by the **mononucleosis spot test.**

–can also be diagnosed by serologic tests involving indirect immunofluorescence procedures on fixed EBV-producing cells or ELISA tests.

b. Burkitt's lymphoma and nasopharyngeal carcinoma

–result in increased antibody titers to EBV.

–have cells that express EBNAs and LMPs and carry multiple copies of viral DNA.

5. Human herpesvirus type 6

–infects and establishes latent infection of the T lymphocyte.

–causes a common **exanthem disease** of children (roseola or exanthem subitum) and mononucleosis.

D. Parvoviruses

1. General characteristics—parvoviruses

–are small, naked viruses with **icosahedral nucleocapsids.**

–contain **single-stranded DNA** and replicate in the nucleus.

–include **human parvovirus** and **adenoassociated virus,** a defective virus of the *Dependovirus* genus that requires adenovirus to replicate.

2. Human parvovirus

–enters the body through the respiratory tract and infects and lyses progenitor erythroid cells.

–causes **febrile illness** in blood recipients, **aplastic crises** in patients with hemolytic anemias, and **erythema infectiosum** (fifth disease) in normal healthy individuals.

E. Papovaviruses

–are naked viruses with an **icosahedral nucleocapsid** that contains **double-stranded, circular DNA.**

–replicate in the nucleus of the cell.

–produce **latent and chronic infections** in their natural host.

–can induce tumors in some animals (see XII B).

–include the animal viruses papillomavirus, polyomavirus, and simian virus 40 (SV40).

1. Human papillomavirus

–replicates in epithelial cells of the skin.

–forms **keilocytotic (vacuolated) cells** during replication.

–is directly transferred from person to person.

–causes **warts and laryngeal papillomas.**

–has been associated with benign cervical tumors and vulvar and penile cancers.

2. Human polyomaviruses

–include the **JC virus** (isolated from patients with progressive multifocal leukoencephalopathy).

–include the **BK virus,** which latently infects the kidney but can cause urinary tract infections in immunocompromised persons.

–are detected by virus isolation from urine (BK virus), Papanicolaou smear of urinary sediment cells, or fluorescent antibody or immunoperoxidase staining of tissues on cells.

F. Poxviruses

–have a complex brick-shaped virion that consists of an outer envelope enclosing a core containing **linear double-stranded DNA** and two **lateral bodies.**

–have more than 100 structural polypeptides, including many enzymes and a **transcriptional system** associated with the virion.

–replicate in the cytoplasm of the cell.

–are unique because **de novo formation of the viral membrane** is required for replication.

–have **post-translational cleavage** of proteins as part of their replication process.

–produce eosinophilic inclusion bodies called **Guarnieri bodies** and membrane **hemagglutinins** in infected cells.

–share a common nucleoprotein (NP) antigen in their inner core.

–may be inhibited by rifampin (which blocks envelope formation) and methisazone (which interferes with late proteins and assembly).

–include the human viruses (**vaccinia, variola,** and **molluscum contagiosum**) and the animal viruses (**cowpox virus, paravaccinia virus** [in cows], and **orf virus** [in sheep]); the animal viruses can cause highly localized occupational infections (usually of the finger).

1. Variola virus

–causes **smallpox,** a generalized viral infection that presumably has been eradicated by a World Health Organization vaccine program.

–grows on the chorioallantoic membrane of eggs, where it forms **pocks,** focal areas of viral-induced cellular necrosis.

–was treated prophylactically with methisazone and by vaccination with the vaccinia virus.

2. Vaccinia virus

–is the variant of variola virus that generally produces only a mild disease and is used as the **immunogen in smallpox vaccination.**

–causes **postvaccinal encephalitis** in a minority (three per million) of vaccinated persons.

–produces a 140-residue polypeptide closely related to epidermal growth factor.

–is being studied as a possible **immunizing vector** containing foreign genes for polypeptides, which would elicit neutralizing antibodies for other viruses (e.g., HSV types 1 and 2).

3. Molluscum contagiosum virus

–infects epithelial cells, where it causes a localized disease that usually resolves spontaneously in several months but may persist for 1 to 2 years.

–causes small, **wart-like lesions** on the face, arms, back, buttocks, and genitals.

–is transmitted by direct or indirect contact.

–can cause a sexually transmitted disease with papular lesions that can ulcerate and mimic genital herpes.

–forms characteristic eosinophilic inclusion bodies in infected cells.

VIII. Positive-Sense RNA Viruses (Table 4–9)

A. Coronaviruses

–are enveloped viruses with a **helical nucleocapsid** that contains **single-stranded RNA** with **positive (messenger) polarity.**

–have distinctive club-shaped surface projections that give the appearance of a **solar corona** to the virion.

–replicate in the cytoplasm and bind to cytoplasmic vesicles; no viral antigens appear on the surface of the infected cell.

–produce the **common cold** in adults (the second most frequent cause) and are implicated in **infant gastroenteritis.**

–usually are not diagnosed in the laboratory, although complement-fixation and neutralization tests are available.

–are represented in humans by **prototype strains 229E and OC43.**

–are represented in mice by **mouse hepatitis virus,** which causes a chronic demyelinating disease used as a model for multiple sclerosis in humans.

B. Flaviviruses

–are enveloped viruses with a **single-stranded, positive-sense RNA** and no discernible capsid structure.

–replicate in the cytoplasm of the cell, where their RNA is translated into a large polyprotein that is subsequently cleaved (by post-translational cleavage) into individual proteins.

–bud into the endoplasmic reticulum.

1. Dengue virus

–is an **arbovirus** transmitted from monkeys to humans by mosquitoes.

–causes characteristic skin lesions as well as fever and muscle and joint pain.

–may be fatal if hemorrhages are associated with the infection.

–is sometimes called **break bone fever.**

2. Hepatitis C virus (HCV)

–is also known as **non-A, non-B hepatitis virus.**

–infects the body after parenteral entry, causing hepatitis after a 14- to 20-day incubation period.

–causes 90% of blood transfusion–associated or blood product administration–associated hepatitis.

–can cause **chronic infections;** therefore, individuals with the virus are in a **carrier state.**

–is diagnosed by ELISA for the antigen.

3. St. Louis encephalitis virus

–is an **arbovirus** with a mosquito vector that transfers the virus from wild birds to humans.

–usually causes inapparent infections but may produce encephalitis.

4. Yellow fever virus

–is an **arbovirus** that is usually transferred from monkeys to humans by mosquitoes.

–is a **biphasic disease** with clinical signs involving the vascular endothelium during initial virus replication and in the liver during later replication.

–can be diagnosed by eosinophilic hyaline masses called **Councilman bodies** in the cytoplasm of infected liver cells.

–does not occur after immunization with the **attenuated vaccine strains 17D and Dakar.**

–can cause **chronic infections;** therefore, individuals with the virus are in a **carrier state.**

C. Picornaviruses

–are small, naked viruses with an **icosahedral nucleocapsid** that contains **single-stranded, positive-sense RNA covalently linked to a small protein** (VPg in poliovirus).

–replicate in the cytoplasm of the cell, where their RNA is translated into a large polyprotein that is subsequently cleaved (**post-translational cleavage**).

–modify their capsid proteins while in the assembled capsid.

–have cytopathic effects that include the formation of virus crystals in the cytoplasm of infected cells.

–are frequently cytolytic to infected cells.

–are classified as enteroviruses or rhinoviruses.

1. Enteroviruses

–cause a variety of human diseases involving infections of the alimentary tract.

–are stable at acidic pH (3–5).

–include the polioviruses, coxsackie A and B viruses, echoviruses, enteroviruses, and hepatitis A virus.

–that have been isolated since 1969 are classified simply as enteroviruses and given a serotype number instead of being classified as either coxsackieviruses or echoviruses.

a. Poliovirus infections

–are usually subclinical but can occur as **mild illness, aseptic meningitis,** or an acute disease of the CNS (**poliomyelitis**), in which spinal cord motor neurons (anterior horn cells) are killed and flaccid paralysis results.

Table 4–9. Properties of Positive-Sense RNA Viruses

Virus Family	Virus Name	Unique Genes or Gene Products	Associated Acute Diseases	Associated Chronic or Persistent Diseases	Diagnostic Methods
Coronaviridae	Coronaviruses	...	Colds (adults)	...	...
			Gastroenteritis (infants)		
Flaviviridae	Dengue (arbovirus)	...	Break bone fever	...	...
			Hemorrhagic fever		
	Hepatitis C virus	...	Post-transfusion hepatitis	Hepatitis	ELISA test for IgM
	Yellow fever virus (arbovirus)	...	Yellow fever	...	Councilman bodies
	St. Louis encephalitis virus (arbovirus)	...	Encephalitis, frequent inapparent disease	...	...
Picornaviridae	Enteroviruses				
	Poliovirus	...	Inapparent to mild febrile illness (abortive poliomyelitis) to paralytic poliomyelitis	...	Virus isolation
	Coxsackie A viruses	...	Herpangina	...	Occasional rashes
			Hand-foot-and-mouth disease		Virus isolation
			Common cold		
			Aseptic meningitis		
	Coxsackie B viruses	...	Myocarditis	...	Occasional rashes
			Pericarditis		Virus isolation
			Pleurodynia (Bornholm disease)		
			Common cold		
			Aseptic meningitis		
			Juvenile diabetes (B4)		

	Echoviruses	...	Aseptic meningitis / Common cold / Infantile diarrhea / Hemorrhagic conjunctivitis	...	Frequent rashes / Virus isolation
	Hepatitis A virus	...	Infectious hepatitis	...	ELISA test for IgM
	Rhinovirus	...	Common cold	...	
Retroviridae	Human immunodeficiency viruses 1 and 2	Regulatory proteins: TAT, REV, and NEF Envelope glycoproteins: gp41 and gp120 Core proteins: p18, p24, and reverse transcriptase (RT) Regulatory genes: TRE and RRE	Inapparent disease or flu-like syndrome	AIDS AIDS dementia	Syncytia formation / ELISA for p24 / Western blot
	Human T-cell leukemia viruses types 1 and 2	Regulatory proteins: TAX and REX	Adult acute T-cell lymphocytic leukemia; some hairy cell leukemias	...	
Togaviridae	Alphaviruses Eastern equine encephalomyelitis virus (arbovirus)	...	Severe encephalitis	...	
	Western equine encephalomyelitis virus (arbovirus)	...	Encephalitis (usually inapparent disease)	...	
	Rubiviruses Rubella	...	German measles / Congenital rubella syndrome	...	Rash ELISA: IgM for recent infection, IgG for protection
Caliciviridae	Norwalk agent	...	Epidemic gastroenteritis	...	RIA serology

ELISA = enzyme-linked immunosorbent assay; RIA = radioimmunoassay; AIDS = acquired immune deficiency syndrome.

–are caused by **three serotypes** of virus.

–can occur in epidemics.

–begin in the oropharynx and intestine but can travel inside axons to the spinal cord.

–are controlled by immunization with either a **killed vaccine** (Salk vaccine) or a **live attenuated trivalent vaccine** containing the three serotypes (Sabin vaccine).

–are diagnosed serologically by a complement-fixation test or by virus isolation from the throat (early in illness) or feces (later in illness).

b. Coxsackievirus infections

–are caused by 29 serotypes of viruses divided into two groups, based on the type of paralysis observed after inoculation into mice; group A viruses cause flaccid paralysis, group B viruses cause spastic paralysis.

–are the most common cause of **viral heart disease** (type B).

–tend to occur in the summer and early fall.

–can be diagnosed by virus isolation from throat washings, stools, or both or from serologic tests using specific viral antigen if a particular virus strain is suspected.

–are associated with various diseases:

(1) Herpangina (group B)

(2) Hand-foot-and-mouth disease (group A)

(3) Hemorrhagic conjunctivitis (group A)

(4) Pleurodynia, myocarditis, pericarditis, and meningoencephalitis (group B)

(5) Aseptic meningitis and colds (groups A and B)

c. Echovirus infections

–are caused by more than 30 serotypes of viruses that initially infect the human enteric tract but cause diseases ranging from common colds and fevers (with or without rashes) to aseptic meningitis and acute hemorrhagic conjunctivitis.

–may be diagnosed by virus isolation from the throat or stools; however, this is done only in summer outbreaks of **aseptic meningitis** or **febrile illness with rash.**

d. Enterovirus infections

–are associated with various respiratory tract infections, CNS disease (enterovirus type 71), and acute hemorrhagic conjunctivitis (enterovirus type 70).

e. Hepatitis A virus infections

–are caused by an enterovirus that could be called **enterovirus type 72.**

–are called **infectious hepatitis.**

–are distinguished from HBV infections by their abrupt onset, relatively short incubation period (15–45 days), and transfer by the fecal–oral route.

–are acute infections that can occur in epidemics.

−may be treated prophylactically by immune human globulin or prevented by immunization with **killed virus vaccine.**

−are diagnosed serologically by increases in IgM detected by an ELISA test.

2. Rhinoviruses

−cause localized upper respiratory tract infections.

−are the most frequent cause of the **common cold.**

−exist in more than **100 serotypes.**

−are acid-labile.

D. Retroviruses

−are enveloped viruses that probably have an **icosahedral capsid** surrounding a **helical nucleocapsid,** which contains an inverted dimer of **linear, single-stranded positive-sense RNA** (diploid genome).

−are divided morphologically into four types (A, B, C, and D).

−are classified into three groups: **lentiviruses** (visna and maedi viruses of sheep, **HIV**), **spumaviruses,** and **oncoviruses** (types B, C, and D RNA tumor viruses).

−have a virion-associated reverse transcriptase (which makes DNA copies from RNA) and replicate in the nucleus.

−need host-cell transfer RNA to interact with reverse transcriptase before the reverse transcriptase complex can bind to RNA and initiate DNA synthesis.

−have three distinctive genes: **gag (structural proteins), pol (reverse transcriptase),** and **env (envelope glycoproteins),** which are flanked by **long terminal repeat sequences** with regulatory functions.

−use post-translational cleavage processes during the synthesis of gag and env gene products.

−cause mostly "slow" diseases of animals and various cancers (see XII), except for HIV, which causes AIDS.

1. Human immunodeficiency virus (HIV)

a. General characteristics—HIV

−is a member of the lentivirus subfamily.

−initiates infection by interaction of an envelope glycoprotein (gp120) with the cellular T4 (CD4) lymphocyte surface receptor.

−synthesizes core proteins (p18, p24, and RT) and transregulatory proteins (TAT, REV, and NEF).

−has regulatory genes (TRE and RRE).

−infects and **kills helper T cells,** resulting in **depression of both humoral and cell-mediated immunity.**

−travels throughout the body, particularly in macrophages.

−induces a distinctive CPE called **giant-cell (syncytia) formation.**

b. AIDS

−results from suppression of the immune system.

−is characterized by unusual cancers (e.g., Kaposi's sarcoma), severe opportunistic infections (e.g., *Pneumocystis carinii,* CMV), or, frequently, **AIDS dementia complex.**

–is a high-risk disease for homosexuals, bisexual men, and intravenous drug users.

–does not always occur in persons who are seropositive for HIV.

–is diagnosed by clinical symptoms and serologic assays, including ELISA and Western blot tests.

2. Endogenous type C retroviruses

–are viruses of type C RNA tumor virus morphology (see XII C 2).

–have a provirus that is a constant part of the genome of an organism and whose expression is regulated by the host cell.

–are transmitted genetically to all offspring.

–are not pathogenic for their hosts.

–are frequently induced to replicate when cells are placed in tissue culture.

–are called **ecotrophic** if they multiply in cells of the species in which they were induced, **xenotrophic** if they cannot infect cells from the species in which they were induced but infect other species, and **amphotrophic** if they grow in cells of the species from which they were induced as well as in cells from other species.

E. Togaviruses

–are enveloped viruses with an **icosahedral nucleocapsid** containing **single-stranded, positive-sense RNA.**

–have **hemagglutinins** associated with their envelope.

–replicate in the cytoplasm and post-translationally process the polyproteins they synthesize.

–cause generalized infections.

–are divided into four groups of which two (alphaviruses and rubiviruses) are human pathogens.

1. Alphavirus

–bud from the cell surface.

–are **arboviruses** with mosquito vectors and animal reservoirs.

–produce encephalitis or moderate systemic disease following the bite of a mosquito that has fed on an animal viral reservoir.

–lead to more serious encephalitis than do flaviviruses.

–are diagnosed by serologic tests, usually ELISA for IgM, because virus isolation is difficult.

–include **eastern equine encephalitis virus, western equine encephalitis virus,** and **Venezuelan equine encephalitis virus.**

2. Rubiviruses

a. General characteristics–rubiviruses

–bud into the endoplasmic reticulum and the cell surface.

–include **rubella virus.**

b. Rubella virus infections

–cause **German measles,** a systemic infection characterized by lymphadenopathy and morbilliform rash.

–are often subclinical in adults.

–can produce **congenital infections,** which can cause serious damage to the infected fetus during the first 10 weeks of pregnancy and lead to rubella syndrome.

–are difficult to diagnose clinically but can be diagnosed by serologic tests for IgM antibodies, including hemagglutination inhibition or ELISA.

–can be prevented by immunization with the **live attenuated vaccine strains HPV77** or **RA 27/3.**

F. Norwalk virus

–is most likely a member of the *Caliciviridae* family.

–is a naked virus with an **icosahedral nucleocapsid** containing **single-stranded, positive-sense RNA.**

–replicates in the cytoplasm.

–causes **epidemic gastroenteritis.**

–has never been grown in tissue culture.

–may be demonstrated by a radioimmunoassay blocking test or immune adherence methods.

IX. Negative-Sense RNA Viruses (Table 4–10)

A. Bunyaviruses

1. General characteristics—bunyaviruses

–are enveloped viruses with **three circular helical nucleocapsids,** each containing a unique piece of **single-stranded, negative polarity RNA** (L, M, and S segments), viral nucleoprotein, and transcriptase enzyme.

–replicate with cytoplasm and bud from the **membranes of the Golgi apparatus.**

–can interact with viruses that are closely related serologically to produce **recombinant viruses by genetic reassortment.**

–are arboviruses that have rodent hosts and infect humans during an arthropod bite.

–produce mosquito-borne encephalitis (**California** and **LaCrosse encephalitis viruses**), sandfly and mosquito-borne fever (**sandfly fever virus** and **Rift Valley fever virus**), rodent-borne hemorrhagic fever (**Hantaan virus**), or respiratory distress syndrome (**Hantavirus**).

2. Bunyavirus encephalitis

–is caused by the California and LaCrosse viruses, which occur mainly in the Mississippi and Ohio River valleys.

–has a small forest rodent reservoir for the virus and a mosquito vector.

–is usually mild (sometimes causing only meningitis), with an excellent prognosis and rare sequelae.

3. Hantavirus pulmonary syndrome

–is caused by inhaling Hantavirus contained in dried deer mouse saliva, urine, or feces.

–may evolve to a fatal disease (> 50%) characterized by respiratory insufficiency.

Table 4–10. Properties of Negative-Sense RNA Viruses

Virus Family	Virus Name	Unique Genes or Gene Products	Associated Acute Diseases	Associated Chronic or Persistent Diseases	Diagnostic Methods
Bunyaviridae	California encephalitis virus (arbovirus) LaCrosse encephalitis virus (arbovirus) Hantavirus	...	Mild febrile illness Encephalitis Severe respiratory distress	...	Serology
Orthomyxoviridae	Influenza A, B, and C viruses	Hemagglutinin neuraminidase Nucleoprotein Matrix protein	Influenza Reye's syndrome (type B virus)	...	Clinical manifestations Virus isolation
Paramyxoviridae	Newcastle disease virus Measles virus	Hemagglutinin only Fusion factor Matrix protein	Mild conjunctivitis (poultry workers) Measles Giant-cell pneumonia Encephalitis	SSPE	Koplik's spots Warthin-Finkeldey cells ELISA for IgM

			Clinical manifestations
Mumps virus	Hemagglutinin neuraminidase	Mumps	...
	Fusion factor	Orchitis	
	Matrix protein	Aseptic meningitis	...
Parainfluenza virus (types 1–4)	Hemagglutinin neuraminidase	Croup (types 1–3)	IF of respiratory secretions
	Fusion factor	Pharyngitis	Virus isolation
	Matrix protein	Upper and lower respiratory tract infections	
Respiratory syncytial virus	Fusion factor	Bronchiolitis and pneumonia in infants	...
	Matrix factor	Nosocomial infections	Viral antigen in nasal washing by FA
		Colds in adults	
Rhabdoviridae	...	Rabies	...
Rabies			Negri bodies
Vesicular stomatitis virus		Foot and mouth disease in cattle	FA staining of tissue sections

ELISA = enzyme-linked immunosorbent assay; FA = fluorescent antibody; IF = immunofluorescence; SSPE = subacute sclerosing panencephalitis.

B. Orthomyxoviruses

–are enveloped, spherical, or filamentous viruses with **eight helical nucleo-capsids** containing a unique **single-stranded, negative-sense RNA.**

–have a **hemagglutinin (H)**, a **neuraminidase (N)**, and a **matrix protein (M)** associated with the envelope, a **transcriptase (P)** that is nucleocapsid-associated, and an **NP** associated with the RNA.

–form **defective interfering (DI) particles** that lack a segment of RNA necessary for productive replication.

–are assembled in the cytoplasm but depend on host nuclear functions, including RNA polymerase II, for transcription.

–are **influenza viruses** and are classified as type A, B, or C, depending on a nucleocapsid antigen.

–have the capacity to undergo **genetic reassortment** due to the segmented nature of the genome.

–do not replicate well in tissue culture and are grown in animals or embryonated eggs.

–are designated by the nomenclature, which indicates virus type, species isolated from (unless human), site of isolation, strain number, year of isolation, and hemagglutinin and neuraminidase subtype, for example, A/swine/New Jersey/8/76 (H1N1) and A/Phillippines/2/82 (H3N2).

1. Glycoproteins

a. Influenza virus hemagglutinin

–is an envelope glycoprotein containing a **virus receptor** that binds to the cellular receptor site.

–agglutinates many species of red blood cells.

–induces neutralizing antibodies.

–has **fusion activity** that allows the virion envelope to fuse with the host-cell plasma membranes.

–is responsible for influenza epidemics when it changes antigenically.

–undergoes frequent minor mutations that result in antigenic changes leading to **antigenic drift.**

–undergoes **antigenic shift** when major antigenic changes follow reassortment between the hemagglutinin-coding RNA segments of animal or human viruses.

b. Influenza virus neuraminidase

–is an envelope glycoprotein that removes terminal sialic acid residues from oligosaccharide chains.

–is involved in the **release of virions** from infected cells.

–can undergo antigenic shift and drift mutations; however, epidemics do not result from these changes.

2. Influenza

–is a localized infection of the respiratory tract.

–is usually not serious, except in the elderly or in patients with a secondary bacterial pneumonia.

–is associated with Guillain-Barré syndrome (influenza virus types A and B) and Reye's syndrome (influenza virus type B).

–can be diagnosed by virus isolation or a hemagglutination inhibition serologic test.

–may be treated prophylactically with amantadine or rimantadine if type A virus is involved or with a polyvalent killed vaccine containing the prevailing type A and type B strains.

C. Paramyxoviruses

–are spherical, enveloped viruses with a **single helical nucleocapsid** containing **single-stranded, negative-sense RNA.**

–have a **hemagglutinin–neuraminidase** (HN), a **fusion protein** (F), and a **matrix protein** (M) associated with the envelope and a nucleocapsid-associated **transcriptase** (P).

–replicate in the cytoplasm of the cell.

–form **DI particles** by segment deletions within the genome.

–form **heteroploid particles** (two nucleocapsids from unrelated paramyxoviruses in the same envelope) or **polyploid particles** (multiple copies of the same nucleocapsid in a large envelope).

–cause acute and persistent infections.

–are divided into three genera on the basis of chemical and biologic properties: **paramyxoviruses** (parainfluenza and mumps viruses), **morbilliviruses** (measles virus), and **pneumoviruses** (respiratory syncytial virus).

–exist in few antigenic types.

1. Glycoproteins

a. Paramyxovirus hemagglutinin–neuraminidase

–is a large surface glycoprotein with both **hemagglutinating** and **neuraminidase activity,** except in measles virus, which lacks neuraminidase activity, and in respiratory syncytial virus, in which both activities have been lost.

–is responsible for **virus adsorption.**

–stimulates the production of neutralizing antibodies.

b. Paramyxovirus fusion protein

–is a surface glycoprotein with **fusion and hemolysin activities,** except in respiratory syncytial virus, in which hemolysis activity is lost.

–is responsible for **virus penetration** into the cell.

–is composed of two subunits, F_1 and F_2, formed by proteolytic cleavage of precursor F_0 by a host enzyme.

2. Parainfluenza virus infections

–are caused by **parainfluenza type 1 virus (Sendai virus).**

–cause a variety of upper and lower respiratory tract illnesses, usually occurring in the fall and winter.

–cause **croup** (parainfluenza type 2 virus) in infants.

–can be diagnosed using hemagglutination inhibition or complement fixation tests.

3. Mumps virus infections

–are frequently subclinical and occur in winter or early spring.

–result in generalized disease characterized by enlargement of one or both parotid glands.

–may affect the testes and ovaries, causing swelling and pain.

–cause 10% to 15% of aseptic meningitis cases.

–are most frequently diagnosed by clinical observation, although the virus can be isolated from the saliva, cerebrospinal fluid, or urine.

–are inhibited by a **live attenuated vaccine** containing the Jeryl Lynn strain of virus (usually included with live attenuated measles and rubella virus strains).

4. Measles virus infections

–cause an acute generalized disease characterized by a maculopapular rash, fever, respiratory distress, and **Koplik's spots** on the buccal mucosa.

–can produce **Warthin-Finkeldey cells** (large multinuclear cells) in nasal secretions.

–can progress to **encephalomyelitis** (in 1 of every 1000 cases) or **giant-cell pneumonia.**

–cause temporary depression of cell-mediated immunity (due to viral infection of lymphocytes), which sometimes leads to secondary bacterial infections.

–can produce **subacute sclerosing panencephalitis,** a slowly progressive degenerative neurologic disease of children and young adults.

–can be prevented by a **live attenuated measles vaccine** (Moraten strain) that is part of the trivalent (measles, mumps, and rubella) vaccine given to children.

5. Respiratory syncytial virus infections

–are localized virus infections that are most often confined to the upper respiratory tract but can involve the lower respiratory tract.

–are the major cause of **serious bronchiolitis** and **pneumonia** in infants.

–may be treated with ribavirin if infection is severe.

–may have an immediate hypersensitivity component.

–are caused by an extremely labile virus that produces a characteristic **syncytial effect (cell fusion)** in infected cells.

–may be rapidly diagnosed by a direct immunofluorescent test on exfoliated cells in nasopharyngeal smears.

–may be diagnosed by demonstration of viral antigens in nasal washings by fluorescent antibody or immunohistochemical techniques.

6. Newcastle disease virus infections

–are caused by a paramyxovirus that is a natural respiratory tract pathogen of birds, particularly chickens.

–occur as an **occupational disease** of poultry workers.

–are observed clinically as a **mild conjunctivitis** without corneal involvement.

D. Rhabdoviruses

–are enveloped, **bullet-shaped** viruses with a **helical nucleocapsid** containing **single-stranded, negative-sense RNA.**

–have a virion-associated transcriptase and replicate in the cytoplasm.

–generate deletion mutants that form **DI particles.**

–establish persistent infections in cell cultures.

–are represented by the human pathogen **rabies virus** and the bovine pathogen **vesicular stomatitis virus.**

1. Rabies virus

–produces specific cytoplasmic inclusion bodies, called **Negri bodies,** in infected cells.

–can travel throughout the nervous system in nerve fibers.

–has a predilection for the hippocampus (Ammon's horn cells).

–is called **street virus** if it is freshly isolated and **fixed virus** if it is serially passaged in a rabbit brain so that it no longer multiplies in extraneural tissue.

–produces disease after inoculation by an animal bite or, occasionally, by inhalation.

–causes fatal disease unless the infected person previously received immunization or receives postexposure prophylaxis consisting of passive immunization with human rabies immune globulin and immunization with a vaccine.

–is identified in suspected tissues by a direct immunofluorescence test.

–is grown in rabbit brain (**Semple's vaccine**), embryonated eggs (**duck embryo vaccine**), or W1-38 cells (**human diploid cell vaccine**) before inactivation and use as a vaccine.

–has been attenuated by growth in chick embryo for use as an animal, not human, vaccine (**Flury's vaccine**).

2. Vesicular stomatitis virus

–causes foot-and-mouth disease in cattle.

–is well known for its ability to produce DI particles and persistent infections.

E. Marburg and Ebola viruses

–belong to a virus family called *Filoviridae.*

–are enveloped viruses with a **helical nucleocapsid** containing **single-stranded, negative-sense RNA.**

–cause **African hemorrhagic fevers,** which often lead to death.

X. Other RNA Viruses (Table 4–11)

A. Arenaviruses

–are enveloped viruses with **two string-of-beads nucleocapsids,** each containing a unique **single-stranded, circular RNA.**

–have one molecule of genomic RNA (L, or large) with negative polarity and one molecule (S, or short) that is **ambisense** (i.e., has both a negative and a positive sense).

–replicate in the cytoplasm and have **host-cell ribosomes** in their virion.

Table 4–11. Properties of Other RNA Viruses

Virus Family	Virus Name	Unique Genes or Gene Products	Acute Diseases	Chronic or Persistent Diseases	Diagnostic Methods
Arenaviridae	Junin, Machupo, and Lassa viruses	...	Hemorrhagic fevers	...	...
	Lymphocytic choriomeningitis virus	...	Flu-like illness	...	...
Reoviridae	Reoviruses	σ-Hemagglutinin	Mild upper respiratory infections Gastroenteritis	...	...
	Colorado tick fever virus (arbovirus)	...	Colorado tick fever	...	FA staining of erythrocytes
	Rotaviruses	...	Infantile diarrhea Gastroenteritis in children	...	Enzyme immunoassay for viral antigen in stool
Unknown	Delta agent	Delta antigen	Hepatitis	Hepatitis	ELISA for IgM

ELISA = enzyme-linked immunosorbent assay; FA = fluorescent antibody.

–infect mice, rats, or both as their natural hosts.

–are initially passed from rodents to humans but can be transferred by direct human contact.

–cause highly contagious hemorrhagic fevers (**Junin, Machupo,** and **Lassa viruses**) that are not endemic to the United States and meningitis or flu-like illness (**lymphocytic choriomeningitis virus**) that is endemic.

B. Reoviruses

–are naked viruses with a **double-shelled** (outer shell and core) **icosahedral capsid** containing **10 or 11 segments of double-stranded RNA.**

–replicate in the cytoplasm.

–have a core-associated transcriptase.

–are classified into three groups: reoviruses, rotaviruses, and orbiviruses.

1. Reoviruses

–have **10 segments of double-stranded RNA.**

–have an **outer shell–associated hemagglutinin** (σ 1) that agglutinates human 0 or bovine erythrocytes, is the **viral receptor,** therefore determining tissue trophism, and is the determinant for the three serotypes of reoviruses.

–form distinctive eosinophilic inclusion bodies.

–replicate their RNA **conservatively,** not semiconservatively.

–produce **minor upper respiratory tract infections** and **gastrointestinal disease,** but also are frequently recovered from healthy people.

–are diagnosed by a complement fixation test and serotyped by hemagglutination inhibition assays.

–may be isolated from feces and throat washings.

2. Rotaviruses

–have **11 segments of double-stranded RNA.**

–exist in at least four serotypes, with type A being involved in most human infections.

–cause **infantile diarrhea** and are the most common cause of **gastroenteritis in children.**

–are frequent causes of **nosocomial infections.**

–are diagnosed by demonstrating virus in the stool or by serologic tests, particularly ELISA.

3. Orbiviruses

–have **10 segments of double-stranded RNA.**

–infect insects, which transfer the virus to humans.

–cause mild fevers in humans.

–are represented by **Colorado tick fever virus,** which is carried by the wood tick *Dermacentor andersoni.*

C. Hepatitis D virus (delta-associated virus)

–is a virus with **circular, single-stranded RNA** molecules (viroid-like) and an **internal core δ antigen** surrounded by an **HBV envelope.**

–is **defective** and can replicate only in the presence of HBV.

–is associated with both acute and chronic hepatitis and always with HBV.

–causes more severe hepatitis than does HBV alone.

–may be diagnosed serologically with an ELISA test.

XI. Slow Viruses and Prions

A. Subacute sclerosing panencephalitis virus

–is a variant or close relative of measles virus.

–causes **subacute sclerosing panencephalitis,** a rare, fatal, slowly progressive demyelinating CNS disease of teenagers and young adults.

–may result from improper synthesis or processing of the matrix (M) viral protein.

B. JC virus

–is a papovavirus that frequently infects humans but rarely produces disease unless the host is immunosuppressed.

–has been isolated from patients with **progressive multifocal leukoencephalopathy,** a rare CNS disease.

–causes demyelination by infecting and killing oligodendrocytes.

C. Animal lentiviruses

–are retroviruses that cause slow, generalized infections of sheep (**visna** and **progressive pneumonia virus**) and goats (**caprine arthritis virus**).

–produce minimal amounts of infectious virus in their hosts.

–undergo considerable **antigenic variation** in their host due to mutations in envelope glycoproteins.

D. Prions

–are not viruses but are proteinaceous material lacking nucleic acid.

–are associated with four degenerative CNS diseases (**subacute spongiform virus encephalopathies**): kuru and Creutzfeldt-Jakob disease of humans, scrapie of sheep, and transmissible encephalopathy of mink.

–have a **prion protein (PrP)** that is associated with their infectivity but is encoded by a cellular gene.

XII. Oncogenic Viruses (Table 4–12)

A. General characteristics—oncogenic viruses

–are classified as DNA or RNA tumor viruses.

–produce tumors when they infect appropriate animals.

–transform infected cells by altering cell growth, cell surface antigens, and biochemical processes.

–introduce "transforming" genes or induce expression of quiescent cellular genes, which results in the synthesis of one or more transforming proteins.

B. DNA tumor viruses

–cause **transformation** in **nonpermissive cells** (infected cells that do not support total virus replication).

–form **proviruses.**

Table 4–12. Oncogenic Viruses

Virus	Proteins or Process Implicated in Transformation	Associated Disease
DNA tumor viruses		
Simian virus 40	Large tumor antigen	Hamster sarcomas
Polyoma viruses (JC and BK viruses)	Tumor antigen	Hamster brain tumors
Human papillomaviruses types 16 and 18	E6 and E7 protein	Cervical dysplasia and neoplasia
Adenovirus (types 12, 18, and 31)	E1A and E1B	Hamster sarcomas
Epstein-Barr virus	EBNA and LMP proteins	Burkitt's lymphoma Nasopharyngeal carcinoma
Hepatitis B virus	X protein	Primary hepatocellular carcinoma
Molluscum contagiosum virus	. . .	Benign skin lesions
Herpes simplex virus type 2	. . .	Cervical carcinoma
RNA tumor viruses		
Human T-cell leukemia virus type 1	Transactivating gene products (e.g., TAX)	Adult acute T-cell lymphocytic leukemia
Human T-cell leukemia virus type 2		Atypical hairy cell leukemia
Oncovirus type B (mouse mammary tumor virus)	Proximal activation of growth genes	Mouse adenocarcinoma and mammary cancers
Oncoviruses type C (avian and murine sarcoma and leukemia viruses)	Oncogenes, insertional mutagenesis, or proximal activation of growth genes	Avian and murine sarcomas and leukemias

EBNA = Epstein-Barr nuclear antigen, LMP = latent membrane proteins.

—include human papillomaviruses: adenoviruses, HBV, EBV, molluscum contagiosum virus, JC and BK viruses, and possibly HSV-2.

—include animal viruses: chicken **Marek's disease virus** (a herpesvirus), mouse **polyomavirus** (a papovavirus), and monkey **SV40 virus** (a papovavirus).

—have protein products (e.g., adenovirus, papillomavirus, and polyomavirus) that interact with cellular **tumor suppressor gene** or **antioncogene** products that suppress oncogene expression.

1. **SV40 virus**

—undergoes productive replication in monkey cells but transforms nonpermissive hamster and mouse cells.

—synthesizes an early protein called **large tumor (T) antigen,** which associates with two antioncogene proteins, p53 and p110^{Rb}, and the retinoblastoma gene product, and establishes and maintains **SV40-induced transformation.**

–synthesizes two other tumor antigens, middle T and small T antigens.

2. Polyomavirus

–grows permissively in mouse cells but transforms nonpermissive hamster and rat cells.

–synthesizes a **transforming large T antigen.**

3. Human adenovirus

–may be highly oncogenic (types 12, 18, and 31) or weakly oncogenic (types 3, 7, 14, 16, and 21) when injected into hamsters.

–synthesize an **E1A** protein that binds to cellular p53 and **E1B** protein that binds to cellular p110^{Rb} if highly oncogenic.

4. Human papillomavirus

–may have a strong association (types 16 and 18) or a moderate association (types 31, 33, 35, 45, 51, 52, and 56) with cervical carcinoma.

–synthesizes an **E6 protein** that binds to cellular p53 and **E7 protein** that binds to cellular p110^{Rb}.

5. Epstein-Barr virus (EBV)

–is a cofactor in the etiology of **Burkitt's lymphoma** and **nasopharyngeal carcinoma.**

–can immortalize and transform B lymphocytes due to specific EBNA and LMP proteins.

6. Hepatitis B virus (HBV)

–is associated with primary hepatocellular carcinoma.

–synthesizes an x protein, which binds to cellular p53.

C. RNA tumor viruses

–are **retroviruses** (oncovirus group).

–infect permissive cells but transform rather than kill.

–cause tumors of the reticuloendothelial and hematopoietic systems (leukemias), connective tissues (sarcomas), or mammary gland.

–are also called **oncornaviruses.**

1. Type B tumor viruses

–have an eccentric electron-dense core structure in their virion.

–are best exemplified by **mouse mammary tumor virus,** also called **Bittner virus.**

2. Type C tumor viruses

–have electron-dense cores in the center of the virion.

–include most RNA tumor viruses.

–are classified as nondefective or defective based on replicative ability.

–contain a cellular-derived **oncogene** (which codes for a cancer-inducing product) as well as **virogenes** (gag, pol, and env); however, a few nondefective murine leukosis viruses (AKR and Moloney viruses) lack oncogenes.

a. Oncogenes

–are genes that cause cancer.

–have copies in viruses (**v-***onc*) and cells (**c-***onc* or **proto-oncogene**).

–are "switched off" or downregulated in normal cells by antioncogene proteins (e.g., p53 and p110^{Rb}).

–have products that are essential to normal cell function or development.

–may code for proteins, which can be:

(1) Tyrosine protein kinases (*src* gene-Rous sarcoma virus, abl gene-Abelson leukemia virus)

(2) Guanine-nucleotide–binding proteins (Ha-*ras*-Harvey sarcoma virus)

(3) Chromatin-binding proteins (*myc*-MC29 myclocytomatosis virus and *fos*-FBJ osteosarcoma virus)

(4) Cellular surface receptors such as epidermal growth factor receptor (*erb*-B product of avian erythroblastosis virus)

(5) Cellular growth factors such as platelet-derived growth factor (SIS gene product of simian sarcoma virus)

b. Nondefective viruses

–have all their virogenes and can therefore replicate themselves.

–have high oncogenic potential if they also contain an oncogene (e.g., **Rous chicken sarcoma virus**).

–have low oncogenic potential if they do not have an oncogene (e.g., **AKR** and **Moloney murine leukemia viruses** and **human T-cell leukemia viruses [HTLV] I and II**).

c. Defective viruses

–have a virogene or part of a virogene replaced by an oncogene.

–need **helper viruses** to provide missing virogene products for replication.

–have high oncogenic potential, for example, murine sarcoma viruses (**Kirsten** and **Harvey viruses**) and murine leukemia viruses (**Friend** and **Abelson viruses**).

d. Human T-cell leukemia viruses (HTLV)

–are nondefective, exogenous retroviruses.

–replicate and transform T4 antigen-positive cells.

–produce giant multinucleated cells.

–have no identifiable oncogene.

–are associated with human adult acute HTLV (HTLV-1) and some forms of hairy cell leukemia virus (HTLV-2).

Review Test

Directions: Each of the numbered items or incomplete statements in this section is followed by answers or by completions of the statement. Select the **one** lettered answer or completion that is **best** in each case.

1. Which statement pertaining to persistent virus infections is correct?

(A) They are usually confined to the initial site of infection.
(B) They are preceded by acute clinical disease.
(C) They elicit a poor antibody response.
(D) They may involve infected carrier individuals.

2. Which of the following statements concerning antiviral nucleoside analogues is correct?

(A) They are effective only against replicating viruses.
(B) They include foscarnet.
(C) They inhibit replicases.
(D) They may block viral penetration.

3. Which of the following statements concerning localized viral disease is correct?

(A) It is a major feature of congenital viral infections.
(B) It is associated with a pronounced viremia.
(C) It can be associated with carrier individuals.
(D) It may have systemic clinical features such as fever.

4. Which of the following statements concerning viral transcription is correct?

(A) It occurs in a specific temporal pattern for most RNA and DNA viruses.
(B) It involves a virion transcriptase for negative-sense, enveloped RNA viruses.
(C) It occurs in the nucleus for poxviruses.
(D) It may be inhibited by amantadine hydrochloride.

5. Which one of the following statements concerning clinical viral disease is correct?

(A) It is most frequently due to toxin production.
(B) It usually follows virus infection.
(C) It can result without infection of host cells.
(D) It is associated with target organs in most disseminated viral infections.

6. The eclipse period of a one-step viral multiplication curve is defined as the period of time

(A) between the uncoating and assembly of the virus.
(B) between the start of the infection and the first appearance of extracellular virus.
(C) between the start of the infection and the first appearance of intracellular virus.
(D) between the start of the infection and uncoating of the virus.

Directions: Each of the numbered items or incomplete statements in this section is negatively phrased, as indicated by a capitalized word such as NOT, LEAST, or EXCEPT. Select the **one** lettered answer or completion that is **best** in each case.

7. Which of the following host defense mechanisms is NOT viral specific?

(A) Neutralizing antibodies
(B) Sensitized T cells
(C) Complement-fixing antibodies
(D) Interferon

8. All of the following diseases are associated with human adenoviruses EXCEPT

(A) acute respiratory disease.
(B) pinkeye.
(C) pharyngoconjunctival fever.
(D) generalized systemic disease with a rash.

Directions: Each group of items in this section consists of lettered options followed by a set of numbered items. For each item, select the **one** lettered option that is most closely associated with it. Each lettered option may be selected once, more than once, or not at all.

Questions 9–13

Match each description with the virus it best characterizes.

(A) Varicella-zoster virus
(B) Coronavirus
(C) Parainfluenza virus
(D) Influenza virus
(E) Epstein-Barr virus
(F) Cytomegalovirus
(G) Parvovirus
(H) Poxvirus
(I) Respiratory syncytial virus
(J) Papovavirus

9. Contains single-stranded DNA *G*

10. Stimulates anti-VCA antibodies *E*

11. Contains circular, double-stranded DNA *J*

12. Is latent in human neurons ~~F~~ *A*

13. Has a genome of positive-sense RNA *B*

Questions 14–17

Match each description with the type of infection it best describes.

(A) Congenital infections
(B) Acute infections
(C) Disseminated infections
(D) Persistent infections
(E) Latent infections
(F) Localized infections
(G) Subclinical infections

14. Frequently involves a primary and secondary viremia *C*

15. Occurs when a virus does not reach its target organ *G*

16. May produce carriers *D*

17. Involves the periodic conversion of a noninfectious form to an infectious form *E*

Questions 18–21

Match each description with the vaccine it best describes.

(A) Live, enveloped virus vaccine
(B) Naked virus capsid, subunit vaccine
(C) Recombinant viral receptor, polypeptide vaccine
(D) Inactivated, whole naked virus vaccine

18. Uses attenuated virus strains *A*

19. Stimulates antibodies to nucleocapsid antigens *A*

20. Exemplified by Salk poliovirus vaccine *D*

21. Induces the widest spectrum of antibodies and cytotoxic cells *A*

Questions 22–25

Match each virus with its distinguishing characteristic.

(A) Dane particle
(B) Infectious hepatitis
(C) Double-shelled capsid
(D) Diploid genome

22. Hepatitis B virus *A*

23. Hepatitis A virus *B*

24. Human immmunodeficiency virus *E ?*

25. Reovirus *C ?*

Questions 26–29

Match each description with the laboratory testing method to which it best applies.

(A) Dot blot
(B) Enzyme-linked immunosorbent assay (ELISA)
(C) Fluorescence-activated cell sorter
(D) Fluorescent antibody staining
(E) High-performance liquid chromatography

26. Is the most sensitive method of detecting viral antigens *B*

27. Detects viral nucleic acid sequences *A*

28. Is used to detect viral antigens in tissue slices D

29. Is used to detect antiviral antibodies B

Questions 30–33

Match each infection with the appropriate diagnostic feature.

(A) Australian antigen
(B) Cowdry type A inclusions
(C) Owl's eye inclusions
(D) Koplik's spots
(E) Heterophile antibodies

30. Cytomegalovirus infection C

31. Herpes simplex virus infection B

32. Epstein-Barr virus infection E

33. Measles virus infection D

Questions 34–37

Match each phrase with the appropriate genetic term.

(A) Phenotypic mixing
(B) Complementation
(C) Phenotypic masking
(D) Genetic reassortment

34. Occurs in some segmented RNA viruses D

35. Results in a surface antigen "mosaic" A

36. Occurs with different mutants of the same DNA virus B

37. Results in a stable genetic change D

Questions 38–42

Match each disease or condition with the virus that most likely causes it.

(A) Coronavirus
(B) Flavivirus
(C) Hantavirus
(D) Echovirus
(E) Respiratory syncytial virus
(F) Newcastle disease virus
(G) Norwalk agent
(H) Rotavirus
(I) Human immunodeficiency virus
(J) Parvovirus

38. Aseptic meningitis D

39. Colds A

40. Conjunctivitis F

41. Infantile diarrhea H

42. Encephalitis B

Questions 43 and 44

Match each description with the virus to which it best applies.

(A) Simian virus 40 (SV40)
(B) Orbivirus
(C) Rous sarcoma virus
(D) JC virus

43. Contain oncogenes C

44. Is a DNA virus that produces transforming proteins that bind to tumor suppressor gene products A

Answers and Explanations

1–D. Some persistent virus infections, such as serum hepatitis caused by hepatitis B virus, have carriers who may not have clinical signs of the disease.

2–A. Nucleoside analogues inhibit viral replication by inhibiting viral DNA synthesis or function; they do not affect replicases or block penetration.

3–D. Although localized infections are not associated with pronounced viremia, they can have clinical features similar to the viremic systemic infections.

4–B. Specific temporal patterns of transcription occur only with DNA viruses. Poxviruses are synthesized in the cytoplasm. Amantadine hydrochloride inhibits penetration and uncoating of influenza A virus.

5–D. Many viral infections are asymptomatic or subclinical. Clinical disease, however, is often associated with viral replication in target organs during disseminated viral infections.

6–C. The period of time between the adsorption and penetration of the virus until the first appearance of intracellular virus is the eclipse phase.

7–D. Interferon, a host-cell glycoprotein produced in response to virus infection, is relatively host specific, but it is not virus specific.

8–D. A generalized systemic disease with a rash is not associated with human adenoviruses. Acute respiratory diseases, pinkeye, and pharyngoconjunctival fever are all associated with human adenoviruses.

9–G. Parvoviruses are very small naked viruses with a single-stranded DNA genome.

10–E. Epstein-Barr virus produces a viral capsid antigen (VCA) early during active replication, but not in non–virus-producing B lymphocyte cell lines transformed by the virus.

11–J. Papovaviruses, naked viruses with a double-stranded circular DNA genome, can induce tumors in some animals.

12–A. Varicella-zoster virus, which can become latent in neurons within the brain, is sometimes reactivated to cause shingles.

13–B. Coronaviruses are enveloped viruses with a genome consisting of a single-stranded positive-sense RNA molecule.

14–C. In disseminated infections, a primary viremia results following virus multiplication at the initial site of infection, and a secondary viremia frequently occurs during virus multiplication in the target organ.

15–G. Subclinical or inapparent infections occur when the virus does not reach its target organ.

16–D. Infected individuals who may or may not have clinical signs of disease are associated with persistent infections.

17–E. Latent virus infections have a phase during which the virus persists in a noninfectious state that can periodically be reactivated to an infectious state.

18–A. Attentuated, avirulent virus strains are used in live virus vaccines.

19–A. Live virus vaccines can induce antibodies to internal virion antigens such as the nucleocapsid; killed virus vaccines induce only antibodies to surface viral antigens.

20–D. Salk polio vaccine is a chemically inactivated virus preparation.

21–A. Because live virus vaccines are the only ones that progress through a natural course of infection, they produce the widest spectrum of antiviral antibodies.

22–A. The 42-nm hepatitis B virus virion is also called the Dane particle.

23–B. Infectious hepatitis is caused by hepatitis A virus, a member of the picornavirus family.

24–E. Human immunodeficiency virus has a genome that contains two linked copies of single-stranded, positive-sense RNA.

25–C. Reoviruses have a unique double-shelled capsid that contains a segmented double-stranded RNA genome.

26–B. ELISA tests can detect viral antigens at the nanogram level.

27–A. Dot blot tests use either single-stranded nucleic acid probes or enzyme-linked antibodies to detect viral nucleic acid sequences or protein antigens in specimens.

28–D. Specific antibodies labeled with fluorescein dyes are used in staining techniques for the detection of viral antigens in tissue slices.

29–B. ELISA tests using anti–human immunoglobulin antibodies are used to detect levels of human antiviral antibodies.

30–C. Cells with owl's eye inclusions are frequently found in the urine of individuals with cytomegalovirus infections.

31–B. Herpes simplex virus frequently produces eosinophilic nuclear inclusion bodies classified as Cowdry type A in infected cells.

32–E. Infection with Epstein-Barr virus can cause infectious mononucleosis, which may be characterized by the appearance of heterophile antibodies.

33–D. Koplik's spots (exanthems of the buccal mucosa) appear during the prodromal period of measles.

34–D. Genetic reassortment involves the exchange of homologous segments of RNA between two related segmented RNA viruses.

35–A. Phenotypic mixing results in the production of virions with surface antigens from two different viruses.

36–B. Complementation can occur when two different mutants of the same virus infect a cell and each one supplies the replicating virus with the functional protein that the other one is lacking.

37–D. Genetic reassortment involves a one-for-one genetic exchange of segments of an RNA genome; the resultant genetic change is passed on to succeeding viral generations.

38–D. Echoviruses are a type of picornavirus that can cause summer epidemics of aseptic meningitis.

39–A. Coronaviruses (as well as rhinoviruses) are frequently associated with colds in adults.

40–F. Newcastle disease virus is a respiratory tract pathogen of chickens that can be transferred to poultry workers; it causes a mild conjunctivitis.

41–H. Rotaviruses, a member of the reovirus family, are a major cause of infantile diarrhea.

42–B. St. Louis encephalitis virus, a flavivirus with a mosquito vector, causes an important arboviral encephalitic disease in the United States.

43–C. Rous sarcoma virus is a nondefective retrovirus that contains the *src* oncogene.

44–A. The large T antigen synthesized by SV40 virus, a DNA tumor virus, binds to p53 and $p110^{Rb}$, which are tumor suppressor gene or antioncogene proteins.

5

Mycology

I. **Fungi**

–are **eukaryotic.**

–are commonly called **yeasts, molds,** and **mushrooms.**

–have a complex cell wall.

–reproduce typically by asexual and sexual mechanisms.

–belong to a kingdom, the Fungi, which is separate from plants and bacteria.

A. **Fungal cell wall**

–protects cells from osmotic shock and determines shape.

–is a **multilayered, fibrillar structure** that is refractile under light microscopy.

–is composed primarily of polysaccharides, notably **chitin,** but also **glucans**
and **mannans.**

–is **antigenic.**

B. **Fungal cell membrane**

–has a typical eukaryotic **bilayered** membrane.

–has **ergosterol** as the dominant sterol rather than cholesterol (dominant in
mammalian membranes).

C. **Fungal cellular components**

–include eukaryotic **nuclei, mitochondria,** and numerous **vacuoles.**

–do not include chloroplasts.

D. **Fungal forms**

1. **Hyphae**

–are **filamentous** subunits of molds and mushrooms.

–may lack septa (cross-walls); these forms are referred to as nonseptate,
aseptate (without regularly occurring cross-walls), or coenocytic (multi-
nucleate) [Figure 5–1*A*].

–may be septate (see Figure 5–1*B*).

–may be dematiaceous (dark colored, typically olive brown to black) or
hyaline (colorless).

–grow apically and, in a mass, are referred to as **mycelium,** or, in an
organized body, are referred to as a fruiting body (e.g., a mushroom).

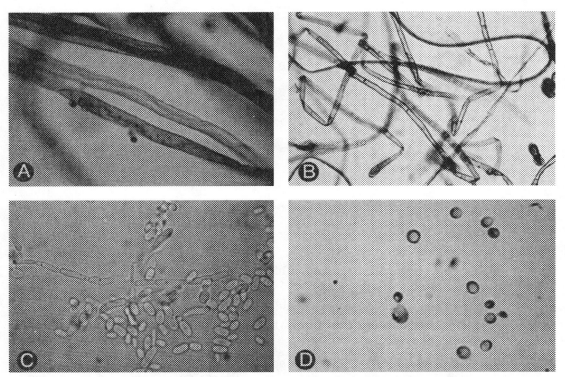

Figure 5–1. Fungal subunits. *(A)* Aseptate hyphae, *(B)* septate hyphae, *(C)* pseudohyphae, and *(D)* yeasts. (Reprinted with permission from Koneman EW, Roberts GD: *Practical Laboratory Mycology,* 3rd ed. Baltimore, Williams & Wilkins, 1985, pp 69 and 71.)

2. Yeasts

–may elongate in some species to develop into pseudohyphae (see Figure 5–1*C*).

–are **single-celled** fungi, generally round- to oval-shaped (see Figure 5–1*D*).

–generally reproduce by budding (**blastoconidia**).

–may have a capsule (e.g., *Cryptococcus*).

3. Dimorphic fungi

–are capable of **converting from a yeast** or yeast-like form **to a filamentous form** and vice versa.

–are stimulated to convert by environmental conditions such as temperature and availability of nutrients.

–usually exist in the yeast or yeast-like form in a mammalian body.

–usually exist as the filamentous form in the environment (e.g., *Coccidioides* hyphae and arthroconidia in the desert soil).

–include the major pathogens *Blastomyces, Histoplasma, Coccidioides,* and *Sporothrix* in the United States. *Candida,* an opportunist, is often referred to as a yeast, but also forms pseudohyphae and hyphae.

4. Pseudohyphae

–are a series of elongated blastoconidia that remain attached to each other and form a hyphal-like structure, with constrictions at the septations (see Figure 5–1*C*).

–are characteristic of most *Candida* species.

5. Fungal spores or propagules

–may be formed either asexually (without nuclear fusion) or by a sexual process involving nuclear fusion and then meiosis. Most important in clinical isolates are the asexual spores:

a. Conidia—asexual spores formed on the outside of a specialized fruiting structure called a **conidiophore** (Figure 5–2*A*)

b. Blastoconidia—**buds** from a mother yeast cell (see Figure 5–2*B*)

c. Arthroconidia—**conidia** formed by the fragmentation of the hyphal strand (see Figure 5–2*C*)

d. Chlamydoconidia—thick-walled **resting spores,** generally spherical in shape and occurring terminally or within the hyphae (see Figure 5–2*D*)

e. Sporangiospores—spores formed on the inside of a specialized fruiting structure called a **sporangium** (see Figure 5–2*E*)

II. Fungal Diseases—Overview

A. Fungal allergies

–are common; molds grow on any damp organic surface, and spores are constantly in the air. Spores and volatile fungal toxins may play a role in "sick building syndrome."

–generally occur in individuals with other allergies.

B. Mycotoxicosis

–may result from ingestion of fungal-contaminated foods (e.g., St. Anthony's fire from ingestion of bread made with ergot-contaminated grain). This is generally an animal problem (e.g., turkey X disease caused by ingestion of feed contaminated with aflatoxin, a carcinogen).

–may be a mycetismus, that is, ingestion of a psychotropic (e.g., *Psilocybe*) or toxic (e.g., *Amanita*) mushroom.

C. Fungal infections (mycoses)

–range from superficial infections to overwhelming infections that are rapidly fatal in the compromised host.

–are increasing in frequency as a result of increased use of antibiotics, corticosteroids, and cytotoxic drugs.

–are commonly classified as superficial, cutaneous, subcutaneous, and systemic infections; the systemic infections are subdivided into those caused by pathogenic fungi and those caused by opportunistic fungi (Table 5–1).

D. Diagnosis of fungal infections

1. Clinical manifestations suggestive of fungal infection

a. Flu-type infection that has lasted longer than or is more severe than a viral flu

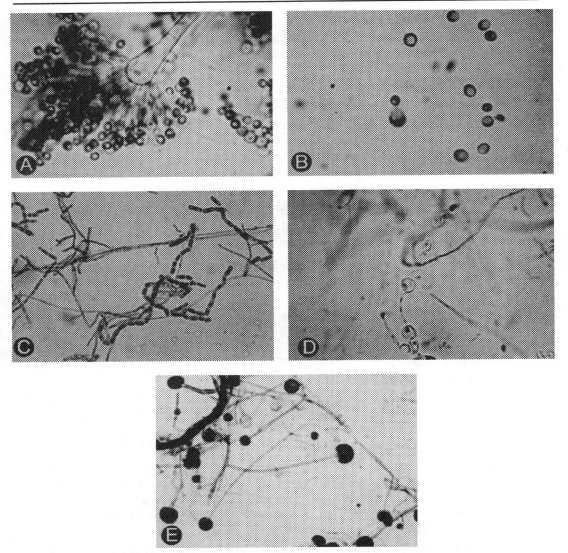

Figure 5–2. Asexual spores. *(A)* Conidia, *(B)* blastoconidia (buds), *(C)* arthroconidia, *(D)* chlamydoconidia, and *(E)* sporangiospores inside sporangial head. (Reprinted with permission from Koneman EW, Roberts GD: *Practical Laboratory Mycology,* 3rd ed. Baltimore, Williams & Wilkins, 1985, pp 71 and 73.)

   b. Chronic respiratory problem with weight loss and night sweats

   c. Fever of unknown origin that does not respond to antibacterial agents or initially responds and then worsens; mixed infections occur commonly in severely compromised patients

   d. Any **infection with negative bacterial cultures** that does not respond to antibiotics and that does not appear viral

   e. Signs of meningitis

   f. Exposure to dust (e.g., a cave explorer) **with bird or bat guano**

Table 5–1. Fungal Infections Commonly Found in the United States

Type	Disease	Causative Organism
Superficial mycoses	Tinea nigra	*Exophiala werneckii*
	Pityriasis versicolor	*Malassezia furfur*
	Piedra	*Trichosporon beigelii* (white)
		Piedraia hortae (black)
Cutaneous mycoses	Dermatophytosis	Dermatophytes (*Microsporum, Trichophyton, Epidermophyton*), and
	Candidiasis	*Candida*
Subcutaneous mycoses	Sporotrichosis	*Sporothrix schenckii*
	Chromyoblastocosis	*Fonsecaea, Phialophora, Cladosporium*
	Eumycotic mycotic mycetoma	*Pseudallescheria boydii, Madurella*
Systemic mycoses	Pathogenic fungus infections	
	Coccidioidomycosis	*Coccidioides immitis*
	Histoplasmosis	*Histoplasma capsulatum*
	Blastomycosis	*Blastomyces dermatitidis*
	Paracoccidioidomycosis	*Paracoccidioides brasiliensis*
	Opportunistic fungus infections	
	Cryptococcosis	*Cryptococcus neoformans*
	Malassezia fungemia	*Malassezia furfur*
	Aspergillosis	*Aspergillus fumigatus, Aspergillus* sp.
	Zygomycosis (phycomycosis)	*Mucor, Absidia, Rhizopus, Rhizomucor*
	Candidiasis, systemic and local	*Candida albicans, Candida* sp.
	Pseudallescheriasis	*Pseudallescheria boydii*

(Reprinted and modified with permission from Rippon JW: *Medical Mycology: The Pathogenic Fungi and Pathogenic Actinomycetes*, 3rd ed. Philadelphia, WB Saunders, 1988, p 3.)

or to **desert sand** (e.g., southwestern United States) and subsequent respiratory infection

2. **Microscopic examination—rapid methods**

   a. **Potassium hydroxide (KOH)** breaks down the human cells in a mount of skin scrapings, hair and nail clippings, lesion exudates, or sputum, but the fungus is unaffected.

   b. **Nigrosin or India ink** mount of cerebrospinal fluid (CSF) demonstrates the encapsulated yeast *Cryptococcus neoformans* in 50% of patients with cryptococcal meningitis.

   c. **Giemsa** or **Wright's stain** of thick blood or of a bone marrow smear may detect the intracellular *Histoplasma capsulatum*.

   d. **Calcofluor white stain with Evans blue** used as a counterstain shows fungal elements in exudates and small skin scales under a fluorescent microscope.

3. Histologic staining—special fungal stains

–are necessary because fungi are not distinguished by color with hematoxylin and eosin (H and E) stain.

   a. Gomori methenamine–silver stain (fungi are stained dark gray to black)

   b. Periodic acid–Schiff reaction (fungi are stained hot pink to red)

   c. Gridley fungus stain (fungi are stained purplish rose with a yellow background)

   d. Calcofluor white stain (may be used on tissue sections)

4. Laboratory cultures for fungi

–must be specially ordered.

–use special media (e.g., **Sabouraud's dextrose medium**), enriched media (e.g., **blood agar**) with antibiotics to inhibit bacterial growth, and enriched media with both **antibiotics and cycloheximide** (which inhibits many saprophytic fungi).

   a. Identification of yeast cultures

     –is based on **morphologic characteristics** (presence of capsule, formation of germ tubes in serum, and morphology on cornmeal agar) and **biochemical tests** (urease, nitrate reduction, and carbohydrate assimilations and fermentations).

   b. Identification of filamentous fungal cultures

     –is based on morphologic criteria or uses an immunologic method called **exoantigen testing,** in which antigens extracted from the culture to be identified are immunodiffused against known antisera.

5. Serologic testing

–is used to identify antibodies specific to the fungi.

–is complicated by some cross-reactivity among pathogenic fungi.

–may use known antibodies to identify circulating fungal antigens in a patient's serum, CSF, or urine.

E. Treatment with antifungal drugs

1. Amphotericin B

–is a **polyene** antifungal agent administered **intravenously** (IV).

–causes nephrotoxicity.

–is the drug of choice in most life-threatening fungal infections.

2. 5-Fluorocytosine (5-FC, flucytosine)

–is an **antimetabolite** that is administered **orally.**

–is used primarily in combination with amphotericin B in the treatment of cryptococcal meningitis or alone at high strength to irrigate the bladder in the treatment of yeast infections. Some fungal infections develop a resistance to the drug.

3. Miconazole

–is an **imidazole** requiring **IV** administration and exhibiting greater toxicity than ketoconazole.

–is used **topically** for mucocutaneous infections.

4. Ketoconazole

–is an **orally** administered **imidazole** that is useful in non–life-threatening systemic fungal infections and in chronic mucocutaneous candidiasis and in many other cutaneous infections. It is ineffective against *Aspergillus*.

–is used in AIDS patients to reduce recurring fungal infections such as *Cryptococcus*.

–is administered orally to treat mucocutaneous infections.

5. Fluconazole

–is a **systemic triazole** antifungal drug.

–is used in candidal infections, for coccidioidomycoses including coccidioidal meningitis in AIDS patients, and as maintenance therapy after cryptococcal meningitis.

6. Itraconazole

–is an imidazole drug administered orally.

–may be used for treatment of *Aspergillus* infection, moderate or severe histoplasmosis, or blastomycosis.

7. Potassium iodide (KI)

–is given **orally in milk** in the treatment of subcutaneous sporotrichosis.

8. Griseofulvin

–is an **inhibitor of microtubules;** it is administered orally and localizes in the stratum corneum epidermidis.

–is effective against **dermatophytes** but may worsen yeast infections.

9. Nystatin

–is a **polyene** drug that is not absorbed from the gastrointestinal tract. It is used topically, intravaginally, or orally to treat **yeast infections** or reduce yeast growth in the gastrointestinal tract of compromised patients.

10. Tolnaftate, miconazole, clotrimazole, ciclopirox, olamine, naftifine, and econazole

–are antifungals used in the treatment of tinea cruris or pedis.

11. Haloprogin

–is a **topical** antifungal used in the treatment of dermatophytes and yeast infections.

III. Superficial Mycoses

–affect the outermost layer of **skin** and **hair.**

–generally do not induce a cellular response to the infection.

–have primarily cosmetic symptoms.

–include pityriasis versicolor, tinea nigra, and white or black piedra.

A. Pityriasis versicolor

–is a fungal infection of the **stratum corneum epidermidis** that manifests as hypopigmented or hyperpigmented skin patches, usually on the trunk of the body. The color of the patch varies with pigmentation of skin, exposure to sun, and severity of disease.

–is caused by *Malassezia furfur*, which is found in skin scales as short, curved, septate hyphae and yeast-like cells ("spaghetti and meatballs" appearance).

–is diagnosed by KOH mount of skin scales; Wood's lamp fluoresces yellow.

–is treated most easily with **selenium sulfide.**

B. Tinea nigra

–is a superficial infection of the **stratum corneum epidermidis** on the palmar surfaces causing benign, flat, dark, melanoma-like lesions.

–is caused by *Exophiala werneckii*, a dematiaceous fungus producing melanin.

C. Piedra

–is a fungal infection of the **hair shaft** that produces hair breakage.

–has two different forms: **white piedra** (caused by *Trichosporon beigelii*) and **black piedra** (caused by *Piedraia hortae*).

IV. Cutaneous Mycoses

–may be a **dermatophytosis** caused by any of the dermatophytes, a homogeneous group of filamentous fungi with three genera, *Epidermophyton, Microsporum,* and *Trichophyton,* or may be a **yeast infection** caused by some of the yeasts, primarily *Candida* (Table 5–2).

–may give rise to a hypersensitive state known as the **dermatophytid,** or "id," reaction, which is a result of circulating fungal antigens.

–may involve the **skin, hair,** or **nails.**

–are classified by the area of the body involved.

––may be acquired from animals (**zoophilic**), in which case the lesions are quite inflammatory. Two common zoophilic species are *Microsporum canis* and *Trichophyton rubrum.*

–may be acquired from humans (**anthropophilic**), in which case there is less inflammation. Two common anthropophilic species are *Epidermophyton floccosum* and *Microsporum audouinii.*

–may fluoresce under a Wood's lamp when the infecting agent is *Microsporum.*

–are diagnosed primarily by microscopic examination of skin, hair, or nail material mounted in 10% KOH.

A. Tinea capitis (ringworm of the scalp)

–is an infection of the **skin and hair** of the head.

–has **pediatric and adult** forms.

Table 5–2. Tissues Infected by Dermatophytes and *Candida*

Group	Genus	Hair	Skin	Nails	Fluoresces
			**Tissue Infected**		
Dermatophytes	*Trichophyton*	yes	yes	yes	. . .
	Epidermophyton	. . .	yes	yes	. . .
	Microsporum	yes	yes	. . .	yes
Yeasts	*Candida*	. . .	yes	yes	. . .

−is diagnosed by Wood's lamp examination (most species of *Microsporum* fluoresce) and microscopic examination of KOH mount of skin and plucked hairs.

1. **Epidemic tinea capitis**

   −occurs in **children** and is **anthropophilic.**

   −is caused by *M. audouinii.*

   −is usually **noninflammatory** and produces **gray patches** of hair.

   −is contagious through headbands, hats, and so on; can be epidemic in schools and day-care facilities.

   −may heal spontaneously at puberty.

   −is treated with **oral griseofulvin and a topical fungistatic agent,** such as boric acid, to reduce infectivity.

2. **Zoophilic tinea capitis (nonepidemic)**

   −occurs primarily in **children.**

   −is usually transmitted by **pets** and occasionally by **farm animals,** which also need to be treated.

   −is most commonly caused by *M. canis* or by *Trichophyton mentagrophytes.*

   −is more **inflammatory** and occurs with kerion in *T. mentagrophytes* infections.

   −may result in temporary alopecia, kerion, keloid, and inflammation.

   −may heal **spontaneously** but usually is treated with **oral antifungals** because it is often tender to the touch.

3. **Black-dot tinea capitis**

   −occurs in **adults** and is a **chronic infection** characterized by **hair breakage,** followed by filling of follicles with dark conidia.

   −is caused by *T. tonsurans.*

   −is usually treated with **oral griseofulvin** or **oral ketoconazole.**

4. **Favus (tinea favosa)**

   −occurs in both **children and adults.**

   −is caused by *T. schoenleinii.*

   −is a severe form of tinea capitis with scutula formation and **permanent hair loss** caused by scarring.

   −is treated with **griseofulvin and by removal of debris;** family members should be treated concurrently.

B. Tinea barbae

   −is an acute or chronic **folliculitis** of the beard, neck, or face.

   −is most commonly caused by *T. verrucosum* (the most common causative agent in dairy areas, acquired from animals), *T. mentagrophytes,* and *T. rubrum.*

   −results in **pustular or dry, scaly lesions.**

   −may be superinfected with bacteria.

   −must be treated with an oral antifungal agent, such as **griseofulvin,** because the hair follicle is infected.

C. Tinea corporis

–is a fungal infection of the **glabrous skin.** Where the infection is limited to inside skinfolds, it is usually a **yeast infection** rather than a dermatophytic infection.

–is most commonly caused by *T. rubrum, T. mentagrophytes,* or *M. canis.*

–is characterized by **annular lesions** with an active border that may be pustular or vesicular.

–is treated with **topical or antifungal agents,** except in recalcitrant infections (usually caused by *T. rubrum*).

D. Tinea cruris

–is an acute or chronic fungal infection of the **groin,** commonly called jock itch.

–is often accompanied by athlete's foot, which also must be treated.

–is caused by *E. floccosum, T. rubrum, T. mentagrophytes,* or *Candida* species or other yeasts.

–is treated with **topical antifungal agents** such as tolnaftate, econazole, or miconazole.

E. Tinea pedis

–is an acute to chronic fungal infection of the **feet,** commonly called athlete's foot.

–is most commonly caused by *T. rubrum, T. mentagrophytes,* or *E. floccosum.*

–may be superinfected with bacteria, which may require antibiotic treatment before tinea pedis is treated.

1. Chronic intertriginous tinea pedis

–results in white macerated tissue between the **toes** (the most common form).

–is treated with **imidazoles or tolnaftate** and by keeping the feet dry (using **aluminum chloride**) and aerated. If infection persists, griseofulvin or oral ketoconazole is used.

2. Chronic dry, scaly tinea pedis

–results in hyperkeratotic scales on the **heel, sole, or sides of the feet.**

–is treated with **keratolytic agents** such as Whitfield's ointment and griseofulvin.

3. Vesicular tinea pedis

–is characterized by vesicles and vesiculopustules.

–is treated gently to avoid massive dermatophytid reaction. **Permanganate or Burow's solution** is used to open vesicles and release antigens to the surface. **Griseofulvin** is the treatment of choice.

V. Subcutaneous Mycoses

–are mycoses that generally begin with **traumatic implantation** of normally saprobic fungi and remain localized in the cutaneous and subcutaneous tissues. In some cases, there is limited, slow spread via the lymphatics.

–are uncommon in the United States. Sporotrichosis, mycetoma (eumycotic and actinomycotic), and chromomycosis have been reported.

A. Sporotrichosis

–is caused by *Sporothrix schenckii*, which is a dimorphic fungus that grows at 37°C as a cigar-shaped, budding yeast and at 25°C as a sporulating hyphae.

–*S. schenckii* is found in or on plant materials such as rose thorns, sphagnum moss, and mine timbers.

B. Lymphocutaneous sporotrichosis

–is a subcutaneous, nodular, fungal disease that spreads via the **lymphatics.**

–is generally not painful.

–classically presents with a **chain of lesions;** lower lesions are often ulcerating and follow the lymph nodes along a limb.

–most commonly **appears on extremities**.

–is known as "the rose gardener's disease" in the United States.

–is diagnosed by culture; histologic findings are generally negative.

–is treated with **KI drops** in a milk menstruum.

C. Eumycotic mycetoma

–is a subcutaneous fungal disease that is characterized by swelling, sinus tract formation, and presence of sulfur granules (microcolonies).

–is caused by *Pseudallescheria boydii* and *Madurella*, which are filamentous true fungi found in **soil or on vegetation;** entry is by **traumatic implantation.**

–usually occurs in rural, third-world agricultural workers in the **tropics.**

D. Chromoblastomycoses

–is one **group of infections** (the phaeohyphomycoses) all caused by dematiaceous fungi.

–begins with **traumatic implantation** of the spores, usually on a **limb or shoulder.**

–has **colored lesions** that start out scaly and become raised, cauliflower-like lesions.

VI. Systemic Mycoses

–affect internal organs and may disseminate to multiple sites of the body; are sometimes known as the **deep mycoses.**

–are caused by **pathogenic fungi,** which can invade and cause disease in healthy or compromised hosts.

–in the United States, are caused by the **dimorphic fungal pathogens** *Histoplasma, Coccidioides*, and *Blastomyces*, which have specific environmental associations, produce airborne spores, and are endemic to specific geographic regions.

–occur in three disease forms: **acute self-limited pulmonary** (asymptomatic to severe); **chronic** (pulmonary or disseminated); and **disseminated.**

–patients are primarily people who are exposed to large amounts of **airborne dust or sand** containing the fungus.

A. Histoplasmosis

–must be differentiated from influenza and other pneumonias.

–infections are most often **(95%) inapparent, subclinical, or self-resolving;** the disease often leaves residual calcification in the lungs.

–infection type depends on the health, lung structure, and immune system of the host and on the dose of the inoculum.

–can be classified as local or disseminated, and as acute, chronic, or fulminant.

–is a granulomatous fungal infection caused by *Histoplasma capsulatum.*

1. ***H. capsulatum***

   –is a small, **dimorphic** fungus that is a **facultative intracellular yeast,** localizing in monocytic cells that circulate throughout the reticuloendothelial system (RES).

   –does not have a capsule.

   –is found as a filamentous form, with microconidia and large tuberculate macroconidia, in **soil enriched with bat or bird guano.**

   –can be isolated from most areas of the world; the major endemic regions are in the drainage areas of the Ohio, Missouri, and Mississippi rivers and the St. Lawrence Seaway.

2. **Laboratory diagnosis**

   a. **Microscopic examination** for **small intracellular yeasts** in thick blood, bone marrow smear, buffy coat, or liver biopsy, stained with Wright's or Giemsa stain

   b. **Microscopic stain of KOH** mount of sputum

   c. **Culture** of sputum or bronchial washings and blood for dimorphic fungus

      (1) At 25°C in the laboratory or in nature, *H. capsulatum* is found as a filamentous form with round, tuberculate macroconidia and small, tear-shaped microconidia.

      (2) Inside human cells or at 37°C on enriched medium, *H. capsulatum* is a small, nondescript budding yeast.

   d. **Serologic testing,** including complement fixation, immunodiffusion, and radioimmunoassay

   e. **Skin testing**

      –**cannot be used** to diagnose active disease.

      –can be used to demonstrate previous exposure to the antigen.

      –if negative, is a poor prognostic sign in a patient with known active histoplasmosis.

      –can boost antibody levels if performed before serology testing.

3. **Forms of histoplasmosis**

   a. **Acute histoplasmosis**

      –is known as the **"fungus flu."**

      –ranges from an asymptomatic to a severe flu-like but **self-resolving** disease.

      –is almost always a pulmonary disease; however, a transient, hematogenous spread of the fungal cells occurs via the macrophages.

      –shows a highly variable x-ray pattern with hilar lymphadenopathy; calcification is extremely common on healing, especially in young persons. Characteristically, **both lungs** are involved.

      –is treated in healthy persons with bed rest and good nutrition.

b. Disseminated histoplasmosis (chronic to fulminant)
  (1) Symptoms
    (a) Mucous membrane lesions or focus of infection other than the lungs
    (b) Prominent hepatosplenomegaly
    (c) Decrease in white blood cell count, hemoglobin level, and number of platelets; disseminated intravascular coagulation
    (d) Pulmonary symptoms (these may be lacking)
    (e) Anemia and leukopenia
    (f) Weight loss
    (g) Addison's disease (in approximately 50% of fulminant cases)
  (2) Epidemiology—disseminated histoplasmosis
    –occurs in individuals with underlying **immune cell defects** (e.g., patients with AIDS, T-cell deficits, or lymphoma).
    –occurs in children younger than age 1 year who appear to have an **RES defect** (fulminant disease of childhood).
  (3) Treatment must be aggressive, usually with **amphotericin B;** prognosis is poor.

B. Blastomycosis (North American)
  –is a **pulmonary, disseminated, or cutaneous** fungal disease that is caused by the dimorphic fungus *Blastomyces dermatitidis.*
  –type of infection depends on the patient's underlying state of health.

  1. *B. dermatitidis*
    –is a **thermally dimorphic fungus.**
    –is found in the **tissues** as a **large,** mainly free, **yeast with a double refractile wall** and **broad-based buds.**
    –is most likely **inhaled** as **conidia** and is transformed into the yeast form in the lung.
    –is endemic mainly to the St. Lawrence, Mississippi, and Ohio riverbeds and to the southeastern United States (excluding Florida).
    –has been environmentally associated with rotting wood including beaver dams.

  2. Laboratory diagnosis of blastomycosis
    a. Radiology—infiltrative pattern, nodular pattern, and single lesion resembling a neoplasm are most common. Generally there is no calcification.
    b. Direct microscopic examination—pus, skin scrapings, or sputum is examined after KOH ingestion for the presence of **double-walled, large yeasts with broad-based buds.**
    c. Culture for dimorphic fungi—is performed in the laboratory at or below 30°C to grow the filamentous form, with conversion to yeast at 37°C, or DNA probes are used to confirm identification.
    d. Pathology—*B. dermatitidis* may be extracellular or may be found in giant cells; suppurative reaction is most common.
    e. Serologic testing—is performed by complement fixation and immu-

nodiffusion, although cross-reactions are still a problem; radioimmuno-assay is more sensitive.

3. Forms of blastomycosis

a. Acute pulmonary blastomycosis

–may resolve without treatment; however, **itraconazole** is often used.

b. Chronic pulmonary blastomycosis

–usually has suppurative or granulomatous **lesions** in the upper lobe.

–is often misdiagnosed as carcinoma.

–most often occurs with an **infiltrative pattern** without cavitation or calcification.

–is treated successfully with **itraconazole.**

c. Disseminated blastomycosis

–generally occurs in individuals with a low stimulation index to the antigen and a negative skin test.

–is caused by **organisms** carried by macrophages to remote sites, most commonly skin and bones.

–is often diagnosed by the demonstration of broad-based budding **yeasts** in KOH mounts of scrapings of skin lesion edges.

–is treated with **itraconazole.**

C. Coccidioidomycosis

–is an acute or chronic pulmonary or disseminated fungal infection caused by *Coccidioides immitis.*

–is commonly known as **"valley fever."**

1. *C. immitis*

–is a **thermally dimorphic** fungus.

–is found in the human body as large **spherules** within which endospores develop; spherules break and release **endospores,** which enlarge to form new spherules.

–is found in **sand** as **arthroconidia,** which are inhaled.

–is highly endemic in the San Joaquin Valley and the Lower Sonoran Desert of the **southwestern United States.**

2. Laboratory diagnosis of coccidioidomycosis

a. Direct examination—is made of scrapings of any lesions, specimens of sputum, or bronchial washings.

b. Culture—is of sputum, bronchial washings, biopsy, or scrapings; this highly infectious agent grows in the laboratory at or below 30°C as a filamentous form.

c. Serologic testing

(1) Tube precipitin test measures **IgM.**

(2) Complement fixation test measures **IgG.**

(3) Latex particle **agglutination and immunodiffusion tests** are used as screening tools in endemic areas and can detect 93% of cases.

    d. Skin test—becomes **positive** early in the infection; anergy is a poor prognostic sign.

   3. Forms of coccidioidomycosis

    a. Acute self-limiting coccidioidomycosis

     –is similar to acute histoplasmosis except that erythema nodosum or multiforme is more likely to be present.

     –usually requires no treatment.

    b. Chronic coccidioidomycosis

     –does not self-resolve.

     –usually requires treatment with ketoconazole if the infection is not life-threatening.

    c. Disseminated coccidioidomycosis

     –is similar to disseminated histoplasmosis with dissemination to the meninges occurring in many AIDS patients in the endemic region.

     –requires treatment with itraconazole or fluconazole, or, if the infection is disseminated to the brain, requires treatment with fluconazole.

VII. Opportunistic Mycoses (Table 5–3)

–range from annoying or painful **mucous membrane or cutaneous infections** in mildly compromised patients **to serious disseminated infections** in severely compromised patients.

–are caused by endogenous or ubiquitous organisms of low inherent virulence that cause infection in debilitated, compromised patients.

–are caused most commonly by *Candida, Cryptococcus, Geotrichum, Aspergillus, Rhizopus, Mucor,* and *Absidia.*

–may be caused by any fungus if a patient is immunocompromised.

–are increasing as the number of compromised patients increases.

–are rarely serious in well-nourished, drug-free, healthy persons.

A. Candidiases

–are acute to chronic fungal infections involving the mouth, vagina, skin, nails, bronchi or lung, alimentary tract, bloodstream, urinary tract, and, less commonly, the heart or meninges.

–are caused by *Candida albicans* or other species of *Candida.*

–are predisposed by extremes of age, wasting and nutritional diseases, excessive moisture, pregnancy, diabetes, long-term antibiotic and steroid use, indwelling catheters, immunosuppression, and AIDS.

–are generally treated with imidazoles, polyenes, or both.

   1. *C. albicans*

    –is part of the normal flora of the skin, mucous membranes, and gastrointestinal tract, along with other *Candida* species. Normal colonization must be distinguished from infection.

    –forms elongated "budding forms" called **pseudohyphae,** which are often seen in clinical material along with true hyphae, blastoconidia, and yeast cells.

Table 5–3. Symptoms and Conditions Associated With Opportunistic Mycoses

Symptoms	Common Underlying Condition	Fungal Disease
Vaginitis	Antibiotic use; pregnancy	*Candida* vaginitis
Facial swelling; lethargy	Diabetes, leukemia	Rhinocerebral mucormycosis
Fever without pulmonary symptoms	Indwelling catheter; lipid supplements	Fungemia
Fever; pain on urination	Urinary catheter	Urinary candidiasis
Difficulty in swallowing	AIDS	Esophageal candidiasis
Meningeal symptoms	AIDS	Cryptococcal meningitis, *Histoplasma* or coccidioidal meningitis, *Candida* cerebritis
	Severe neutropenia	*Aspergillus* central nervous system infection
	Hodgkin's disease; diabetes	Cryptococcal meningitis
Pulmonary symptoms	Immunocompromised patient, particularly if neutropenic	Invasive *Aspergillosis*
	AIDS	*Pneumocystis* pneumonia Histoplasmosis, coccidioidomycosis
	Alcoholism (urban)	Sporotrichosis (pulmonary)
Hemoptysis	Previous lung damage, especially cavities	Aspergilloma
Endocarditis	Intravenous drug abuse	*Candida* endocarditis
Enteritis (often with anal pruritis)	Antibiotic use	*Candida* enteritis (irritable bowel syndrome)
Whitish covering in mouth	Premature infants, children on antibiotics	*Candida* thrush
Corners of mouth sore	Elderly suffering from malnourishment	Perlèche
Sore gums	Dentures	Denture stomatitis or allergy to antifungal used in treatment of denture stomatitis
Skin lesions; endophthalmitis	Indwelling catheter	Candidemia

2. **Laboratory diagnosis of candidiases**

   a. **KOH mount** of skin or nail scrapings or exudate

   b. Demonstration of the **presence of pseudohyphae or true hyphae** in the tissues

   c. **Cultures** of normally sterile parts of the body (such as CSF), with cultures identified by germ tube formation and morphologic and chemical tests

   d. **Serologic testing** demonstrating high levels of *Candida* precipitins or antigens

   e. **Chromatographic methods** to detect fungal products

3. **Forms of candidiases**

   a. **Oral thrush**

      –is a yeast infection of the oral **mucocutaneous membranes.**

      –manifests as **white curd-like patches** in the oral cavity.

      –occurs in premature infants, older infants being treated with antibiotics, immunosuppressed patients on long-term antibiotics, and AIDS patients.

   b. **Vulvovaginitis or vaginal thrush**

      –is a **yeast infection** of the vagina that tends to recur.

      –manifests with a **thick yellow-white discharge,** a burning sensation, curd-like patches on the vaginal mucosa, and inflammation of the peritoneum.

      –is predisposed by diabetes, antibiotic therapy, oral contraceptive use, and pregnancy.

   c. **Cutaneous candidiasis**

      –involves the **nails, skin folds (visible as creamy growth), or groin.**

      –may be eczematoid or vesicular and pustular.

      –is predisposed by **moist conditions.**

   d. **Alimentary tract disease**

      –is usually an extension of oral thrush and may include **esophagitis** and, ultimately, the **entire gastrointestinal tract.**

      –is found in patients with AIDS or other **immunosuppressive disorders,** particularly those patients on long-term antibiotic therapy.

      –is reduced in highly susceptible populations by fungal prophylaxis.

   e. **Candidemias or blood-borne infections**

      –occur most commonly in patients with indwelling catheters; these infections are manifested by fever, macronodular skin lesions, and endophthalmitis.

   f. **Endocarditis**

      –occurs in patients who have manipulated or damaged valves or in IV drug abusers.

   g. **Bronchopulmonary infection**

      –occurs in patients with chronic lung disease; it is usually manifested by persistent cough.

   h. Cerebromeningeal infection

   –may occur in compromised patients.

   i. Chronic mucocutaneous candidiasis

   –is a chronic, often disfiguring, infection of the **epithelial surfaces** of the body.

   –is diagnosed microscopically and by the lack of cell-mediated immunity to *Candida* antigens.

B. *Malassezia furfur* **septicemia**

   –is a **blood-borne infection** caused by the lipophilic skin organism *M. furfur.*

   –occurs in patients (primarily neonates) who are on **IV lipid emulsions.**

   –is diagnosed by culturing blood on fungal medium that is either lightly overlaid with sterile olive oil or has lipids incorporated into the medium.

   –may resolve by halting the lipid supplements.

C. Cryptococcoses

   –include subacute or chronic fungal infections involving the lungs, meninges, or, less commonly, the skin, bones, and other tissues.

   –most commonly occur as cryptococcal meningitis (often occurring in AIDS patients).

   –are caused by *C. neoformans.*

   1. *C. neoformans*

   –is a **yeast** that possesses an **antigenic polysaccharide capsule.**

   –may be isolated from fruit, milk, vegetation, and soil.

   –is also associated with **pigeon feces;** infection is an occupational hazard to pigeon handlers.

   –is considered to be an **opportunist** in the presence of underlying disease in patients with Hodgkin's disease, leukemias, or leukocyte enzyme deficiency diseases.

   2. Forms of cryptococcoses

   –most often presents as **meningitis.**

   a. Pulmonary infections

   –are usually asymptomatic and self-resolving.

   –are most common in pigeon breeders.

   b. Meningitis or meningoencephalitis

   –occurs most commonly with a headache of increasing severity, usually with fever, followed by typical signs of meningitis.

   –occurs in AIDS patients.

   3. Laboratory diagnosis

   a. Detection of the **capsular material in the CSF** by the cryptococcal antigen **latex agglutination test**

   b. Demonstration of **encapsulated yeast in CSF sediment** on a wet mount in nigrosin or **India ink** (However, India ink in the mount misses approximately 50% of the culturally proven cases of cryptococcal meningitis.)

   c. Confirmation by isolation of *C. neoformans* in culture of CSF

   4. Treatment of meningitis

   a. Amphotericin B is used in conjunction with 5-FC or fluconazole.

   b. Maintenance therapy with an imidazole is necessary for AIDS patients.

D. Aspergilloses

   –are a variety of **infections** and **allergic** diseases that are caused by *Aspergillus fumigatus* and a variety of other species of *Aspergillus*.

   1. *A. fumigatus*

   –is a ubiquitous filamentous fungus whose **airborne spores** are constantly in the air.

   –is recognized both in tissue and in culture by its characteristic septate hyphae with dichotomous branching.

   –produces conidial heads with numerous conidia.

   –is an **opportunistic** organism.

   –*A. fumigatus* and *Aspergillus flavus* are the most common species.

   2. Forms of aspergilloses

   a. Allergic bronchopulmonary aspergillosis

   –is an **allergic disease** in which the organism colonizes the mucous plugs formed in the lungs but does not invade lung tissues.

   –is diagnosed by the finding of high titers of IgE antibodies to *Aspergillus*.

   b. Aspergilloma

   –is a roughly spherical growth of *Aspergillus* in preexisting lung cavities; growth does not invade the lung tissues.

   –occurs clinically as **recurrent hemoptysis.**

   –is diagnosed by radiologic methods.

   c. Invasive aspergillosis

   –occurs most commonly during severe **neutropenia** in leukemia and in transplant patients.

   –most commonly occurs as fever of unknown origin in patients with fewer than 500 neutrophils/mm^3 and pneumonia. It may begin as sinusitis; from either the sinuses or the lungs, it disseminates to any part of the body, most frequently the brain.

   –is diagnosed by microscopy and culture of lung biopsy material.

   –is treated aggressively with amphotericin B or itraconazole.

   –has a high fatality rate unless neutrophil numbers become elevated.

E. Zygomycoses

   –are also known as **phycomycoses or mucormycoses.**

   –are infections most commonly caused by the genera *Rhizopus, Absidia, Mucor,* and *Rhizomucor,* which belong to the phylum Zygomycota (**the nonseptate fungi**).

   1. Zygomycota

   –have **nonseptate** hyphae.

   –grow rapidly.

   –have a predilection for invading blood vessels and the brain.

2. **Forms of zygomycoses**

a. **Rhinocerebral infection**

–is the most common form; it occurs in patients with **acidotic diabetes.**

–presents with facial swelling and blood-tinged exudate in the turbinate bones and eyes, mental lethargy, and fixated pupils.

–is a fatal infection that spreads rapidly.

–must be diagnosed rapidly, usually by a KOH mount of necrotic tissue or exudates from the eye, ear, or nose.

–is rarely treated successfully; treatment consists of **control of diabetes, surgical débridement,** and aggressive treatment with **amphotericin B.**

b. **Thoracic infection** occurs in leukemia and lymphoma patients.

c. **Abdominal–pelvic infection** occurs in malnourished patients.

d. **Cutaneous infection** occurs in patients with leukemia.

F. *Pneumocystis* **pneumonitis and pneumonia**

–are infections cause by *Pneumocystis carinii.*

1. *Pneumocystis carinii*

–is considered a fungus, based on molecular biological techniques such as ribotyping and DNA homology.

–is an obligate parasite of humans (cannot be grown in vitro) but is extracellular, growing on the surfactant layer over the alveolar epithelium.

–colonizes most humans early in life, without apparent disease.

–causes severe disease only in malnourished infants, immunosuppressed patients, and AIDS patients with low $CD4^+$ cell counts.

–is seen in the alveolar spaces as both small trophozoites and larger cysts. Cysts are seen in methenamine silver or calcofluor stains to contain 4–8 intracystic bodies (called nuclei or sporozoites).

2. **Forms of disease**

a. **Interstitial plasma cell pneumonitis**

–occurs in malnourished infants, transplant patients, patients on antineoplastic chemotherapy, and patients on corticosteroid therapy.

–is characterized on radiographs by a patchy, diffuse appearance, sometimes referred to as having a ground-glass appearance.

–is diagnosed as for pneumocystis pneumonia.

b. **Pneumocystis pneumonia**

–was the major cause of death in AIDS patients and is currently responsible for approximately 30% of deaths in AIDS patients.

–causes morbidity and mortality when $CD4^+$ counts decrease to less than $200/mm^3$ unless prevented with prophylaxis.

–lacks plasma cells in the alveolar spaces of AIDS patients.

–has a P_{O_2} decline that is out of proportion to radiologic appearance.

–is characterized on radiographs as having a ground-glass appearance.

Table 5–4. Symptoms and Clues to Diagnosis of Fungal Diseases in Generally Healthy Patients With Superficial, Cutaneous, Mucocutaneous, Subcutaneous, or Allergic Fungal Diseases*

Presenting Symptoms	Possible Disease	Clues†	Most Common Fungal Agent
Hyperpigmented or hypopigmented skin macules with little inflammation	Pityriasis versicolor	KOH: yeast-like cells and short curved septate hyphae	*Malassezia furfur*
Hair breakage with nodules	Piedra	Cream-colored soft nodules on hair	*Trichosporon beigelii* (white piedra)
		Hard, black nodules on hair	*Piedraia hortae* (black piedra)
Cutaneous lesions with various degrees of inflammation	Tineas	KOH: hyphae and arthroconidia	Dermatophytes: *Epidermophyton, Trichophyton, Microsporum*
Candidiasis of skin	Candidiasis of skin	KOH: pseudohyphae and true hyphae and yeasts	*Candida albicans* and related species
Mucocutaneous lesion (vaginitis, diaper rash)	Candidiasis	KOH: pseudohyphae and true hyphae and yeast	*Candida albicans* and related species
Subcutaneous lesions following lymph nodes or solitary nodule	Sporotrichosis	KOH: cigar-shaped yeast in tissue Hyphae and conidia at 25°C	*Sporothrix schenckii* (most likely in the United States)
Colorful subcutaneous lesions, often pedunculated	Chromoblastomycosis	KOH: sclerotic bodies in giant cells	*Fonsecaea pedrosoi* and related forms
Subcutaneous swelling with sinus tracts and granules in exudate	Mycotic mycetoma	Granules that are microcolonies of fungus	*Pseudallescheria boydii*
Allergic reactions	Allergic bronchopulmonary aspergillosis	High IgE levels against *Aspergillus*	*Aspergillus* sp.

* See Table 5–3 for causes for infections in immunocompromised patients.
† Examination of skin scrapings or other tissue mounted in and cleared with potassium hydroxide (KOH) and examined microscopically.

Table 5–5. Symptoms and Clues to Diagnosis of Fungal Diseases in Generally Healthy Patients With Systemic Symptoms

Presenting Symptoms	Possible Disease	Clues	Most Common Fungal Agent
Acute pulmonary disease (cough, fever, night sweats)	Histoplasmosis	Exposure to soil/dust contaminated with bird (especially chicken and starling) or bat feces Endemic region: Ohio, Mississippi, Missouri riverbeds Tissue: small, intracellular yeast 25°C culture: hyphae with microconidia and large tuberculate macroconidia	*Histoplasma capsulatum*
	Blastomycosis	Exposure to rotting wood Endemic region: as for *Histoplasma* plus southeastern seaboard of the U.S. Tissue: large budding yeast with double refractile wall 25°C culture: hyphae with microconidia	*Blastomyces dermatitidis*
	Coccidioidomycosis	Exposure to desert sand with arthroconidia Endemic region: deserts of the southwestern U.S. Tissue form: spherules with endospores 25°C culture: hyphae with arthroconidia	*Coccidioides immitis*
Chronic pulmonary disease (cough, fever, night sweats, weight loss, protracted)	Histoplasmosis; blastomycosis; coccidioidomycosis	Same as for acute pulmonary disease; sedimentation rate elevated	Same as above
Disseminated disease (extrapulmonary sites such as skin, mucous membrane lesions, brain)	Histoplasmosis; blastomycosis; coccidioidomycosis	Same as acute pulmonary disease; once diagnosed, anergy (negative skin test)	Same as above

–is diagnosed by microscopy of biopsy specimen or alveolar fluids (Giemsa, specific fluorescent antibody, toluidine blue, methenamine silver, or calcofluor stains). Presence of serum antibodies is not a useful indicator of infection because almost all healthy and immuno-compromised individuals have antibodies to *Pneumocystis*.

–is treated prophylactically with trimethoprim–sulfamethoxazole or trimethoprim and dapsone.

VIII. Review Chart

–Table 5–4 summarizes superficial, cutaneous, mucocutaneous, and subcutaneous allergic fungal diseases in a format useful for solving case-history questions on the USMLE.

–Table 5–5 summarizes systemic infections in immunocompetent patients.

Review Test

Directions: Each of the numbered items or incomplete statements in this section is followed by answers or by completions of the statement. Select the **one** lettered answer or completion that is **best** in each case.

1. A florist presents with a subcutaneous lesion on the hand, which she thinks resulted from a jab wound she received while she was making a sphagnum moss–wire frame for a floral wreath. The lesion has not healed despite use of antibacterial cream and has begun to spread up her arm with the next lymph node raised and red and beginning to look like it might ulcerate, like the original lesion. The lymph node above is also beginning to redden and is slightly raised. Which treatment is most likely to be appropriate for this wound?

(A) Potassium iodide (KI) in milk
(B) Miconazole cream
(C) Cortisone cream
(D) Oral griseofulvin
(E) Penicillin

2. Which of the following stains allows differentiation of fungus from the human tissues by staining the fungus a pink-red color?

(A) Calcofluor white stain
(B) Gomori methenamine silver stain
(C) Periodic acid–Schiff reaction
(D) Hematoxylin and eosin stain

3. Which of the following statements reflects most accurately the human medical conditions under which the Zygomycota (Phycomycetes) infect and the resulting pathology?

(A) They cause serious infection, primarily in AIDS patients; the yeast form of this dimorphic fungus can be demonstrated easily intracellularly in blood or pulmonary tissues.
(B) They cause serious infection in ketoacidotic diabetic patients; their broad, nonseptate hyphae can be seen penetrating blood vessels and necrotic tissues in the swollen rhinocerebral tissues.
(C) They cause serious infections, primarily in neutropenic patients; their septate dichotomously branching hyphae can be seen in the lungs and often in the brain of these patients.
(D) They cause serious fungemias in AIDS patients; the yeasts, pseudohyphae, and true hyphae can be found in the bloodstream and in other tissues in disseminated cases.

Directions: Each of the numbered items or incomplete statements in this section is negatively phrased, as indicated by a capitalized word such as NOT, LEAST, or EXCEPT. Select the **one** answer or completion that is **best** in each case.

4. Skin lesions are common in all of the following fungal diseases EXCEPT

(A) piedra.
(B) chronic mucocutaneous candidiasis.
(C) disseminated blastomycosis.
(D) disseminated candidiasis.

5. Fungi have all of the following components EXCEPT

(A) 80S ribosomes.
(B) cell walls composed of complex carbohydrates.
(C) ergosterol as the major membrane sterol.
(D) enzymes that allow them to use CO_2 as their sole carbon source.

Directions: Each group of items in this section consists of lettered options followed by a set of numbered items. For each item, select the **one** lettered option that is most closely associated with it. Each lettered option may be selected once, more than once, or not at all.

Questions 6–8

Match each description with the fungal form.

(A) Pseudohyphae
(B) Dimorphic fungus
(C) Hypha
(D) Mycelium
(E) Septum
(F) Yeast

6. A mass of fungal filaments

7. Cross-wall

8. A filamentous fungus subunit

Questions 9–11

Match each description with the antifungal.

(A) Amphotericin B
(B) Griseofulvin
(C) Ketoconazole
(D) Miconazole
(E) Nystatin

9. Oral antifungal that inhibits microtubule formation and is used to treat dermatophytic infections

10. Polyene antifungal that is used for many life-threatening fungal infections

11. Fungistatic imidazole that is used orally or systemically for systemic or superficial fungal infections

Questions 12 and 13

Match the description of the infection to the proper genus.

(A) *Candida*
(B) *Trichosporon*
(C) *Trichophyton*
(D) *Malassezia*
(E) *Microphyton*

12. Causes splotchy hypopigmentation or hyperpigmentation, most commonly of the chest or back

13. Causes yeast skin infections, some of which may resemble dermatophytic infections

Questions 14–17

Match each description to the disease to which it best applies.

(A) Actinomycotic mycetoma
(B) Chromomycosis
(C) Eumycotic mycetoma
(D) Sporotrichosis
(E) Paracoccidioidomycosis

14. Subcutaneous fungal disease characterized by swelling of the sinus tracts and the presence of sulfur granules

15. Subcutaneous fungal disease presenting with raised, colored, cauliflower-like lesions; finding of sclerotic bodies in tissue is of diagnostic importance

16. Subcutaneous or lymphocutaneous disease treated with potassium iodide (KI)

17. A disease caused by *Sporothrix schenckii*

Questions 18–20

Match the description with the microorganism that it best describes.

(A) *Aspergillus fumigatus*
(B) *Blastomyces dermatitidis*
(C) *Coccidioides immitis*
(D) *Histoplasma capsulatum*
(E) *Sporothrix schenckii*

18. Small nondescript yeast form is found inside monocytic cells

19. Environmental form consists of hyphae that break up into arthroconidia

20. Tissue form is large yeast with a thick cell wall and broad-based buds

Questions 21–23

Match each disease with the organism that causes it.

(A) *Aspergillus*
(B) *Cryptococcus*
(C) *Candida*
(D) *Malassezia*
(E) *Sporothrix*

21. Causes septicemias that are found primarily in neonates on intravenous lipid emulsions

22. Causes meningitis in patients with AIDS

23. Invasive fungal disease in patients with severe neutropenia; tissue sections show dichotomously branching (generally with acute angles), filamentous fungi.

Answers and Explanations

1–A. This is a classic case of lymphocutaneous sporotrichosis in which a gardener or florist receives a puncture wound. The drug of choice is potassium iodide given in milk. Topical antifungals are not effective, and the cortisone cream would probably enhance the spread of the disease. Griseofulvin localizes in the keratinized tissues and would not halt the subcutaneous spread of this infection. Penicillin would have no effect because *Sporothrix* is not a bacterium.

2–C. Calcofluor, the Gomori methenamine silver, and the periodic acid–Schiff are all differential stains, but only the periodic acid–Schiff stains the fungi a pink-red. The hematoxylin and eosin stains fungi a pink-red also, but does not differentiate.

3–B. Zygomycota cause serious infection, primarily in ketoacidotic diabetic patients. *Histoplasma* cause serious infection in patients with AIDS; *Aspergillus* causes infections in neutropenic patients, particularly those who have had bone marrow transplants; and *Candida* causes fungemias in patients with AIDS.

4–A. Piedra is an infection of the hair that results in hair breakage. It does not have skin lesions associated with it. Chronic mucocutaneous candidiasis occurs in individuals who have an endocrine defect that results (without treatment) in overwhelming cutaneous lesions and anergy to *Candida* antigens. When *Blastomyces* disseminates, it frequently disseminates to the skin or brain. Fungemias with *Candida* may also lead to maculonodular or maculopapular skin lesions.

5–D. Fungi are heterotrophic rather than autotrophic and thus cannot use CO_2 as their carbon source. Instead, fungi break down organic carbon compounds. Ergosterol is the major fungus membrane sterol, and its presence is important in chemotherapy of fungal infections; for example, amphotericin B binds to ergosterol, producing pores that leak out cellular contents, and imidazole drugs inhibit the synthesis of ergosterol.

6–D. A mycelium is a mass of hyphae.

7–E. The cross-wall of hyphae is called a septum or septation.

8–C. The fungal subunit, called a hypha, is a filamentous structure with or without cell walls.

9–B. Griseofulvin, which localizes in the keratinized tissues, inhibits the growth of dermatophytes by inhibiting microtubule assembly.

10–A. Amphotericin B, a polyene, is the most effective treatment for many life-threatening fungal infections.

11–C. Ketoconazole is an imidazole that can be used either orally or intravenously. Miconazole, also an imidazole, is available in topical or intravenous preparations.

12–D. *Malassezia furfur* is the causative agent of pityriasis or tinea versicolor, which causes pigmentation disturbances.

13–A. *Candida* may cause skin infections that resemble some dermatophytic infections. It may also cause serious infections in immunocompromised patients.

14–C. The disease syndrome is mycetoma and the fungal disease is eumycotic. (*Actinomyces* are bacteria.)

15–B. The finding of dematiaceous yeast-like forms with sharp planar division lines with the clinical presentation is characteristic of chromomycoses.

16–D. Sporotrichosis spreads along lymphatics but rarely disseminates in healthy, well-nourished adults. It is treated with potassium iodide.

17–D. *Sporothrix* causes sporotrichosis. Chromomycosis is caused by the dematiaceous fungi such as *Phialophora, Fonsecaea,* or *Cladosporium.* Eumycotic mycetoma most commonly is caused by *Pseudallescheria* or *Madurella* (true fungi). Actinomycotic mycetoma is caused by actinomycetes such as *Nocardia* or *Actinomadura.*

18–D. *Histoplasma* is a facultative intracellular parasite circulating in the reticuloendothelial system.

19–C. *Coccidioides* is found in desert sand, primarily as arthroconidia and hyphae.

20–B. *Blastomyces* has a double refractile wall and buds with a broad base of attachment to the mother cell.

21–D. *Malassezia furfur* is a lipophilic fungus that is found on skin; it causes septicemia.

22–B. *Cryptococcus* is the major causative agent of meningitis in patients with AIDS.

23–A. *Aspergillus* spores are commonly airborne. Invasive infections with *Aspergillus* are controlled by phagocytic cells. In severe neutropenia, risk of infection is high.

6

Parasitology

I. Characteristics of Parasites and Their Hosts

A. Parasites

–are classified as **ectoparasites** if they live on the skin or hair (e.g., lice) or as **endoparasites** if they live in the host.

–may be obligate (entirely dependent on the host) or facultative (free living or associated with the host).

–rival malnutrition as the major cause of morbidity and mortality worldwide.

B. Hosts

–may be one of three types:

1. **Definitive,** in which the adult parasite reaches sexual maturity

2. **Intermediate,** in which the larval or intermediate parasite stages develop

3. A **reservoir,** which is essential to parasite survival and a focus for spread to other hosts (e.g., swine for *Trichinella* organisms)

C. Vectors

–are living transmitters of disease.

–may be one of two types:

1. **Mechanical,** or nonessential to the life cycle of the parasite

2. **Biological,** serving as the site of some developmental events in the life cycle of the parasite

II. Protozoan Parasites

A. General characteristics—protozoan parasites

–are single-celled animals.

–may cause infections.

B. Classification

1. **Amebas**

–move by **pseudopods.**

–have two distinctive forms:

    a. Trophozoite, the actively motile form

    b. Cyst, the resting stage (the stage most often transmitted from host to host)

2. Flagellates

    —move by the action of **flagella.**

3. Ciliates

    —move by the action of **cilia.**

C. Important intestinal and urogenital protozoans (Table 6–1)

    —include *Entamoeba histolytica, Giardia lamblia, Cryptosporidium* species, *Balantidium coli,* and *Trichomonas vaginalis.*

    1. *Cryptosporidium* is gaining importance in the United States because of its increased frequency in patients with AIDS, in whom it can cause severe diarrhea. Furthermore, because of its resistance to chlorination, there have been major outbreaks of *Cryptosporidium* infection in immunocompetent people exposed to high-level contamination in swimming pools or drinking water.

    2. *Entamoeba histolytica,* a pathogen, must be differentiated from *Entamoeba coli,* a nonpathogenic commensal. *E. histolytica* has a nucleus that looks like a wagon wheel with a sharp central dot (karyosome), fine radiating "spokes" of nucleoplasm, and a fine peripheral rim of nucleoplasm. *E. histolytica* ingests both white cells and red cells, which may be seen inside the cytoplasm as dark dots. (This also accounts for fecal polymorphonuclear counts not being as high as would be expected from this highly invasive organism.)

D. Important tissue or blood protozoans

    —include *Plasmodium, Toxoplasma, Pneumocystis, Babesia, Trypanosoma,* and *Leishmania.*

    1. *Plasmodium* **species** (Table 6–2)

        —are transmitted by the bite of an infected *Anopheles* mosquito. Sporozoites are injected in the new human host.

        —cause disease by a wide variety of mechanisms, including hemoglobin metabolism and lysis of infected red blood cells, leading to **anemia** and agglutination of infected red blood cells.

        —cause **paroxysms** (chills, fever, and malarial rigors) when infected red cells are lysed, liberating a new crop of merozoites.

        —have **two distinct hosts:**

        a. A **vertebrate** (e.g., a human) acts as the intermediate host; the asexual phase of the parasite's life cycle (schizogony) takes place in the liver and red blood cells.

        b. An **arthropod** (e.g., *Anopheles* mosquito) is the site of the sexual phase (sporogony) (Figure 6–1).

    2. *Toxoplasma* **and** *Babesia*

        a. *Toxoplasma gondii*

        —can cause severe disease in immunosuppressed patients, such as those with AIDS, and can cause mononucleosis-like symptoms in healthy adults.

        —can cross the placenta (generally in women with no or low antibody levels)

Table 6–1. Intestinal and Urogenital Protozoan Parasites and Associated Diseases

Species	Morphology	Associated Diseases	Mode/Form of Transmission	Diagnosis	Treatment
Entamoeba histolytica		Amebiasis (dysentery with dissemination)	Fecal–oral by water, fresh fruits and vegetables; via cysts	Trophozoites Cysts in stool; serologic testing Pathologic appearance (inverted flask-shaped lesions)	Metronidazole followed by iodoquinol
Giardia lamblia		Giardiasis (diarrhea with malabsorption)	Fecal (e.g., human, beaver, muskrat) by water, food, oral–anal intercourse, day care; via cysts	Trophozoites Cysts in stool	Quinacrine hydrochloride or metronidazole
Cryptosporidium species		Cryptosporidiosis (transient diarrhea in healthy persons; severe diarrhea in immunocompromised persons)	Undercooked meat; via cysts	Acid-fast oocysts in stool Biopsy: dots (cysts) in intestinal glands	Under study
Balantidium coli		Dysentery; colitis; diarrhea to severe dysentery	Contaminated food or water; via cysts	Trophozoites Cysts in feces	Tetracycline
Trichomonas vaginalis		Trichomoniasis (asymptomatic or vaginal discharge associated with burning or itching, or, in males, urethral discharge)	Sexual contact; via trophozoites	Motile trophozoites and excessive neutrophils in methylene blue wet mount	Metronidazole

Illustrations are not to scale.

Table 6–2. Plasmodial Organisms and Associated Diseases

Species*	Associated Diseases	Diagnosis	Treatment
Plasmodium vivax	Tertian malaria	Oval-shaped host cells with Schüffner's granules and ragged cell walls, seen on thick and thin blood examination	Chloroquine phosphate then primaquine
Plasmodium malariae	Quartan malaria	Bar and band forms; rosette schizonts	Chloroquine
Plasmodium falciparum	Malignant tertian malaria†	Multiple ring forms and crescents (gametocytes); schizonts rare in peripheral blood	Chloroquine-resistant strains with quinine sulfate with doxycycline

Plasmodium ovale is rare and can cause benign tertian or ovale malaria. Transmission, diagnosis, and treatment are identical to those for *P. vivax*.
† Constitutes a medical emergency.

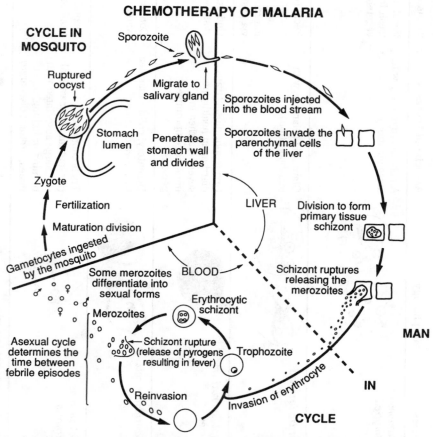

CHEMOTHERAPY OF MALARIA

Figure 6–1. Schematic diagram of the life cycle of the malarial parasite. (Reprinted with permission from Pratt WB, Fekety R: *The Antimicrobial Drugs.* New York, Oxford University Press, 1986, p 357.)

and can cause congenital infections, characterized by intracerebral calcifications, chorioretinitis, hydrocephaly or microcephaly, and convulsions.

–is acquired primarily from the ingestion of undercooked or raw meat.

–may be acquired from cat feces, although a wide variety of animals carry *Toxoplasma.* Pregnant women should not change litter boxes, or they should wear gloves and change the box daily because the infectious form takes more than 24 hours to develop in the soil.

b. *Babesia microti*

–is a malaria-like parasite.

–causes disease primarily in cattle.

–is transmitted by the *Ixodes* tick.

–rarely causes a malaria-like disease in humans (babesiosis).

–is diagnosed by the presence of multiple ring-like forms in the red blood cells.

3. *Trypanosoma* and *Leishmania*

–are **hemoflagellates.**

–infect blood and tissues.

–have life cycles involving several hemoflagellate forms (amastigotes, promastigotes, epimastigotes, and trypanomastigotes).

–cause various diseases (Table 6–3). For example:

a. *Leishmania braziliensis* causes mucocutaneous leishmaniasis. Reservoirs, transmission, diagnosis, and treatment are the same as for *Leishmania donovani.*

b. *Trypanosoma cruzi* affects cardiac muscle, liver, and brain tissue. Romaña's sign (unilateral eyelid swelling) is a sign of Chagas' disease.

4. Free-living amebas

–include *Naegleria* and *Acanthamoeba.*

a. *Naegleria fowleri*

–is the major causative agent of primary amebic meningoencephalitis.

–has both ameba and biflagellated forms.

–is most commonly acquired while diving and swimming during hot weather in brackish or fresh water including (rarely) in swimming pools.

–causes a purulent spinal fluid with motile ameba.

b. *Acanthamoeba*

–causes keratitis, acquired from trauma and contact lens wear, and characterized by severe ocular pain.

–may cause a chronic central nervous system infection called **granulomatous amebic encephalitis** (GAE), generally in debilitated or immunocompromised patients.

–infections do not appear to be associated with swimming. The ameba causing GAE appear to come from some other site in the body.

III. Cestodes

A. General characteristics—cestodes

–are commonly called **tapeworms.**

–have three basic portions:

Table 6–3. Hemoflagellates and Associated Diseases

Species	Associated Diseases	Reservoir Host	Mode of Transmission	Diagnosis	Treatment
Trypanosoma cruzi	Chagas' disease (American trypanosomiasis)	Cat, dog, armadillo, possum	Passage of trypomastigote in feces at site of reduviid bug bite	Blood films; blood or lymph node culture; serologic testing	Nifurtimox
Trypanosoma brucei gambiense; Trypanosoma brucei rhodesiense	African sleeping sickness (African trypanosomiasis)	Gambia: mostly humans; Rhodesia: wild animals	Contamination of bite site by trypomastigote in saliva of tsetse fly	Blood films; lymph node aspiration; cerebrospinal fluid; serologic testing	Suramin (acute therapy); melarsoprol (chronic therapy)
Leishmania donovani	Visceral leishmaniasis (kala-azar, Dumdum fever)	Urban areas: humans; rural areas: rodents and wild animals	Sandfly* bite	Aspiration or culture of bone marrow, liver, or spleen; serologic testing	Stibogluconate sodium
Leishmania tropica; Leishmania mexicana; Leishmania peruviana	Dermal leishmaniasis	(Same as *L. donovani*)	(Same as *L. donovani*)	Scrapings or biopsies of lesion or skin test	Stibogluconate sodium
Leishmania braziliensis	Mucocutaneous leishmaniasis	(Same as *L. donovani*)	(Same as *L. donovani*)	(Same as *L. donovani*)	Stibogluconate sodium

* *Phlebotomus* sandfly genus carries Old World *Leishmania*; *Lutzomyia* sandfly genus carries New World *Leishmania* in South and Central America (*L. mexicana, L. braziliensis,* and *L. donovani* in the Americas).

1. **Head,** or scolex

2. **Neck,** which produces the segments, or proglottids

3. **Proglottids,** which mature as they move away from the scolex (collectively, the neck and proglottids are termed the **strobila**)

–are **hermaphroditic,** with both male and female reproductive organs developing in each proglottid and mature eggs developing in the most distal proglottids.

–adhere to the mucosa via the **scolex,** a knobby structure with suckers or a sucking groove for attachment to the small intestine.

–**lack a gastrointestinal tract**; instead they absorb nutrients from the host's gastrointestinal tract.

–cause infections that can be diagnosed by demonstration of eggs or proglottids in the feces.

–typically have complex life cycles involving:

   a. Extraintestinal **larval** forms in **intermediate hosts**

   b. **Adult tapeworms** found in **definitive hosts**

B. **Clinical manifestations**

   1. When humans are the definitive host, the presence of the **adult tapeworm in the small intestine** is generally **without symptoms** but it may affect nutrition. Human adult tapeworms include *Taenia saginata* (beef), *Taenia solium* (pork), *Diphyllobothrium latum* (fish), *Hymenolepis nana* (humans and rodents), and *Dipylidium caninum* (dogs and cats).

   2. When humans serve as the intermediate host, more serious disease results (Table 6–4). Symptoms depend on the **migration of the larval forms.** These infections include:

      a. **Cysticercosis,** which is caused by the larvae of *T. solium,* whose eggs are ingested from contaminated water or vegetables and hatch in the gastrointestinal tract; larvae migrate into the blood and then the tissues. Cysticerci in the eye and brain have the most serious consequences; calcifications occur when cysticerci die.

      b. **Sparganosis** (*Diphyllobothrium*). The early larval forms of relatives of *D. latum* in crustaceans may be ingested by drinking pond water; because humans are dead-end hosts, only the subcutaneous or eye lesions of sparganosis develop.

      c. **Unilocular hydatid cyst disease**, which occurs when eggs of *Echinococcus granulosus* are ingested; oncospheres escape the intestine and enter the blood, liver, and lung, where cysts containing brood capsules develop. This is most common in sheep-raising areas.

      d. **Alveolar hydatid cyst disease** (*Echinococcus multilocularis*). Transmission occurs via ingestion or inhalation of cat, wolf, or dog feces; progression usually resembles that for diseases caused by *E. granulosus.*

IV. Nematodes

A. **General characteristics—nematodes**

   –are called **roundworms.**

Table 6–4. Important Cestodes

Cestode	Common Intermediate Host	Disease When Human Is Intermediate Host	Treatment When Human Is Intermediate Host	Adult Host	Associated Disease	Treatment When Human Is Definitive Host
Taenia saginata (beef tapeworm)	Cattle	Extremely rare		Humans	Intestinal tapeworm	Praziquantel
Taenia solium (pork tapeworm)	Pork	Cysticercosis	Praziquantel; surgery in some sites	Humans	Intestinal tapeworm	Praziquantel
Diphyllobothrium latum (fish tapeworm)[†]	Microscopic crustaceans; fish	Sparganosis	Surgery, praziquantel, or both	Humans	Intestinal tapeworm	Praziquantel
Echinococcus granulosus	Herbivores: mainly sheep	Hydatid cyst disease	Albendazole; ± surgery	Carnivores	Dog tapeworm (not humans)	
Echinococcus multilocularis	Rodents	Alveolar hydatid cyst disease	Albendazole; ± surgery	Carnivores	Cat, dog, or wolf tapeworms (not humans)	

† Species associated with cool lake regions.

Table 6–5. Nematodes Transmitted by Eggs

Species	Associated Diseases/Symptoms	Mode of Transmission	Diagnosis	Treatment
Enterobius vermicularis (pinworm)*	Enterobiasis (perianal itching)	Ingestion of eggs from dust or autoinfection	Microscopic detection of eggs from perianal area	Pyrantel pamoate given to entire family; damp mop dusting
Trichuris trichiura (whipworm)	Trichuriasis (generally asymptomatic; severe: abdominal pain, bloody diarrhea, appendicitis, rectal prolapse)	Ingestion of eggs (e.g., use of human feces as vegetable fertilizer, contaminated food and water)	Microscopic detection of barrel-shaped eggs with bipolar plugs	Mebendazole
Ascaris lumbricoides†	Ascariasis (Pneumonitis [larvae in lungs]; asymptomatic to heavy bowel infections; anesthetics, fever, drugs may induce adult worms to migrate to places such as the bile ducts or pancreas. Intestinal blockage may occur in children with heavy worm burden.)	Ingestion of eggs (e.g., use of human feces as vegetable fertilizer, contaminated food and water)	Bile-stained knobby eggs or 6–12-inch long roundworms seen on radiograph or cholangiogram; serologic test shows some cross-reaction with *Trichuris*	Supportive therapy during pneumonitis; surgery for ectopic migrations; mebendazole
Toxocara canis; Toxocara cati‡	Toxocariasis (visceral larva migrans)	Ingestion of eggs (e.g., handling puppy or eating dirt [pica])	Clinical findings; serologic testing	Diethylcarbamazine or thiabendazole§

* Most common helminth in the United States. Worm is 2–5 mm long.
† Most common helminth worldwide. Adult worms are 20–35 cm long.
‡ Affects approximately 80% of puppies; high transmission rate to children in household.
§ Disease usually is self-limiting; therefore, treatment may not be needed.

–have round, unsegmented bodies covered by tough cuticle.

–are transmitted in several ways:

1. **Ingestion of eggs** (*Enterobius, Ascaris, Trichuris,* and *Toxocara*)

2. **Direct invasion** of skin by larval forms (*Necator, Ancylostoma,* and *Strongyloides*)

3. **Ingestion of larvae** (*Trichinella*)

4. **Larvae transmission via insect bite** (*Wuchereria, Loa, Mansonella, Onchocerca,* and *Dracunculus*)

B. **Clinical manifestations—nematode**

–cause a wide variety of diseases, including ascariasis, pinworm infection (enterobiasis), whipworm infection (trichuriasis), hookworm infection, trichinosis, strongyloidiasis (threadworm infection), filariasis, and river blindness (onchocerciasis).

–are transmitted by eggs (Table 6–5).

–are transmitted by larval forms (Table 6–6).

V. **Trematodes**

A. **General characteristics—trematodes**

–are called **flukes.**

Table 6–6. Nematodes Transmitted by Larvae

Species	Associated Diseases/ Symptoms	Mode of Transmission	Progression in Humans	Diagnosis	Treatment
Nector americanus (New World hookworm); *Ancylostoma duodenale* (Old World hookworm)	Hookworm infection (ground itch, diarrhea, vomiting, abdominal pain, iron deficiency anemia)	Filariform larvae in soil penetrate intact **skin** of bare feet* (shoes reduce transmission)	Larvae travel from skin to circulation to lungs, then ascend to epiglottis, and are swallowed; adult worms attach and mature in small intestine	Non–bile-staining segmented eggs in stool†; possible occult blood in stools	Mebendazole and treat anemia
Ancylostoma braziliense; Ancylostoma caninum	Cutaneous larva migrans	Filariform larvae penetrate intact **skin** (beaches with free roaming dogs; cat feces in sand-boxes)	Larvae migrate from skin to subcutaneous tissues; they do not mature but "creep" in subcutaneous tissues	Usually a presumptive diagnosis from clinical symptoms; no reliable test exists	Thiabendazole
Strongyloides stercoralis	Strongyloidiasis (skin pruritis, mild pneumonitis; asymptomatic to severe diarrhea with malabsoprtion)	Filariform larvae penetrate intact **skin** of bare feet; free-living cycle occurs outside host	Larvae migrate from skin to blood to lung to small intestine as do *Necator* and *Ancylostoma*; autoinfection also occurs	Larvae in stool; serologic testing	Thiabendazole
Trichinella spiralis	Trichinosis (asymptomatic to gastritis, then fever, muscle aches and eosinophilia)	Consumption of encysted larvae in **undercooked meat** (bear, pork, horse meat)	Larvae leave meat in small intestine and mature into adult worms, which migrate into bloodstream and muscle tissue	Splinter hemorrhages beneath nails; muscle biopsy; marked eosinophilia; serologic testing	Steroids for severe symptoms and mebendazole
Wuchereria bancrofti; Brugia malayi	Filariasis (asymptomatic to elephantiasis)	Infective larvae enter in **mosquito** bite	Larvae migrate to lymphatics and mature; adult worms live in lymph nodes, producing elephantiasis	Blood films, clinical findings	Diethylcarbamazine
Loa loa (African eye worm)	Filariasis (subcutaneous migration, Calabar swellings)	Infective larvae in *Chrysops* (mango fly) bite	Adult *Loa loa* migrate through subcutaneous tissue, often crossing conjunctiva	Calabar swelling; worms in eye; eosinophilia; blood films	Diethylcarbamazine and surgical removal
Onchocerca volvulus	River blindness (subcutaneous nodules, dermatitis, wrinkled skin, eye infections)	Larvae-infected black fly bite	Adult worms develop in subcutaneous nodules, migrate to skin and other tissues	Microfilariae seen on skin examination	Surgical removal of subcutaneous nodules and ivermectin
Dracunculus medinensis (Guinea worm)	Dracunculosis (subcutaneous nodules with systemic symptoms: nausea, vomiting, or diarrhea; asthma.)	Consumption of water contaminated with *Cyclops* organisms containing larvae or direct contact as in step wells	Ingested larvae exit the small intestine and develop into adults; females migrate to surface, causing ulcers, and release motile larvae	Clinical symptoms or flood ulcer to induce worm release	Slow worm removal; metronidazole

* Rhabditiform stage initially released is noninfective and feeds on bacteria and detritus in soil.
† The two species cannot (and need not) be distinguished by eggs.

–are generally flat and fleshy.

–are **hermaphroditic,** except for *Schistosoma*, which has separate males and females.

–have complicated life cycles occurring in two or more hosts.

–have **operculated** eggs (except for *Schistosoma*); these eggs:

1. Contaminate water, perpetuating the life cycle.

2. Are used to diagnose infections.

3. Produce a swimming ciliated larval form, called a **miracidium,** when they hatch.

Table 6–7. Trematodes

Organism	Associated Diseases	Reservoir Host*	Mode of Transmission	Progression in Humans
Schistosoma japonicum; Schistosoma mansoni	Intestinal schistosomiasis	Cats, dogs, cattle, pigs (*S. japonicum*); primates, marsupials, rodents (*S. mansoni*)	Contact with contaminated water	Cercaria enter skin, then circulation; mature into adults in intrahepatic portal blood†
Schistosoma haematobium	Vesicular schistosomiasis	Primates	Contact with contaminated water	See *S. japonicum*‡
Nonhuman schistosomes	Swimmer's itch	Birds	Contact with contaminated water	Penetration of skin, causing dermatitis without further development; itching is most intense at 2–3 days
Opisthorchis (Clonorchis) sinensis (Chinese liver fluke)	Clonorchiasis	Cats, dogs, humans	Ingestion of contaminated raw fish	Cysts germinate in duodenum, exit through wall into liver, and proceed to bile ducts, where they mature; eggs enter feces in bile
Fasciola hepatica (sheep liver fluke)	Fascioliasis	Sheep, cattle, humans	Ingestion of contaminated aquatic plants	Cysts germinate in duodenum, exit through wall into liver, and proceed to bile ducts, where they mature; eggs enter feces in bile
Fasciolopsis buski (giant intestinal fluke)	Fasciolopsiasis	Pigs, dogs, rabbits, humans	Ingestion of contaminated aquatic plants	Cysts germinate in duodenum; adults attach to mucosa of small intestine, where eggs are produced
Paragonimus westermani (lung fluke)	Paragonimiasis	Humans, pigs, felines, canines	Ingestion of contaminated raw crabs, crayfish	Excyst in stomach, migrate to lung; eggs in sputum or feces

* Snails or clams are the intermediate hosts for all organisms. The second intermediate host for *Clonorchis* is freshwater fish; for *Paragonimus*, freshwater crabs or crayfish.
† Adult forms mate in mesenteric veins.
‡ Adult forms mate in bladder veins.

B. Intermediate hosts

–are **snails or other mollusks.**

–are sometimes two in number.

1. *Clonorchis* goes from the snail host to freshwater fish (to humans who eat infected meat).

2. *Paragonimus* leaves the snail and infects crabs and crayfish, which subsequently are eaten.

C. Clinical manifestations (Table 6–7)

–vary greatly, from none for a light intestinal infection with *Fasciolopsis buski* to systemic symptoms with anemia and hepatomegaly with *Fasciola hepatica.*

D. Therapy

–is with **praziquantel** for serious trematode disease.

–is with calamine, trimeprazine, and sometimes sedatives for swimmer's itch.

Review Test

Directions: Each of the numbered items or incomplete statements in this section is followed by answers or by completions of the statement. Select the **one** lettered answer or completion that is best in each case.

1. Which one of the following organisms causes river blindness?

(A) *Ancylostoma duodenale*
(B) *Wuchereria bancrofti*
(C) *Dracunculus medinensis*
(D) *Fasciolopsis buski*
(E) *Onchocerca volvulus*

2. Which of the following is an infective form of *Ascaris?*

(A) Coracidium
(B) Filariform larvae
(C) Rhabditiform larvae
(D) Embryonated egg
(E) Nonembryonated egg

3. Of the following tapeworms, which one has the largest adult form found in the human intestine?

(A) *Echinococcus granulosus*
(B) *Diphyllobothrium latum*
(C) *Hymenolepis nana*
(D) *Dipylidium caninum*
(E) *Taenia solium*

4. Which of the following protozoans is free living and generally does not indicate fecal contamination?

(A) *Acanthamoeba*
(B) *Dientamoeba fragilis*
(C) *Entamoeba histolytica*
(D) *Entamoeba coli*
(E) *Giardia*

Directions: Each of the numbered items or incomplete statements in this section is negatively phrased, as indicated by a capitalized word such as NOT, LEAST, or EXCEPT. Select the **one** answer or completion that is **best** in each case.

5. All of the following statements concerning *Ancylostoma duodenale* are true **EXCEPT**

(A) anemia may be a symptom.
(B) the organism is ingested when peeling water chestnuts with the teeth.
(C) the worm is commonly called the Old World hookworm.
(D) eggs are non–bile staining and found in stools.
(E) the organisms pass through the lungs before reaching the intestine.

6. All of the following statements concerning *Diphyllobothrium latum* are true **EXCEPT**

(A) incidence is higher in tropical climates.
(B) eggs hatch into a ciliated form (coracidium), which is ingested by copepods and other very small crustaceans.
(C) adult worms may reach 10 meters in length.
(D) the organism may still be viable in smoked fish.

7. All of the following statements concerning *Plasmodium* are correct **EXCEPT**

(A) *Plasmodium vivax* generally produces paroxysms about every 36 hours.
(B) *Plasmodium vivax* is the most common form with the widest geographic distribution.
(C) *Plasmodium malariae* infects only mature erythrocytes.
(D) *Plasmodium falciparum* produces daily and then tertian paroxysms, with a fulminating disease called malignant tertian malaria.

8. All of the following statements concerning *Toxoplasma gondii* are true **EXCEPT**

(A) it crosses the placenta.
(B) congenital disease generally is not severe.
(C) it is treated with pyrimethamine.
(D) undercooked meat and cat feces play major roles in dissemination of the disease.
(E) it causes serious disease in patients with AIDS.

Directions: Each group of items in this section consists of lettered options followed by a set of numbered items. For each item, select the **one** lettered option that is most closely associated with it. Each lettered option may be selected once, more than once, or not at all.

Questions 9–12

Match the statement below to the tapeworm associated with it.

(A) *Diphyllobothrium*
(B) *Dipylidium*
(C) *Echinococcus granulosus*
(D) *Hymenolepis nana*
(E) *Taenia saginata*
(F) *Taenia solium*

9. A dog may transmit by licking a child's mouth

10. Mice and flour beetles may play a role in transmission

11. Larva causes hydatid cyst disease

12. Crustaceans act as the intermediate host

Questions 13 and 14

Match the mode of transmission to the roundworm associated with it.

(A) *Ascaris lumbricoides*
(B) *Enterobius vermicularis*
(C) *Necator americanus*
(D) *Toxocara canis*
(E) *Trichuris trichiura*

13. Perianal deposition of eggs contaminates bedding and clothing

14. Larval penetration of skin

Questions 15–18

Match the disease, or sign, and vector with the protozoan that causes it.

(A) *Leishmania braziliensis*
(B) *Leishmania donovani*
(C) *Trypanosoma brucei gambiense*
(D) *Trypanosoma cruzi*
(E) *Leishmania tropica*

15. Romaña's sign—Reduviidae bug

16. Winterbottom's sign—tsetse fly

17. Mucocutaneous leishmaniasis—*Lutzomyia* sandfly

18. Kala-azar—*Phlebotomus* sandfly

Answers and Explanations

1–E. *Onchocerca volvulus* causes river blindness, also known as onchocerciasis.

2–D. Eggs are fertilized before release and embryonate to the second stage (larval stage) inside the egg, which is then ingested by a new host to start a new infection.

3–B. Of this group, *Diphyllobothrium* is the largest adult tapeworm found in humans. Humans are intermediate hosts for *Echinococcus*, so adult forms are not produced in humans.

4–A. *Acanthamoeba* is a free-living organism that generally lives in contaminated waters. A common way of acquiring these infections in the United States is through homemade saline solutions for soft contact lenses.

5–B. *Ancylostoma duodenale* enters the skin as a rhabditiform larvae. *Fasciolopsis buski* is ingested during peeling of water chestnuts.

6–A. These fish tapeworms, particularly *Diphyllobothrium latum,* are more commonly associated with cold water lakes.

7–A. *Plasmodium vivax* generally produces paroxysms every 48 hours.

8–B. Congenital disease is often severe with intracerebral calcification, chorioretinitis, hydrocephaly or microcephaly, and convulsions, which can be fatal.

9–B. *Dipylidium caninum* is the common tapeworm of both cats and dogs. It may be transmitted by ingestion of fleas harboring cysticercoid larvae. This usually occurs in humans when crushed fleas, harboring the disease, are transmitted from a pet by the pet licking the child's mouth.

10–D. *Hymenolepis nana* is a parasite of both humans and mice. It occasionally develops its cysticercoid stage in beetles; humans or mice may acquire the infection by ingestion of infected flour. Humans may be reinfected without passage through another host. This may occur in places such as day-care centers.

11–C. Hydatid cyst disease in humans, in which unilocular hydatid cysts occur, may be caused by *Echinococcus granulosus*, or, when sterile alveolar hydatid cysts occur, it may be caused by *Echinococcus multilocularis*.

12–A. Fish become infected with *Diphyllobothrium latum* by ingesting infected crustaceans.

13–B. *Enterobius vermicularis* is the pinworm; it deposits eggs in the perianal area. Reinfection by hand contamination is common. Eggs survive outside the body and are transmitted via clothing and bedding.

14–C. *Necator americanus* is the New World hookworm that is transmitted by filariform larvae penetrating the skin of the feet.

15–D. The organism that causes Romaña's sign is *Trypanosoma cruzi*. A chagoma occurs at the site of the initial Reduviidae (kissing bug) bite, which commonly occurs around the eye, resulting in unilateral eyelid swelling, or Romaña's sign.

16–C. Winterbottom's sign is enlarged posterior cervical lymph nodes, as seen in African sleeping sickness. The disease is caused by *T. brucei gambiense* and is carried by the tsetse fly.

17–A. Mucocutaneous leishmaniasis begins with a cutaneous sandfly bite, which may become enlarged with mucous membrane lesions developing several years later. It is caused by *Leishmania braziliensis*.

18–B. Visceral leishmaniasis, which is also known as kala-azar or Dumdum fever, is caused by *Leishmania donovani*. It is transmitted by the bite of the *Phlebotomus* sandfly.

7
Immunology

I. Overview
A. Immunity
–is defined as an "enhanced state" of responsiveness to a specific substance, induced by prior contact with that substance.

1. **Natural immunity**

   –is present from birth and is nonspecific.

   –consists of various barriers to external insults, for example, skin, mucous membranes, macrophages, monocytes, neutrophils, eosinophils, and the contents of these cells.

2. **Acquired immunity**

   –is expressed after exposure to a given substance and is **specific.**

   –involves specific receptors on lymphocytes and the participation of macrophages for its expression.

   –consists of:

   a. **Humoral immunity,** mediated by antibodies

   b. **Cell-mediated immunity,** mediated by lymphocytes

B. Immune system
–consists of the cellular and molecular components derived from the central and peripheral lymphoid organs.

1. **Central lymphoid organs**

   –consist of the bone marrow and thymus.

   –are the location of maturation of lymphoid cells.

2. **Peripheral lymphoid organs**

   –consist of the spleen, lymph nodes and lymphatic channels, the tonsils, adenoids, Peyer's patches, and appendix.

   –are the location of reactivity of lymphoid cells.

3. **Cells of the immune system**

   –include the white blood cells (approximately 8000/mm^3 of blood), which are composed of:

   a. **Granulocytes**—50% to 80% of white blood cells

213

  b. Lymphocytes—20% to 45% of white blood cells

  c. Monocytes and macrophages--3% to 8% of white blood cells

 4. Molecules of the immune system

  a. Antibodies (immunoglobulins) are protein products of certain lymphocytes with a precise specificity for a particular antigen.

  b. Lymphokines are soluble lymphocyte products that play a role in the activation of the immune response.

C. Development of the immune system

 –involves the maturation of pluripotential stem cells in the bone marrow or thymus into B cells and T cells, respectively.

 –includes the generation of specific receptors on the cell surface of B cells and T cells.

 1. Pluripotential stem-cell sources

  a. Embryonic yolk sac

  b. Fetal liver

  c. Adult bone marrow

 2. B cells

  –mature in the bursa (hence the name "B" cells) of Fabricius in birds and in the fetal liver and adult bone marrow in humans (bursal equivalents).

  –are involved in the generation of humoral immunity.

  –have specific receptors (**immunoglobulins**) on their surface for antigen recognition.

  –mature into antibody-producing plasma cells.

  –are sessile and located predominantly in the germinal centers of the lymph nodes and spleen.

 3. T cells

  –mature in the thymus.

  –are involved in "helping" B cells become antibody-producing plasma cells.

  –have specific receptors (T-cell receptors) on their surface for antigen recognition.

  –are involved in cell-mediated immunity.

  –participate in suppression of the immune response.

  –are the predominant (95%) lymphocytes in the circulation.

  –are found in the paracortical and interfollicular areas of the lymph nodes and spleen.

D. Physiology of immunity

 –involves the following series of events that culminate in B-cell or T-cell activation (or both) and response to the introduction of a foreign entity into the circulation:

 1. "Processing" of the foreign entity by a macrophage or B cell

 2. Recognition of this foreign entity by specific, preformed receptors on certain B cells and T cells

3. **Proliferation** of these B cells and T cells, as stimulated by soluble signals (interleukins) between macrophages, B cells, and T cells

4. **Blast transformation** and a series of mitotic divisions leading to the generation (from B cells) of **plasma cells that produce immunoglobulins** and (from T cells) of **sensitized T cells**—all capable of interacting with the original foreign stimulus

II. Antigens (Immunogens)

A. Characteristics

1. **Immunogenicity**—the capacity to stimulate production of specific, protective humoral or cellular immunity.

2. **Specific reactivity**—the capacity to be recognized by the antibodies and T cells produced.

3. **Foreignness**—the recognition of a body as nonself (foreign proteins are excellent antigens).

4. **Size**—at least approximately 10 kilodaltons to be recognized.

5. **Shape**—of tertiary and quaternary structures the extent of antigenicity.

B. Definitions

1. **Epitope**

   –is the restricted portion of an antigen molecule that determines the specificity of the reaction with an antibody.

   –is the antibody-binding site on an antigen for a specific antibody.

   –generally contains four to six amino acid or sugar residues.

2. **Hapten**

   –is a small foreign molecule that is not immunogenic by itself but can bind to an antibody molecule already formed to it.

   –can be immunogenic if coupled to a sufficiently large carrier molecule.

III. Antibodies (Immunoglobulins)

A. Characteristics—antibodies

–are a heterogeneous group of proteins that contain carbohydrate.

–have sedimentation coefficients ranging from 7S to 19S.

–are found predominantly in the gamma (γ) globulin fraction of serum; some antibodies are also found in the alpha (α) and beta (β) globulin fractions.

–consist of **polypeptide chains** linked by disulfide bonds, such that each antibody contains a minimum of two identical heavy (H) chains and two identical light (L) chains.

–have interchain disulfide bonds holding the chains together, that is, L to H and H to H.

–have antigen-binding capacity defined by their specific H and L chains.

B. Enzymatic treatment of antibody molecules

1. **Reduction of disulfide bonds**

   –breaks disulfide bonds between polypeptide chains.

–produces two identical H chains and two identical L chains per antibody molecule.

–destroys antibody-binding activity.

–shows that H chains have a molecular weight of approximately 50 kilodaltons.

–shows that L chains have a molecular weight of approximately 25 kilodaltons.

2. Papain treatment

–produces two identical antigen-binding fragments (Fab) per antibody molecule.

–produces one crystallizable fragment (Fc) per antibody molecule.

–shows that Fab has univalent binding capability (i.e., can bind to antigen but cannot precipitate antigen).

3. Pepsin digestion

–yields a large fragment [(Fab′)$_2$] that can precipitate antigen.

–shows that (Fab′)$_2$ fragments have bivalent binding capacity.

C. Structure of antibody molecules (Figure 7–1)

1. H chains

–are polypeptide chains of 440 to 550 amino acid residues in length.

–have intrachain domains of approximately 110 amino acid residues, formed by intrachain disulfide bonds.

–have an amino-terminal variable domain, followed by three to four constant domains.

–are structurally different for each of the defined classes of antibody (mu [μ], gamma [γ], alpha [α], delta [δ], and epsilon [ϵ]).

2. L chains

–are polypeptide chains of approximately 220 amino acid residues in length.

–have intrachain domains of approximately 110 amino acid residues, formed by intrachain disulfide bonds.

–have an amino-terminal variable domain and a carboxy-terminal constant domain.

–have two structurally distinct classes: kappa (κ) chains and lambda (λ) chains.

3. Variable domains

–exist in both H and L chains.

–are involved in antigen specificity of the antibody.

–contain the **hypervariable regions** (complementarity-determining regions, or CDRs), which:

a. Exist in both H- and L-chain variable domains

b. Appear approximately at amino acid positions 25 to 35, 50 to 58, and 95 to 108

c. Define the paratope (antigen-binding site) of the antibody, which binds to the epitope of the antigen

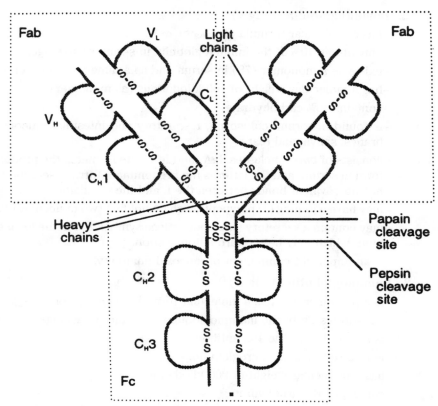

Figure 7–1. Diagrammatic representation of a typical IgG molecule. *L* = light chain; *H* = heavy chain; V_L = variable domain of L chain; *S-S* = disulfide bonds; C_L = constant domain of L chain; V_H = variable domain of H chain; C_H1, C_H2, C_H3 = constant domains of H chains; *Fab* = antigen-binding fragment; *Fc* = crystallizable fragment.

D. Classes (isotypes) of antibody molecules

–are found in all species and all individuals.

–are defined by the type of H chain, of which there are five: γ, μ, α, ϵ, δ.

1. Immunoglobulin G (IgG)

–has a molecular formula of $\gamma_2\kappa_2$ or $\gamma_2\lambda_2$.

–constitutes 73% of the immunoglobulin in serum on average.

–is referred to as 7S antibody.

–has a molecular weight of 150 kilodaltons.

–crosses the placenta (except for subclass IgG_4).

–fixes complement (except for IgG_4).

–contains 3% carbohydrate.

–consists of four subclasses (isotypes): IgG_1, 70% of IgG; IgG_2, 19%; IgG_3, 8%; and IgG_4, 3%; each has an antigenically and chemically distinct H chain defined primarily by the number and type of disulfide bridges.

–is the predominant antibody in the secondary immune response (anamnesis).

2. **Immunoglobulin A (IgA)**

   –has a molecular formula of $\alpha_2\kappa_2$ or $\alpha_2\lambda_2$.

   –constitutes 19% of the immunoglobulin in serum on average.

   –exists as a monomer (7S) in serum and as a dimer (9S) in secretions.

   –has a molecular weight of 160 kilodaltons (as monomer).

   –contains 10% carbohydrate.

   –is found in serum, colostrum, respiratory and intestinal mucous membranes, saliva, and tears.

   –consists of two subclasses: IgA_1 and IgA_2; the former is the predominant form in serum, and the latter is the predominant form in secretions. IgA_2 has no covalent bonds between the L and the α_2 chains.

   –may have a joining (J) polypeptide chain holding two molecules together.

   –may contain a secretory (transport) piece synthesized in the local epithelium, which may help retard autodigestion.

   –is an important component of mucosal immunity.

3. **Immunoglobulin M (IgM)**

   –is a pentamer and has a molecular formula of $(\mu_2\kappa_2)_5$ or $(\mu_2\lambda_2)_5$.

   –constitutes 7% of the immunoglobulin in serum on average.

   –is referred to as the 19S antibody.

   –is referred to as a macroglobulin.

   –has a molecular weight of 900 kilodaltons.

   –contains 15% carbohydrate.

   –is the first immunoglobulin to appear in phylogeny (the lamprey eel has IgM).

   –is the first immunoglobulin to appear in ontogeny.

   –is the first immunoglobulin to appear in response to antigen stimulation.

   –has a J polypeptide chain that holds the IgM pentamer together.

   –has four constant domains on each H chain: $C\mu1$, $C\mu2$, $C\mu3$, and $C\mu4$.

4. **Immunoglobulin D (IgD)**

   –has a molecular formula of $\delta_2\kappa_2$ or $\delta_2\lambda_2$.

   –constitutes 1% of the immunoglobulin in serum on average.

   –has a molecular weight of 150 kilodaltons.

   –contains 18% carbohydrate.

   –has an unknown function in serum.

   –serves as a receptor on the B-cell surface.

5. **Immunoglobulin E (IgE)**

   –has a molecular formula of $\epsilon_2\kappa_2$ or $\epsilon_2\lambda_2$.

   –constitutes less than 0.01% of serum immunoglobulin.

   –has a molecular weight of 200 kilodaltons.

   –contains 18% carbohydrate.

   –is referred to as **reaginic** antibody.

   –is involved in allergic reactions.

—has four constant domains on each H chain (three in the Fc region, as in IgM): $C\epsilon 1$, $C\epsilon 2$, $C\epsilon 3$, and $C\epsilon 4$.

—has an Fc region that binds to receptors on basophils and mast cells.

E. Allotypes of immunoglobulins

—are defined as small, regular structural differences among molecules of a particular immunoglobulin isotype.

—are genetically defined and codominantly expressed.

—may be as simple as a single amino acid substitution in the H or L chains.

—may be detected by immunologic means.

—exist in IgG molecules as Gm_1–Gm_{20}, in IgA molecules as Am_1–Am_3, and in κ chains as Km_1–Km_3.

F. Idiotype of antibody molecules

—is the antibody paratope to the antigenic epitope.

—is defined by the hypervariable regions (CDRs) of the variable domain of the L and H chains.

—involves those determinants that define the binding capability of a given antibody.

—can be defined by immunologic means.

—number in the 10^6 range.

G. Idiotypic–anti-idiotype network

—is the concept that a given antibody idiotype can evoke the generation of an anti-idiotypic antibody; this process may control the generation and level of the antibody response.

IV. Immunoglobulin Genetics

A. Exons

—are defined as minigenes or gene segments.

—encode for distinct parts of polypeptide chain.

—of immunoglobulin genes are:

1. **L exon**--leader segment

2. **V exon**—variable segment

3. **D exon**—diversity segment

4. **J exon**—joining segment

5. **C exon**—constant segment

B. Introns

—are intervening sequences between exons.

—are spliced out via messenger RNA (mRNA) transcription.

C. L chain formation

—is genetically determined on human chromosome 2 (κ) or 22 (λ).

—involves selection, at the germline level, of genes for the L, V, J, and C segments.

—is preceded by DNA arrangement and deletion of "unused" minigenes (exons) at the germline level and by RNA splicing to remove intervening sequences (introns) in translation for the secreted L chain.

D. H chain formation

–is genetically determined on human chromosome 14.

–involves selection, at the germline level, of 1 of 300 L and V exons, 1 of 4 J exons, 1 of 12 D exons, and 1 C exon, as indicated below.

–is preceded, as in L chain formation, by DNA rearrangement and deletion of unused minigenes and by RNA splicing to remove introns before translation into the completed H chains.

E. Isotype formation

–is defined by expression of one of the C exons on the H chain encoding for μ, δ, $\gamma 3$, $\gamma 1$, $\alpha 1$, $\gamma 2$, $\gamma 4$, ϵ, or $\alpha 2$, in that order, on chromosome 14.

–occurs after the determination of idiotype (i.e., the assembly of the V-D-J exons).

F. Immunoglobulin assembly

–is initiated by the formation of a functional L chain from either chromosome 2 (κ) or chromosome 22 (λ).

–has as its second major step the assembly of a specific H-chain isotype.

–has as its final stage the joining of H chains and the joining of L chains to H chains by disulfide bonding.

–ends with secretion of the completed immunoglobulin molecule.

G. Antibody diversity

–is genetically determined and independent of antigen availability.

–allows for the expression of more than 10^6 different idiotypes.

–is generated by:

1. Random joining of V and J genes in L chains

2. Random joining of V, D, and J genes in H chains

3. Random assembly of H and L chains

4. "Errors" in recombination of the V, D, and J genes

5. Somatic mutations

V. Antigen–Antibody Reactions

A. Forces holding antigen–antibody complexes together

–are identical to any protein–protein interaction.

–are not covalent.

–include the following:

1. **Ionic bonds**—attraction of oppositely charged groups (e.g., NH_3+ and -OOC)

2. **Hydrogen bonds**—sharing of hydrogen by hydrophilic groups

3. **Hydrophobic interactions**—exclusion of water by such amino acids as valine, leucine, and phenylalanine

4. **Van der Waals forces**—weak magnetic field

B. Definitions

1. Affinity

–is the tendency to form a stable complex.

–applies to a specific antibody directed against a specified epitope (i.e., a single antibody–antigen reaction).

–is defined by the formula:

$$\text{Affinity} = \frac{k}{k'} = \frac{[SL]}{[S][L]}$$

where

k = association constant
k' = disassociation constant
S = binding site of antibody (paratope)
L = ligand (epitope of antigen)
[ ] = concentration
which is derived from the standard protein (enzyme) formula: S + L = SL

2. Avidity

–is the sum of the affinities.

–refers to the total antibody response to all of the epitopes associated with a given antigen.

3. Lattice theory

–states that a precipitate will form in a lattice arrangement under optimum relationships between antibody and antigen.

–states that antibody or antigen excess will diminish a lattice network and decrease the amount of precipitate.

C. Types of antigen–antibody reactions

1. Quantitative precipitin curve

–is generated by a series of reactions usually involving a constant amount of antibody titrated against increasing amounts of antigen.

–is set as follows:

a. Nine test tubes are prepared, each with 0.1 mL of antiserum to ovalbumin (i.e., anti-OA antibody).

b. Each tube receives increasing amounts of antigen (tube 1 = 0 μg OA; tube 2 = 10 μg OA; tube 3 = 20 μg OA; and so on through tube 9 = 80 μg OA).

c. Upon incubation, there is a zone of antibody excess (tubes 1–3); a zone of equivalence (tubes 4–6); and a zone of antigen excess (tubes 7–9); precipitation occurs in all zones but is greatest at equivalence.

2. Ring test

–is a precipitation reaction that takes place at the interface between two solutions, one containing antigen and one containing antibody.

3. Oudin (single diffusion)

–is a precipitation technique, usually accomplished in a test tube, in which antibody (or antigen) in a gel is allowed to react with soluble antigen (or antibody) diffusing through it from a liquid interface.

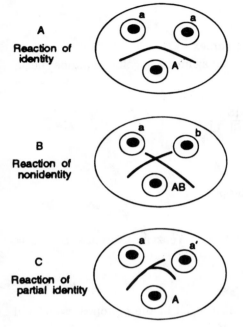

A
Reaction of
identity

B
Reaction of
nonidentity

C
Reaction of
partial identity

Figure 7–2. Ouchterlony double diffusion reactions showing *(A)* reaction of identity, *(B)* reaction of nonidentity, and *(C)* reaction of partial identity. A = antiserum to antigen a; B = antiserum to antigen b; a = antigen a; b = antigen b; a' = antigen with some antigenic determinants similar to a.

4. **Ouchterlony (double diffusion)** (Figure 7–2)

    –is a precipitation technique in agar, usually accomplished in a Petri dish, in which antigen and antibody are allowed to diffuse against each other and permit the formation of a precipitin line between the sample wells.

    –if two or more sample (antigen) wells are diffused against a single antiserum (antibody) well, the following distinctions can be made:

    a. **Lines of identity**—a single precipitin line indicating uniformity and identity of the antigens in the sample wells

    b. **Lines of nonidentity**—two distinct and crossing precipitin lines indicating no cross-reactivity or identity between the antigens in the two sample wells

    c. **Lines of partial identity**—a spur formation, indicating that some of the antigenic determinants (epitopes) are shared between the antigens in the two sample wells

5. **Immunoelectrophoresis (IEP)**

    –is an antigen–antibody reaction technique developed to resolve highly complex mixtures of antigens.

    a. Antigen is placed in agar on a glass slide and subjected to **electrophoresis,** using an electric current, to separate the serum proteins at a given pH (usually pH 8.4) into their constituent parts (albumin, α_1, α_2, β_1, β_2, and γ-globulin fractions).

    b. The separated proteins with their specific antibody are then placed in an antiserum trough, where they form a series of arcs of precipitate.

6. Rocket immunoelectrophoresis

–is a rapid method for estimating antigen concentration.

–uses the following procedure:

a. Sample wells are punched at one end of a gel plate in which antibody to a specific antigen has been dissolved.

b. Samples are applied and electrophoresed.

c. Rocket-like precipitate lines form; their length depends on the initial antigen sample concentration; a reference line is determined.

d. Unknown concentration is determined by the length of the arc relative to the standard reference.

7. Radial immunodiffusion

–is a method for estimating antigen concentration.

–uses the following procedure:

a. Antibody to specific antigen is diffused in an agar gel or slab.

b. Antigen wells are cut, and samples of various known concentrations are applied.

c. The gel is incubated and precipitin rings are developed.

d. The diameter of each precipitin ring is proportional to the initial antigen concentration; a reference line is determined.

e. Unknown concentration is determined by comparison with the reference line.

8. Radioimmunoassay (RIA)

–is a sensitive assay for **antigen** that usually uses a known amount of labeled antigen (Ag*) and a known amount of specific antibody for that antigen.

–uses the following procedure:

a. A standard inhibition ("quench") curve is generated by reacting increasing known amounts of unlabeled antigen with the constant antibody amount and determining the ratio of bound Ag* to free Ag*; the more unlabeled antigen present, the less Ag* will be bound to antibody.

b. Unknown concentration is determined by interpolation of the standard inhibition curve.

9. Radioimmunosorbent test (RIST)

–is an RIA for **total IgE.**

–uses the following procedure:

a. A solid phase surface (e.g., dextran beads) is coupled with anti-IgE antibody.

b. A known concentration of labeled IgE (IgE*) is reacted with the bound antibody along with increasing known concentrations of unlabeled IgE to produce a standard inhibition curve.

c. An unknown serum sample is tested, and its IgE concentration is determined by interpolation of the standard inhibition curve.

10. **Radioallergosorbent test (RAST)**

–is an RIA to determine **specific IgE concentration.**

–uses the following procedure:

a. Solid phase beads are coupled with specific antigen.

b. Known amounts of specific IgE are reacted with the solid phase–antigen complex.

c. Labeled anti-IgE (anti-IgE*) is reacted with the solid phase–antigen complex.

d. Anti-IgE* is added, and the concentration of specific IgE is determined from the standard curve.

11. **Enzyme-linked immunosorbent assay (ELISA)**

–is the same test as RIA (RIST and RAST) except that an enzyme is attached to an antibody instead of a radioactive label, and different immunoglobulins are detected (not just IgE).

–involves measurement of a color change, which results from addition of substrate that is specific for the enzyme; the intensity of the color is proportional to the amount of antigen detected in the sample.

VI. Immunocompetent Cells in the Immune Response

–include macrophages, monocytes, and other antigen-presenting cells (APCs) as well as T cells and B cells.

A. Antigen-presenting cells

–include macrophages and monocytes and their derivatives, including microglial cells, Kupffer's cells, and Langerhans' cells of the skin.

–are characterized by dendritic extensions and by the ability to phagocytose, internalize, and process antigen.

–possess Ia antigens, Fc receptors, and C3b receptors.

–produce interleukin 1 (IL-1).

B. T cells

–are thymus-dependent lymphocytes.

–develop in the thymus.

–have a unique antigen receptor of a specific idiotype (T-cell receptor [TCR]).

–develop a series of thymus-induced differentiation markers labeled as cluster of differentiation (CD) antigens.

–have Fc receptors on some subsets and C3b receptors.

1. **T-cell receptor** (Figure 7–3)

–is the antigen-specific (idiotype) receptor on T cells.

–consists of a heterodimer—usually a 43-kilodalton α chain and a 49-kilodalton β chain, each having two external domains, a transmembrane segment, and a cytoplasmic extension. Most T cells (95%) possess the $\alpha\beta$ TCR.

–may exist as a $\gamma\delta$ heterodimer in a small subset of T cells (5% of total). The $\gamma\delta$ TCR is not usually associated with either CD_4 or CD_8 and may have tumor or microbial antigen specificity.

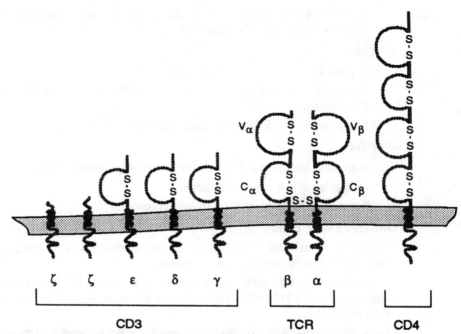

Figure 7–3. The T-cell receptor (TCR) complex consists of the TCR, CD3, and either CD4 or CD8 markers. The TCR is a heterodimer consisting of an alpha (α) and beta (β) chain, each of which has variable (V_α, V_β) and constant (C_α, C_β) domains. The TCR is associated with the CD3 molecule, which consists of five subunits: gamma (γ), delta (δ), epsilon (ϵ), and two zeta (ζ) chains. CD3 transduces the external signal from the TCR to the cell cytoplasm. CD4 appears on T helper cells and binds to the class II histocompatibility antigens on antigen-presenting cells. CD8 is an analogous molecule that appears on T cytotoxic cells and binds the class I histocompatibility antigens found on all nucleated cells.

–α chain is encoded on chromosome 14; β chain is encoded on chromosome 7.

–is encoded by a DNA rearrangement of V, D, and J exons for the V region, and a C gene for the C region.

–is associated with CD3.

2. **CD markers**

–arise on T cells during maturation in the thymus.

–appear on T cells in the following sequence: CD2 (formerly known as T11), CD3 (T3), CD4 (T4), and CD8 (T8).

a. **CD2**

–is the earliest T-cell marker.

–is the sheep red blood cell (SRBC) receptor.

–is an adhesion molecule with a natural ligand of LFA-3 (CD58); the interaction allows T cells to bind to many other cells.

–is present on virtually every peripheral T cell.

–is a 50-kilodalton polypeptide.

b. **CD3**

–is intimately associated with TCR.

–is composed of five molecules (consisting of a γ, δ, ϵ, and two zeta [ζ] polypeptide chains), essentially transmembrane and cytoplasmic, that transduce signals from TCR.

   c. CD4

   –is present mainly on T helper cells.

   –is involved in interaction with human leukocyte antigen (HLA) class II antigens.

   –has a molecular weight of 62 kilodaltons.

   d. CD8

   –is present mainly on T cytotoxic and T suppressor cells.

   –recognizes HLA class I antigens.

   –has a molecular weight of 76 kilodaltons.

3. Ontogeny of T cells

   –occurs as stem cells flow through the thymic cortex, into the medulla, and then out into the general circulation.

   –begins in the thymic cortex with the appearance of CD2, followed by the appearance of CD3 (with TCR), then with concomitant expression of CD4 and CD8.

   –in the thymic medulla, consists of a loss of marker to produce two populations of cells—one CD2$^+$, CD3$^+$, TCR$^+$, CD4$^+$ (65%) and the other CD2$^+$, CD3$^+$, TCR$^+$, CD8$^+$ (35%)—which are then released into the peripheral circulation.

   –is the time when self-recognition via HLA antigens occurs.

C. B cells

–are thymus-independent lymphocytes.

–develop independent of antigen.

–arise from stem cells and mature in the bone marrow (bursa of Fabricius in birds), bursal equivalent, or both.

–have a unique surface immunoglobulin (S-Ig) receptor for antigen.

–develop a series of markers during the differentiation process.

1. Surface immunoglobulin

   –is the antigen-specific idiotype receptor on B cells.

   –is equivalent to an antibody molecule with a transmembrane projection.

   –exists in 100,000 copies per mature B cell.

   –undergoes capping and endocytosis after activation by antigen.

2. Ontogeny of B cells

   –is the process by which a stem cell undergoes differentiation from a pre–B cell, to an immature B cell, to a mature B cell that is driven by antigen to become an activated B cell, and finally becomes a plasma cell that is capable of producing immunoglobulin.

   –is initiated in the fetal liver and adult bone marrow and usually terminates in the germinal centers of the lymph nodes, in the spleen, and in the red pulp of the spleen.

3. **Sequential appearance of B-cell markers in B-cell maturation**

   a. **Stem cell**—HLA class I and class II (HLA-DR) antigens

   b. **Pre–B cell**—cytoplasmic μ chains

   c. **Immature B cell**—membrane-bound IgM subunits, and C3b, Fc, and Epstein-Barr virus (EBV) receptors

   d. **Mature B cell**—membrane-bound IgM, IgD, IgG, IgA, or IgE

   e. **Activated B cell**—"capping" of S-Ig

   f. **Plasma cell**—few S-Ig and HLA-DR molecules; no Fc, C3b, and EBV receptors

VII. Actions and Products of Immune System Cells

A. **Actions of immune system cells**

   1. **Macrophages–antigen-presenting cells (APCs)**

      –phagocytose, process, and degrade the antigen.

      –express antigenic determinants (epitopes) of the antigen on its surface in the context of HLA class II molecules.

      –produce IL-1 and possibly other monokines.

   2. **T helper cells**

      –recognize antigen epitopes in the context of HLA class II molecules by TCR and CD4.

      –use the CD3 molecules to transduce the antigenic signal internally.

      –react with IL-1 from APC.

      –produce interleukin 2 (IL-2) and express IL-2 receptors.

      –become activated when the IL-2 receptors are occupied by IL-2.

      –produce a variety of lymphokines, which have a stimulatory role in B-cell growth and differentiation.

   3. **B cells**

      –recognize antigen epitopes via surface immunoglobulin receptors.

      –cross-link these antigen epitopes on the B-cell surface.

      –undergo capping and internalization (by pinocytosis) of these "occupied" surface receptors.

      –are stimulated to blastogenesis and differentiated into plasma cells by lymphokines produced by T helper cells.

B. **Products of immune system cells** (Table 7–1)

   1. **Interleukin-1 (IL-1)**

      –is produced by many different cell types, with relatively high concentrations being produced by macrophages, monocytes, Langerhans' cells of the skin, and other dendritic cells.

      –was formerly known as lymphocyte-activating factor (LAF).

      –augments the activity of many cell types, especially T cells.

      –is endogenous pyrogen (EP).

      –induces an increase in acute phase reactants.

Table 7–1. Cytokines and Their Actions

Cytokine	Major Cell Source	Major Immunologic Action
IL-1 (α, β)	Macrophages Endothelial cells Dendritic cells Langerhans' cells	Stimulates IL-2 receptor emergency in T cells Enhances B-cell activation Induces fever Induces acute phase reactants Induces IL-6 Increases nonspecific resistance Inhibited by an endogenous IL-1 receptor antagonist
IL-2	Th_1 cells	T-cell growth factor Activates NK cells and B cells
IL-3	T cells	Stimulation of hematopoiesis
IL-4	T cells	Stimulates B-cell synthesis of IgE Down-regulation of interferon-γ
IL-5	T cells	Growth and differentiation of eosinophils B-cell growth factor Enhances IgA synthesis
IL-6	Monocytes T cells Endothelial cells	Induces acute phase proteins Pyrogenic Induces late B-cell differentiation
IL-7	Bone marrow	Stimulates pre-B and pre-T cells
IL-8	Monocytes Endothelial cells Lymphocytes Fibroblasts	Chemotactic factor for neutrophils and T cells
IL-10	Th_2 cells	Inhibits interferon-γ synthesis by Th_1 cells Suppresses other cytokine synthesis
IL-12	Macrophages and B cells	Promotes Th_1 differentiation and interferon-γ synthesis Stimulates NK cells and $CD8^+$ T cells to cytolysis Acts synergistically with IL-2
Tumor necrosis factor α	Macrophages, T cells, B cells, and large granular lymphocytes	Cytotoxic for tumors, causes cachexia, and mediates bacterial shock
Tumor necrosis factor β	T cells	Cytotoxic for tumors
Transforming growth factor β	Almost all normal cell types	Inhibits proliferation of both T and B cells Reduces cytokine receptors Potent chemotactic agent for leukocytes Mediator of inflammation and tissue repair

–is a heat-stable and pH-stable peptide with a molecular weight of 17.5 kilodaltons.

–occurs in two forms: IL-1α and IL-1β.

2. **Interleukin-2 (IL-2)**

–is produced by T cells and large granular lymphocytes (LGLs).

–was formerly known as T-cell growth factor (TCGF).

–augments proliferation of T and B cells.

–enhances activity of T cells and natural killer (NK) cells.

–is a heat-labile glycoprotein with a molecular weight of 15.5 kilodaltons.

3. **Interferon-γ (INF-γ)** (Table 7–2)

–is produced by activated T cells and LGLs.

–increases the expression of HLA class II antigens on B cells, macrophages, and other APCs.

–has antiviral properties.

–provides regulatory control in the immune response.

–has a heat-labile glycoprotein with a molecular weight of 17 kilodaltons.

4. **Interleukin-3 (IL-3)**

–is produced by T cells.

–enhances hematopoiesis.

5. **Interleukin-4 (IL-4)**

–is produced by T cells.

–is mitogenic for B cells.

–promotes a switch to IgE production.

–stimulates mast cells.

Table 7–2. Interferons

Type	Characteristic
Alpha	At least 17 different subtypes
	Produced in B and null lymphocytes, macrophages, and epithelial cells
	Induced by viruses, bacteria, and tumor and foreign cells
	Inhibits viral replication
Beta	Only a single entity
	Produced in fibroblasts, macrophages, and epithelial cells
	Induced by viruses and bacterial products
	Inhibits viral replication
Gamma	Only a single entity
	Produced by Th_1 and NK cells
	Potent activator of macrophages
	Strong immunomodulating agent
	Inhibits IL-4 activation of mast cells and IgE synthesis

6. **Interleukin-5 (IL-5)**

   –is produced by T cells.

   –stimulates B-cell differentiation and maturation.

   –enhances IL-2 receptor expression.

   –enhances IgA synthesis.

7. **Interleukin-6 (IL-6)**

   –is produced by B cells, T cells, monocytes, and fibroblasts.

   –induces acute phase reactants.

   –induces B-cell differentiation.

VIII. Initiators of the Immune Response

A. T-dependent antigens

–are the predominant type of initiator of the immune response.

–necessarily need the presence of an APC and the activation of T helper cells and their concomitant lymphokines to activate and differentiate B cells to become plasma cells and secrete antibody.

B. T-independent antigens

–do not need T helper cell activity, T-cell activation, or the production of lymphokines.

–are polymeric in nature.

–produce a primary (IgM) immune response; they produce neither memory cells nor an anamnestic, secondary (IgG) immune response.

–include endotoxin, lipopolysaccharide, polysaccharide capsules, dextran, polyvinylpyrrolidone, polymerized flagellin, and Epstein-Barr virus.

C. T-cell mitogens

–are polyclonal activators of T cells.

–stimulate general T-cell activation by cross-linking specific sugars on the cell surface.

–include concanavalin A (Con A) and phytohemagglutinin (PHA).

D. B-cell mitogens

–are polyclonal activators of B cells.

–include all of the T-independent antigens.

IX. Immunology of Acquired Immune Deficiency Syndrome (AIDS)

A. AIDS

–is caused by human immunodeficiency virus 1 (HIV-1).

–is characterized by the loss of T helper ($CD4^+$) cells.

–results in an increase in opportunistic infections (e.g., *Pneumocystis carinii*), neoplasms (e.g., Kaposi's sarcoma, a tumor of blood vessel tissue of skin and internal organs), skin disorders, and neurologic disease.

B. History

–the current epidemic has been ongoing since 1981, probably originating in central Africa and moving to the United States and Europe via the Caribbean Islands.

–the causative agent was identified as *l*ymphadenopathy-*a*ssociated *v*irus (LAV) in 1983; in 1984, the human T lymphotropic virus-III (HTLV-III) was identified.

–the virus is now referred to as HIV-1.

–testing for anti–HIV-1 antibody has been available since 1985, a crucial step in ensuring the safety of the blood banking industry.

–in 1988, azidothymidine (**AZT**) was approved as a treatment for AIDS.

–in 1992, didanosine (**ddI**) and dideoxycytidine (**ddC**) were approved as treatments for AIDS.

C. HIV

–is a member of the lentivirus family of retroviruses.

–has an external membrane derived from the host cell.

–has glycoproteins on and in the membrane (gp120 and gp41) that are encoded by the *env* gene.

–has a protein core (p18 and p24) encoded by *gag* genes.

–has two copies of the viral RNA genome and the reverse transcriptase encoded by the *pol* gene within the core.

D. Transmission of HIV

–is most effective via whole infected cells:

1. **By sexual contact**

2. **By drug use,** via shared needles

3. **From blood** and blood products

4. **Perinatally,** from mother to infant

E. Prevalence of AIDS

–was approximately 442,000 cases in the United States as of January 1995; these cases were distributed as follows:

1. Men who have sexual encounters with men: 52%

2. Intravenous drug users: 24%

3. Men who have sexual encounters with men and use intravenous drugs: 7%

4. Heterosexual persons: 7%

5. Undetermined/under investigation: 7%

6. Persons with hemophilia and coagulation disorders: 1%

7. Persons receiving transfer of blood, blood components, or tissues: 1%

8. Children born to infected mothers: 0.1%

F. AIDS testing techniques

1. ELISA

–is the primary test to detect HIV-1 infection.

–detects the presence of anti–HIV antibody (anti-gp120) in the circulation.

–consists of an enzyme-linked antibody, which is specific for the anti-HIV idiotype.

–is approximately 98% accurate.

2. Western blot

  −is the **confirming** test for HIV infection.

  −detects the presence of antibodies to the various protein components of HIV (e.g., anti-p18, anti-p24, anti-gp41).

  −consists of four steps:

  a. Electrophoresis of HIV proteins on cellulose acetate

  b. Reacting putative serum antibodies of the patient with HIV proteins

  c. Reacting conjugated (enzyme or radiolabeled) anti-antibody with the serum antibodies and the HIV proteins

  d. Reading color change or radioactivity for positive result

G. Effect of HIV infection on the immune system

  1. HIV-1 destroys CD4$^+$ (T helper) cells, which are pivotal in the immune response.

  2. The receptor for HIV is the CD4 molecule, probably via gp120 and gp41.

  3. The HIV envelope proteins may mimic parts of HLA class II antigens, leading to binding HIV to CD4 and loss of the immune response.

  4. Macrophages and some brain cells may have low levels of CD4 on the surface, allowing for tropism by HIV and multiplication of HIV within these cells but not destruction of the carrier cells. This would allow HIV to be hidden from the immune system for an indefinite period.

H. Sequential events in HIV infection

  1. After binding to CD4$^+$, the virus is engulfed and uncoated.

  2. RNA is transcribed to DNA by reverse transcriptase (*pol* gene product) and is inserted into human chromosomal DNA by endonuclease (*pol* product) as the provirion.

  3. The provirus is the latent stage.

  4. Activation of the cell causes DNA → RNA → mRNA transcription → protein synthesis → virus → virus budding with destruction of the CD4$^+$ cell and release of the HIV virus.

  5. Death of the cell may be due to formation of **syncytia** by the infected cell gp120 interaction with CD4 of the noninfected cell.

I. Treatment

  1. AZT is the drug treatment of choice. It probably prevents the virus from replicating, interferes with reverse transcriptase, or acts as a false building block in viral DNA assembly.

  2. The drugs **ddI** and **ddC** have similar modes of action and may be used in concert with AZT.

  3. Parenteral injection of gp120 and gp41 proteins to enhance the immune response of HIV-infected persons and as a potential vaccine have thus far had only limited success, which is most likely due to the extensive mutability of the virus envelope.

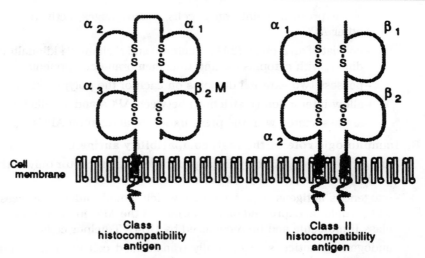

Figure 7–4. Class I and class II histocompatibility antigens α_1, α_2, α_3 are the three external domains of a class I histocompatibility antigen. $\beta_2 M = \beta_2$ microglobulin; α_1 and α_2 = external domains of class II histocompatibility antigen; β_1 and β_2 = external domains of class II histocompatibility antigen.

X. Histocompatibility Antigens

A. Major histocompatibility complex (MHC) (Figure 7–4)

–is located on the short (p) arm of human chromosome 6.

–encodes for the major histocompatibility antigens, known collectively as **HLA.**

–encodes for the class I antigens by the genes HLA-A, HLA-B, and HLA-C.

–encodes for the class II antigens, defined by the genes within the D (immune response) region, HLA-DR, HLA-DP, and HLA-DQ.

–encodes for the class II antigens, which include various complement components such as C2, C4, factor B, and the C3b receptor.

1. HLA class I antigens

–are encoded by HLA-A, HLA-B, and HLA-C genes.

–are expressed on every nucleated cell in the body.

–are associated noncovalently with a 12-kilodalton polypeptide, β_2-microglobulin, which is encoded on chromosome 2.

–consist of a 44-kilodalton polypeptide chain containing transmembrane and cytoplasmic components.

–have three external domains analogous to immunoglobulin domains (β_2-microglobulin defines the fourth domain).

–are involved in recognition (restriction) by T cytotoxic cells, which bear appropriate receptors for the HLA antigens (CD8).

–are associated with the expression of antigen on virus-infected or transformed cells.

2. HLA class II antigens

–are encoded by genes in the HLA-D region: HLA-DR, HLA-DQ, and HLA-DP.

–are expressed mainly on B cells, macrophages, activated T cells, and other APCs.

–consist of an α-chain (29 kilodaltons) and β-chain (34 kilodaltons) heterodimer, with cytoplasmic and transmembrane components.

–possess two external domains on each of the polypeptide chains.

–allow interaction (restriction) between APCs and T cells via CD4.

–are associated with the presentation of antigen on APCs.

B. Immunologic role of the histocompatibility antigens

–antigens are recognized by the appropriate T-cell receptor only in the context of the histocompatibility antigens.

–exogenous antigens (e.g., bacteria), which would undergo processing by an APC, would be expressed on the surface of the APC in the context of an HLA class II molecule and be recognized by $CD4^+$ T helper cells.

–endogenous antigens (e.g., virally transformed cell proteins) would be expressed on the surface of any cell in the context of a class I HLA molecule and be recognized by a $CD8^+$ cytotoxic T (Tc) cell.

C. Histocompatibility antigens in transplantation

–because the HLA gene products, both class I and class II, are cell surface proteins and very antigenic, it is important that tissues be typed before transplantation.

–the histocompatibility antigens are very polymorphic. In the HLA class I, there are at least 24 specificities encoded by HLA-A, 52 by HLA-B, and 11 by HLA-C.

–in the class II HLA, there are at least 20 specificities encoded for HLA-DR, nine for HLA-DQ, and six for HLA-DP.

D. HLA antigens and disease association

–certain diseases have a propensity for persons with a particular HLA antigen.

–relative risk quantifies the chance of an individual with the specific HLA antigen to acquire a specific disease compared with an individual who does not have that HLA antigen.

–Examples are included in Table 7–3.

XI. Tumor Immunology

A. Tumor cells

–are cells that have been transformed by virus or by chemical or physical means.

–are usually not well differentiated.

–lack contact inhibition and usually proliferate uncontrollably.

–have tumor-associated antigen (TAA) expression on their surface.

1. Viral tumors

–are caused by RNA and DNA oncogenic viruses.

–share TAA epitopes with cells transformed by the same or similar viruses and may have cross-reactivity.

Table 7–3. HLA Antigens and Disease Association

Disease	HLA Antigen	Risk*
Ankylosing spondylitis	B27	87
Dermatitis herpetiformis	DR3	56
Reiter's syndrome	B27	40
Insulin-dependent diabetes	DR3/DR4	33
Psoriasis vulgaris	C6	13
Goodpasture's syndrome	DR2	13
Sjögren's syndrome	DR3	6
Behçet's disease	B5	4

* Times more likely to acquire the disease than a person who does not have the specific HLA antigen

2. Chemically induced tumors

–are caused by a variety of chemical carcinogens (e.g., coal tar and 3-methylcholanthrene).

–share virtually no TAA epitopes and have no cross-reactivity.

3. Physically induced tumors

–are caused by physical "insult" such as contact with ultraviolet light, x-rays, or γ-radiation.

–behave akin to chemically induced tumors (i.e., no cross-reactivity).

4. Oncofetal antigens

–are antigenic epitopes that are found in normal fetal development and on some transformed (tumor) cells.

–are not usually present on normal adult cells.

a. Carcinoembryonic antigen (CEA)

–is normally found in the intestine, liver, and pancreas in months 2 to 6 of gestation.

–appears in 90% of pancreatic cancers, 70% of colon cancers, 35% of breast cancers, and 5% of normal persons.

–increases during pregnancy and in recurrence of the relevant tumor.

b. α-Fetoprotein (AFP)

–is the normal α-globulin of embryonic and fetal serum.

–appears in hepatomas, cirrhosis, and hepatitis.

B. Immune mechanisms in tumor-cell destruction

–include both the humoral and the cell-mediated mechanisms elicited by TAAs.

1. Humoral immunity to tumor cells

–starts with antibody binding to tumor cells and can lead to killing of tumor cells by:

    a. Attachment of antibody to Fc receptors on macrophages and neutrophils, followed by phagocytosis

    b. Attachment of antibody to Fc receptors on null (killer) cells, followed by lysis by antibody-dependent cell-mediated cytotoxicity (ADCC)

    c. Activation of the complete complement sequence, causing tumor lysis

    d. Activation of the complement sequence to produce C3b on the tumor-cell surface, which reacts with C3b receptors on macrophages and neutrophils to enhance phagocytosis

2. Cell-mediated immunity to tumor cells

    –leads to killing of tumor cells by:

    a. Production of lymphokines by T helper cells, thereby mobilizing and activating macrophages against tumor cells; these lymphokines include macrophage activating factor, macrophage migration inhibition factor, and macrophage chemotactic factor

    b. Production of monokines by activated macrophages, for example, tumor necrosis factor (TNF)

    c. Activation of $CD8^+$ cytotoxic T cells that recognize TAA on virally transformed cells in association with class I histocompatibility antigens

    d. Killing of tumor cells—spontaneously and without previous sensitization—by NK cells

XII. Blood Group Immunology

A. ABO system

–is defined by the presence of alloantigens A and B on the surface of red blood cells.

–is characterized by natural isohemagglutinins (predominately IgM) in the circulation.

–is determined genetically by the A, B, and O alleles, where A and B are dominant over O.

1. Type (phenotype) A

    –has A alloantigen on red blood cells.

    –has anti-B isohemagglutinin in serum.

    –can be genotype AA (homozygous) or AO (heterozygous).

2. Type B

    –has B alloantigen on red blood cells.

    –has anti-A isohemagglutinin in serum.

    –can be genotype BB or BO.

3. Type AB

    –has both A and B alloantigens on red blood cells.

    –has no isohemagglutinins.

    –is genotype AB.

4. Type O

    –has neither A nor B alloantigens on red blood cells.

    –has both anti-A and anti-B isohemagglutinins.

–is genotype OO; the O allele does not code for any product.

–has H antigen fully expressed.

B. Rh antigens

–are determined by a complex of genes, DCE/dce; the D antigen is the most important medically.

–have codominant expression.

–are called "positive" if the D gene is expressed and "negative" if D is not expressed.

–incompatibility can lead to hemolytic disease of the newborn, which can be prevented if the Rh-negative mother is inoculated with anti-Rh antibody within 72 hours after delivery of an Rh-positive infant.

XIII. The Complement System

A. Complement-mediated cell cytotoxicity

–causes lysis of a target cell.

–may be initiated by antibody fixation to a cell surface antigen.

–may be caused by antigen–antibody complex formation.

–occurs by activation of either:

    1. Classic complement cascade—mediated by IgG, IgG2, IgG3, or IgM antibody

    2. Alternative pathway—initiated by certain antigens (i.e., lipopolysaccharide, endotoxin, zymosan) or antigen–antibody complexes

B. Complement components

–is a collective term for a group of heterogeneous proteins involved in a sequential activation, culminating in target cell lysis.

–are not immunoglobulins.

–are present in normal serum.

–do not increase as a result of antigen stimulation.

–are manufactured early in ontogeny (first trimester).

–are made in macrophages and liver (except C1, which is made and assembled in gastrointestinal epithelium).

–are heat labile.

–are defined by number (C1, C2, C3) and letter (factor B, factor D) designations.

C. Classic activation pathway (Figure 7–5)

    1. A singlet of IgM or a doublet of IgG1, IgG2, or IgG3, very closely spaced on the cell surface, binds C1 by the C1q region via a receptor in the Fc region ($C\mu4$ or $C\gamma3$).

    2. C1 consists of subunits of C1q, C1r, and C1s bound by Ca^{2+} and is activated from a proesterase to an esterase, cleaving both C4 and C2 sequentially.

    3. C4 is cleaved into C4b and C4a, with C4b attaching at the site of antibody fixation and C4a going off in the fluid phase; C4a may act as an anaphylatoxin.

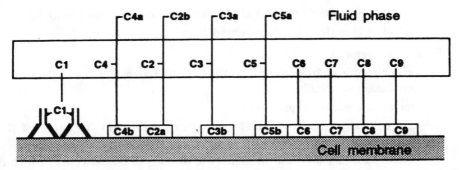

Figure 7–5. Diagrammatic presentation of the classic pathway of complement activation. C1 attaches to a doublet of IgG on cell surface. C4 is cleaved to C4a (goes to fluid phase) and C4b. C2 is cleaved to C2a, which attaches to C4b to yield C3 convertase and C2b (fluid phase). C3 is cleaved to yield C3a (fluid phase) and C3b on cell surface. C5 is cleaved to yield C5a (fluid phase) and C5b on surface. C6, C7, C8, and C9 are then placed on cell surface in equimolar concentrations and probably form a circular channel to allow fluid influx.

4. C2 is cleaved into C2a and C2b, with C2a attaching to C4b via Mg^{2+}; C2b is released in the fluid phase and acts as a kinin.

5. Antibody-C1–C4bC2a complex is C3 convertase.

6. C3 is cleaved into C3a and C3b; C3b has receptors on many cell surfaces, including neutrophils and macrophages; C3a is anaphylatoxin I and attaches preferentially to C3a receptors on mast cells and causes histamine release.

7. C5 is analogous to C3 and is cleaved into C5b and C5a; C5b causes activation of C6 and C7; C5a is anaphylatoxin II, has receptors on mast cells for histamine release, and is chemotactic for neutrophils and macrophages.

8. C6 and C7 are activated by C5b and exist as an activated entity C5b67, which is chemotactic for neutrophils and macrophages.

9. C8 and C9 cause permeability changes and allow water influx, resulting in cell swelling and lysis.

D. Control mechanisms of complement activation

1. **Instability of components**

   –includes the short half-lives of C2a and C5b.

2. **Inhibitors**

   –include C1 inhibitor (C1-INH), which stops continued activation of C1; congenital lack of C1-INH is called hereditary angioedema.

3. **Inactivators**

   –include:

   a. **C3b inactivator**—an enzyme that destroys C3b activity

   b. **C6 inactivator**—destroys C6 activity

   c. **Anaphylatoxin inactivator**—cleaves C-terminal arginine from C3a and C5a

E. Alternative activation pathway

–is caused by the presence of zymosan, endotoxin, or complexes of aggregated human immunoglobulins including $F(ab')_2$ fragments.

–bypasses the need for specific antibody and early components C1, C4, and C2.

1. Low levels of C3b are present in serum under normal circumstances.

2. In the presence of factor D, factor B can be cleaved into Bb and Ba; Bb assembles with C3b.

3. Properdin P stabilizes C3bBb on the surface of zymosan or endotoxin and allows this entity (P.C3b.Bb) to cleave another molecule of C3 to continue the cascade.

XIV. Hypersensitivity Reactions

–are categorized according to the **Gell and Coombs classification.**

A. Type I hypersensitivity—anaphylaxis

–occurs in atopic persons.

–occurs in response to environmental antigens (e.g., allergens) or administered antigens (e.g., penicillin).

–is mediated by IgE (reaginic) antibody bound to the surface of mast cells or basophils.

–may be localized or systemic.

1. **IgE in immediate hypersensitivity**

   –is produced in response to environmental antigens.

   –binds by the Fc portion of IgE to mast cells or basophils.

   –causes release of vasoactive and chemotactic factors from mast cells upon cross-linking of antigen on the surface.

   –can be measured in toto by use of **RIST.**

   –can also be measured for specific idiotypes by **RAST.**

2. **Products released by mast cells upon stimulation of surface IgE**

   a. **Vasoactive mediators**

      (1) **Histamine**—causes smooth muscle contraction in bronchioles and small blood vessels and increased permeability of capillaries; molecular weight is 111 daltons.

      (2) **Platelet-activating factor (PAF)**—activates platelets.

      (3) **Slow-reacting substance of anaphylaxis (SRS-A)**—consists of metabolite of arachidonic acid and includes the leukotrienes LTC4, LTD4, and LTE4.

      (4) **Prostaglandins and thromboxanes**—products of cyclooxygenase metabolism or arachidonic acid; cause erythema and vasopermeability. These metabolites are potent inducers of smooth muscle contractibility, bronchoconstriction, and increased vascular permeability.

   b. **Chemotactic factors**

      (1) **Eosinophil chemotactic factor of anaphylaxis (ECF-A)**—causes influx of eosinophils; molecular weight is 2 kilodaltons.

(2) Neutrophil chemotactic factor—has a high molecular weight (660 kilodaltons); is chemotactic for neutrophils.

3. **Treatment of allergic reactions**

   a. Eliminate or avoid the allergen.

   b. Tie up IgE molecules with haptens of allergens or with monovalent antigens.

   c. Inject patient with solubilized allergen to cause production of IgG, which competes with IgE for allergen (**hypersensitization**).

   d. Administer **cromolyn sodium;** stabilize the mast-cell membrane and decrease the amount of histamine released.

   e. Increase cyclic adenosine monophosphate (cAMP) levels, which stabilizes the mast-cell membrane and decreases the amount of vasoactive and chemotactic molecules released; this may be done by an increase of adenyl cyclase activity (stimulation of β-receptors, isoproterenol) or by a decrease in phosphodiesterase activity (methylxanthines—aminophylline, theophylline).

B. **Type II hypersensitivity—cytotoxic reactions**

   –involve the production of antibody to specific cell-surface epitopes, which cause destruction of the cell.

   1. **Antibody to cell-surface antigen**

      –can cause reduction in cell-surface charges.

      –can cause opsonic adherence via the Fc region of antibody to neutrophils, macrophages, and K cells (the cells responsible for ADCC); enhances cell phagocytosis and promotes cell death.

      –can activate complement to cause cell lysis.

   2. **Examples of type II hypersensitivity reactions**

      a. **Transfusion reactions**—ABO incompatibility involving IgM antibodies against A or B alloantigens

      b. **Rh incompatibility**—IgG antibodies against the D antigen on fetal red cells

      c. **Hemolytic anemia**—antibody to red blood cell epitopes

      d. **Goodpasture's syndrome**—antibody to glomerular and bronchial basement membrane

      e. **Myasthenia gravis**—antibody to muscle acetylcholine receptors

C. **Type III hypersensitivity—immune complex reactions**

   –involve soluble antigen that becomes bound antigen–antibody complexes, which, especially in antigen excess, can cause a series of events that lead to pathologic expression, edema, neutrophil infiltrate, and lesions in blood vessels and kidney glomeruli.

   1. **Consequences of antigen–antibody complex formation**

      a. Platelet aggregation, leading to formation of microthrombi and release of vasoactive amines

    b. Activation of complement and release of anaphylatoxins (causing histamine release) and chemotactic factors (for neutrophils)

    c. Clotting factor XII activation, leading to fibrin, plasmin, and kinin formation

2. Examples of type III hypersensitivity reactions

    a. Arthus reaction—immunization of rabbits with horse serum (classic prototype of type III reaction)

    b. Farmer's lung—antibody to inhaled aspergillus mold

    c. Cheesemaker's lung—antibody to fungi

    d. Pigeon fancier's disease—antibody to pigeon dander

    e. Serum sickness—antibody to "foreign" immunoglobulin injection

    f. Rheumatoid arthritis—rheumatoid factor (IgM) against the Fc portion of self IgG

D. Type IV hypersensitivity—delayed-type hypersensitivity

–is differentiated from immediate-type hypersensitivity reactions (types I, II, and III).

–is an example of cell-mediated immunity; types I, II, and III are mediated by antibody and are examples of humoral immunity.

1. Sequence of events in a type IV reaction

    a. An appropriate antigen (tuberculin, purified protein derivative of *Mycobacterium tuberculosis*, tumor cell, transplanted cell, virally transformed cell) is processed by macrophages; epitopes of antigen are expressed on the macrophage surface via HLA class II antigens; macrophages produce IL-1.

    b. T helper cells react to antigen epitope and class II antigens via TCR and CD4, respectively.

    c. T helper cells are also stimulated by IL-1 from macrophages.

    d. T helper cells produce IL-2, and IL-2 receptors become fully activated and release lymphokines, having an effect on T cells and on macrophages.

2. Lymphokines

–that affect macrophages include macrophage chemotactic factor (MCF), macrophage migration inhibition factor (MIF), and macrophage-activating factor (MAF).

–that affect $CD8^+$ cells include IL-2, which activates them to become fully cytotoxic.

–that are produced by $CD4^+$ and $CD8^+$ cells include **TNF,** osteoclast-activating factor (**OAF**), and histamine-releasing factor (**HRF**).

3. $CD8^+$ cytotoxic cells

–react to viral and tumor antigens and HLA class I antigens via TCR and CD8 molecules, respectively.

–are further stimulated by IL-2 from T helper cells.

–produce IL-2 themselves.

–produce IFN-γ.

XV. Developmental Immunologic Disorders

–are of major concern when considering the immunodeficiency diseases of the neonate and children and the depressed immune response of elderly persons.

–are diagnosed using information concerning the patient's history of multiple infections, which can be verified with quantitative immunoglobulin tests, T- and B-cell ratios, and humoral and cell-mediated responses to common antigens.

A. Transient hypogammaglobulinemia of infancy

–reflects a normal condition resulting from temporal requirements for full development of the infant's immune system.

–occurs in the normal neonate who is born with an adult level of placentally transferred IgG and who possesses antibodies associated with the maternal immune experience; however, the rate of synthesis of secretable immunoglobulin by newborn infants is low and does not reach adequate levels for a number of months.

–is a transient period of physiologic hypogammaglobulinemia, generally from the third to the fifth month, beginning with the disappearance of maternally transferred IgG ($t_{1/2}$ = 22–28 days) and the onset of significant synthesis of IgG by the infant.

–results in increased susceptibility to some microorganisms.

B. Congenital agammaglobulinemia (Bruton's)

–is a sex-linked (male) disorder characterized by recurrent pyogenic infections and digestive tract disorders beginning at age 5 to 6 months.

–is diagnosed by the absence of tonsils, germinal centers, and B cells, and by serum immunoglobulin levels of less than 10%.

–defect may lie in the transition from pre-B to B cells, because the pre-B cells are normal.

–patients have an apparently normal thymus and cell-mediated immunity.

–can be treated by passive transfer of adult serum immunoglobulins to protect the patient.

C. Common variable hypogammaglobulinemia

–can be acquired at any age by either sex.

–patients generally have B cells but do not secrete immunoglobulin.

–patients have depressed serum immunoglobulin to less than 250 mg/dL of IgG and less than 50 mg/dL of IgA and IgM (normal IgG = 800–1400; IgM = 60–200; IgA = 100–300 mg%).

–patients are seen with increased susceptibility to pyogenic infections and autoimmune diseases.

–has multiple causes and diverse treatments.

D. Dysgammaglobulinemia

–patients are seen with a selective immunoglobulin class (one or more, but not all) deficiency.

–commonly results in depressed IgA levels (less than 5 mg/dL; 1 in 600–800 individuals), leading to:

   1. Loss of mucosal surface protection
   2. Patients with normal numbers of IgA cells; however, these cells fail to differentiate into plasma cells
   3. Increased autoimmunity

E. Congenital thymic aplasia (DiGeorge syndrome)

   –is characterized by an absence of T cells, hypocalcemia, and tetany; it is not hereditary.

   –is caused by an intrauterine insult to the third and fourth pharyngeal pouches, resulting in lack of development of the thymus and the parathyroid between the fifth and sixth weeks of human gestation.

   –results in a depressed cell-mediated immunity that permits disease caused by opportunistic organisms (e.g., *Candida*, *Pneumocystis*, viral infections).

   –patients can die from vaccination with live vaccines (e.g., measles, smallpox).

   –patients have apparently normal germinal centers, plasma cells, and serum immunoglobulin.

   –treatment with transplantation of fetal thymus is experimental and may be complicated by a graft-versus-host reaction.

F. Chronic mucocutaneous candidiasis

   –is a highly specific T-cell disorder characterized by an absence of immunity to *Candida*.

   –patients have apparently normal T-cell absolute numbers and other T-cell functions.

   –can include endocrine dysfunctions (hypothyroidism) in about half of these patients.

G. Wiskott-Aldrich syndrome

   –is a sex-linked (male) disease, with patients presenting with a triad of thrombocytopenia, eczema, and recurrent infections.

   –is characterized by a depressed cell-mediated immunity and serum IgM but normal IgG and IgA levels.

   –patients respond poorly to polysaccharide antigens.

   –can include increased lymphoreticular malignancies or lymphomas.

   –may have as its primary defect an absence of specific glycoprotein receptors on both T cells and platelets.

   –patients can receive bone marrow transplantation as an experimental treatment.

H. Severe combined immunodeficiency disease (SCID)

   –is characterized by a genetic defect in stem cells, resulting in absence of the thymus and T and B cells.

   –involves, in half of the patients, a loss in the enzyme adenosine deaminase, resulting in accumulation of toxic deoxyadenosine triphosphate (dATP), which inhibits ribonucleotide reductase and prevents DNA synthesis.

   –results in extreme susceptibility to infections and a very short life span.

I. Chronic granulomatous disease

   –is characterized by a genetic defect in the nicotinamide adenine dinucleotide phosphate (NADPH) oxidase system.

–results in a defective neutrophil bactericidal activity because of depressed superoxide dismutase and decreased hydrogen peroxide levels.

–is diagnosed in the laboratory based on failure of neutrophils and macrophages to reduce a nitroblue tetrazolium (NBT) dye.

–may be treated with interferon-γ with some success.

J. Senescence of the immune response

–is manifest in the elderly by depressed humoral and cellular immune responses.

–is highly variable with chronologic age.

–is characterized primarily by a loss in some T-cell functions.

–includes an increase in occurrence of autoimmune disease.

XVI. Autoimmune Disorders

–are disorders in immune regulation resulting in antibody or cell-mediated immunity against the host's own tissues.

–may or may not result in injury to the host.

–are disorders in which persons are normally unresponsive to self-antigens due to tolerance; however, B-cell clones do exist in persons with idiotypes reacting with self-antigens.

A. Explanatory theories

1. Microbial antigens cross-reacting with host tissues induce an immune response against self

–is not a true autoimmunity because the stimulus is of exogenous origin.

–examples include:

a. Streptococcal antigens cross-react with sarcolemmal heart muscle and kidney.

b. Anti-DNA antibodies reacting with cells in patients with systemic lupus erythematosus (SLE) may be induced by microbial DNA.

c. Deposition of viral antigens on host-cell membranes may involve an immune reaction against the host cell.

2. Host antigens previously sequestered from fetal tolerance–inducing mechanism are released and become immunogenic

–such as for some antigens in thyroid and heart tissue that emerge after tissue damage by microbes or surgery.

3. Alteration of host molecules, exposing new antigenic determinants unavailable at the time of induction of fetal tolerance

–for example, rheumatoid factor (in patients with rheumatoid arthritis), which is mainly an IgM antibody against the Fc fragment of slightly altered IgG.

4. Attachment of foreign hapten to self-molecule, forming a hapten-carrier complex

–for example, when certain drugs (e.g., quinidine and sulfathiazole) attach to platelets, the antibody to the drug reacts with the drug on the platelet membrane and activates complement; then the platelet lyses.

5. Depletion of suppressor cells

–may result in autoantibodies if the normally occurring suppression by T-suppressor cells of B-cell clones with idiotype specificity for self-antigens is lost or diminished.

B. Systemic autoimmune disorders

1. Systemic lupus erythematosus (SLE)

–is an episodic multisystem disease usually in young women, with vasculitis as a major lesion.

–is characterized by multiple autoreactive antibodies, the most dominant of which is antinuclear antibody (ANA).

–cross-reactive ANA may be induced by microbial infection.

–may include nephritis resulting from continuous insult by antigen–antibody complexes in antigen excess and complement activation at the level of the glomeruli.

–can be confused with rheumatoid arthritis, because 30% of SLE patients exhibit serum rheumatoid factor.

2. Rheumatoid arthritis

–is a chronic, systemic inflammatory disease mainly of the joints.

–is characterized by the appearance in serum and synovial fluids of rheumatoid factors (antibodies against immunoglobulin) and complement activation; resulting chemotactic factors attract inflammatory cells into joints, which damage tissues via release of pharmacologically active mediators.

–rheumatoid factor formation may be a response by synovial lymphocytes against microbial antigens.

–may involve a genetic predisposition (HLA-D4 and HLA-DR4) for this condition.

3. Sjögren's syndrome

–is a chronic inflammatory disease, primarily of postmenopausal women, characterized by autoantibodies against salivary duct antigens.

–patients may complain of dryness of the mouth, trachea, bronchi, eyes, nose, vagina, and skin.

–may occur secondary to rheumatoid arthritis and SLE.

–is of unknown etiology.

4. Polyarteritis nodosa

–is one of a number of similar human vasculitides that can be reproduced experimentally by antigen–antibody complexes.

–often involves complexes of hepatitis B antigen with its specific antibody that are found deposited in vessel walls (30%–40% of patients).

C. Organ-specific autoimmune disorders

1. Blood

a. Autoantibodies reacting with blood cells result in anemia; leukopenia and thrombocytopenia can occur (e.g., SLE).

b. Malignant transformation of a single plasma cell clone (mul-

tiple myeloma) results in the appearance of an excess of IgG or other immunoglobulin classes (termed paraproteins); such patients may also secrete Bence Jones proteins (monoclonal light chains) in their urine.

2. Central nervous system

a. Allergic encephalitis

–is a demyelinating disease that can occur after an infection or immunization.

–is characterized immunologically by a perivascular mononuclear cell infiltrate in the white matter of the central nervous system (CNS).

–can be mimicked experimentally by immunization of animals with homologous extracts of brain or a nonapeptide from the basic protein of myelin.

–experimental disease can be transferred with sensitized lymphocytes, thereby complicating cell-mediated immunity in the demyelination process.

b. Multiple sclerosis

–is a chronic, relapsing disease characterized immunologically by mononuclear cell infiltration and demyelinating lesions (plaques) in the white matter of the CNS.

–patients generally have increased IgG in the cerebrospinal fluid, containing elevated titers to measles and other viruses.

–is characterized by a decrease in suppressor T-cell function, which indicates an immunoregulatory disorder.

c. Myasthenia gravis

–is characterized by a defect in neuromuscular transmission, resulting in muscle weakness and fatigue.

–is associated with the presence of an antiacetylcholine receptor antibody, causing loss of the receptor.

–patients often have thymic hyperplasia or thymoma with increased numbers of B lymphocytes.

3. Endocrine

a. Chronic thyroiditis

–is characterized by autoantibodies and cell-mediated immunity to thyroglobulin or thyroid microsomes.

–lesions can be reproduced experimentally by infection of autoantigen with an adjuvant.

–generally is a self-limiting disease of females with a probable genetic basis.

–may involve tissue damage occurring via antibody-dependent cell-mediated cytotoxicity (ADCC).

b. Graves' disease (hyperthyroidism)

–is characterized by autoantibodies to the thyroid-stimulating hormone receptor and infiltration of the thyroid gland with T cells and B cells.

–antibodies may compete with thyroid-stimulating hormone (TSH) for receptor site and mimic TSH activity.

   c. **Diabetes mellitus**
   –is characterized in insulin-dependent (juvenile onset, or type I) diabetes by the destruction of insulin-producing cells through either humoral or cell-mediated anti-islet cell immunity; there is no evidence for autoimmune pathogenesis in non–insulin-dependent (maturity onset, or type II) diabetes.

4. **Gastrointestinal tract**
   a. **Pernicious anemia**
      –is characterized by autoantibodies to the gastric parietal cell and intrinsic factor.
      –results in inability to absorb vitamin B_{12}.
   b. **Ulcerative colitis**
      –is characterized by chronic inflammatory lesions confined to the rectum and colon and by infiltration of monocytes, lymphocytes, and plasma cells.
      –patients' lymphocytes show cytotoxicity against colonic epithelial cells in culture.
      –patients have antibodies that are cross-reactive with *Escherichia coli*, but the disease is of unknown etiology.
   c. **Crohn's disease**
      –is an inflammatory, granulomatous disease usually occurring in the submucosal area of the terminal ileum.
      –is a chronic progressive disease, often suspected, but not established, as being of microbial etiology.
   d. **Chronic active hepatitis**
      –is characterized by infiltration of the liver by T cells, B cells, and monocytes.
      –patients have diminished suppressor cell numbers.
      –may be a disease of faulty immunoregulation.

Review Test

Directions: Each of the numbered items or incomplete statements in this section is followed by answers or by completions of the statement. Select the **one** lettered answer or completion that is best in each case.

1. To which of the following classes of immunoglobulins do the allergy-mediating antibodies belong?

(A) IgA
(B) IgG
(C) IgM
(D) IgD
(E) IgE

2. Which of the following antibody classes is the first to be produced in an immune response to a given antigen?

(A) IgA
(B) IgG
(C) IgM
(D) IgD
(E) IgE

3. In most normal persons, what percentage of the total serum immunoglobulins is IgG?

(A) 10%
(B) 25%
(C) 50%
(D) 60%
(E) Over 70%

4. Which one of the following immunoglobulins is the principal immunoglobulin in exocrine secretions?

(A) IgA
(B) IgG
(C) IgM
(D) IgD
(E) IgE

5. Which of the following statements about IgM is true?

(A) It is the reaginic antibody.
(B) It is important in the first few days of the primary immune response.
(C) It increases in serum concentration after IgG has reached its peak serum concentration.
(D) It is the smallest of the immunoglobulin molecules.
(E) It is involved in allergic reactions.

6. Which of the following fragments are seen when IgG is split by papain?

(A) Two monovalent fractions with antibody activity (Fab)
(B) Two fractions devoid of antibody activity
(C) Fab fragments that contain all the variable (V) sections of the heavy chain but not the light chain
(D) Fab fragments that contain all the variable (V) sections of the light chain but not the heavy chain
(E) Two Fc fractions and one Fab fraction

7. Which of the following findings is seen in neonatally thymectomized mice?

(A) Increased numbers of blood lymphocytes
(B) Depleted T-cell areas in lymph nodes and spleen
(C) Increased ability to reject allografts
(D) Large amounts of antibody produced in response to many antigens
(E) Large amounts of antibody of the IgG class

8. What is the approximate molecular weight of IgG?

(A) 10 kilodaltons
(B) 15 kilodaltons
(C) 150 kilodaltons
(D) 200 kilodaltons
(E) 900 kilodaltons

9. Actively acquired immunity can be caused by all of the following EXCEPT

(A) the specific disease.
(B) exposure to subclinical doses of the disease-causing organism.
(C) vaccination with the appropriate antigen.
(D) injection with immune serum containing appropriate antibodies.

10. All of the following are characteristics of the human immunodeficiency virus (HIV) EXCEPT

(A) it binds to the CD4 molecule preferentially.
(B) it contains gp120 and gp41 envelope proteins.
(C) it is the causative agent of AIDS.
(D) it contains DNA within its core.
(E) it contains a reverse transcriptase within its core.

11. Which of the following substances is not liberated during an anaphylactic reaction?

(A) Histamine
(B) Kinins
(C) C3a anaphylatoxin
(D) Serotonin
(E) Slow-reacting substances (SRS-A)

12. Which of the following components determines the class-specific antigenicity of immunoglobulins?

(A) J chain
(B) T chain
(C) Light chain
(D) Heavy chain
(E) Secretory component

13. The classic complement cascade consists of a series of sequential events that eventually culminates in cell lysis. Which of the following complement components causes the cleavage of C3 into C3a and C3b?

(A) C5b
(B) C5a
(C) C1qrs
(D) C4b2a
(E) C2b

14. Release of mast cell contents can be caused by all of the following EXCEPT

(A) C3a anaphylatoxin.
(B) C5a anaphylatoxin.
(C) cross-linking of IgE on mast cell surface by allergen.
(D) cross-linking of IgE on mast cell surface by anti-IgE antibody.
(E) interleukin-1 (IL-1).

15. Which clinical feature is commonly found in patients with systemic lupus erythematosus (SLE)?

(A) Vasculitis is a basic lesion.
(B) A linear deposition of immunoglobulin in their glomerular basement membrane occurs with nephritis.
(C) Thyroid receptor antibody is present.
(D) Rheumatoid factor is rarely present.

16. Which one of the following statements best describes the rheumatoid factor?

(A) It is the antigen initiating the rheumatoid inflammatory process.
(B) It is an antibody against cellular DNA.
(C) It consists primarily of DNA.
(D) It is an antibody against immunoglobulin.

17. All of the following are immunologic features EXCEPT

(A) increased IgG in the cerebrospinal fluid.
(B) mononuclear infiltration in the brain.
(C) an increase in suppressor T-cell function.
(D) autoantibodies to intrinsic factor and loss of vitamin B_{12} uptake.

18. Susceptibility to the yeast *Candida* can occur in

(A) congenital agammaglobulinemia.
(B) congenital thymic aplasia (DiGeorge syndrome).
(C) common variable hypogammaglobulinemia.
(D) SLE.

19. Which one of the following factors characterizes the immune deficiency in chronic granulomatous disease?

(A) Reduced levels of the fifth component of complement
(B) Inability of polymorphonuclear leukocytes to ingest bacteria
(C) Dysgammaglobulinemia
(D) Inability of polymorphonuclear leukocytes to kill ingested bacteria

20. Which clinical finding is associated with severe combined immunodeficiency disease (SCID)?

(A) Presence of the thymus but absence of the bursal equivalent
(B) Clinical findings in the nicotinamide adenine dinucleotide phosphate (NADPH) oxidase system
(C) Clinical findings in adenosine deaminase, resulting in a loss of this enzyme activity
(D) A transient low level of humoral immunity in neonates

21. Which immunological finding is associated with aging?

(A) Interleukin-2 (IL-2) levels diminish
(B) Suppressor cell function decreases
(C) Cellular immune response increases
(D) Thymus tissue increases

22. Which of the following reactions requires complement?

(A) IgG-mediated anaphylaxis
(B) Killing the cytotoxic T lymphocytes
(C) Development of glomerulonephritis caused by antigen–antibody complexes
(D) Antibody-dependent cell-mediated cytotoxicity

23. All of the following statements describe characteristics of complement EXCEPT

(A) it consists of at least 11 different proteins.
(B) it makes up approximately 10% of the globulins in normal human serum.
(C) it is not an immunoglobulin.
(D) it is increased in concentration by immunization.

24. The first component of complement (C1) would disassemble into its component parts as a result of

(A) conditions that have minimized its polymeric behavior.
(B) autodigestion.
(C) loss of calcium.
(D) loss of magnesium.

25. Which one of the following substances may be passively transferred from the mother to the fetus during the third trimester of pregnancy?

(A) IgG
(B) IgM
(C) Anti-Rh antibody
(D) Natural isohemagglutinins

26. A male heterozygous for Rh factor mates with an Rh-negative female. On the basis of genetic theory, it could be predicted that

(A) no offspring would be Rh positive.
(B) 25% of the offspring would be Rh positive.
(C) 50% of the offspring would be Rh positive.
(D) 100% of the offspring would be Rh positive.

27. All of the following statements accurately describe antibody molecules EXCEPT they

(A) contain two identical H chains.
(B) contain carbohydrate.
(C) contain two identical L chains.
(D) are electrophoretically homogeneous.

28. Pluripotential stem cells arise from each of the following locations EXCEPT the

(A) fetal liver.
(B) embryonic yolk sac.
(C) adult bone marrow.
(D) adult spleen.

29. All of the following statements regarding B cells are true EXCEPT

(A) they mature in the bursa of Fabricius or bursal equivalent.
(B) they are found in the germinal centers of lymph nodes and spleens.
(C) they are progenitors of plasma cells.
(D) they are involved in humoral and cell-mediated immunity.

30. All of the following statements about T cells are correct EXCEPT

(A) they arise in the bone marrow.
(B) they mature in the lymph nodes.
(C) they are predominately recirculating lymphocytes.
(D) they are involved in humoral and cell-mediated immunity.

Directions: Each group of items in this section consists of lettered options followed by a set of numbered items. For each item, select the one lettered option that is most closely associated with it. Each lettered option may be selected once, more than once, or not at all.

Questions 31–36

Match each characteristic with the appropriate immunoglobulin.

(A) IgA
(B) IgG
(C) IgM
(D) IgD
(E) IgE

31. Protects the mucosal surfaces of the respiratory, intestinal, and genitourinary tracts from pathogenic organisms

32. Highest level in normal adult

33. Highest level in normal 1-day-old infant

34. Implicated in atopic response

35. Produced by B cells in response to antigen

36. Longest half-life

Questions 37–45

Match each of the characteristics below with the substance it best describes.

(A) IL-1
(B) IL-2
(C) IL-3
(D) IL-4
(E) IL-5
(F) IL-6
(G) IFN-γ
(H) TNF-β

37. Enhances switch from IgG to IgE production

38. Is produced by macrophages and macrophage-like cells

39. Is a potent stimulator of hematopoiesis

40. Is endogenous pyrogen

41. Increases expression of class II histocompatibility antigens on surface of antigen processing cells

42. Is a factor made by T cells that is cytotoxic to certain tumor cells

43. Is a T-cell growth factor

44. Enhances switch from IgG to IgA production

45. Stimulates IL-2 receptor production on surface of T cells

Questions 46–53

Match each of the characteristics below with the antigen it best describes.

(A) CD2
(B) CD3
(C) CD4
(D) CD8
(E) CD25

46. Is a receptor for the gp120 envelope protein of HIV

47. Is a five-polypeptide transmembrane chain complex

48. Is a receptor for LFA-3

49. Is the structure responsible for T-cell rosettes in the presence of sheep red blood cells

50. Is the receptor for IL-2

51. Binds to class I histocompatibility antigens

52. Binds to class II histocompatibility antigens

53. Is invariably a part of the T-cell receptor complex

Questions 54–60

Match each of the following conditions with the type of hypersensitivity reaction most closely related to it.

(A) Type I (anaphylactic) hypersensitivity reaction
(B) Type II (cytotoxic) hypersensitivity reaction
(C) Type III (immune complex) hypersensitivity reaction
(D) Type IV (delayed) hypersensitivity reaction
(E) None of the above

54. Hives, urticaria, and allergy

55. Farmer's lung

56. Addison's disease

57. Myasthenia gravis

58. Reaction to purified protein derivative of *Mycobacterium tuberculosis*

59. Serum sickness

60. Autoimmune hemolytic anemia

Questions 61–73

Match each of the following characteristics with the autoimmune disease associated with it.

(A) Ulcerative colitis
(B) Multiple sclerosis
(C) Chronic granulomatous disease
(D) Systemic lupus erythematosus (SLE)
(E) Congenital thymic aplasia
(F) Myasthenia gravis
(G) Severe combined immunodeficiency disease (SCID)
(H) Pernicious anemia
(I) Congenital agammaglobulinemia
(J) Wiskott-Aldrich syndrome
(K) Dysgammaglobulinemia
(L) Graves' disease
(M) Chronic mucocutaneous candidiasis

61. Decreased IgA levels; occurs in 1 in 800 persons

62. Characterized by demyelinating lesions, increased IgG in the cerebrospinal fluid, chronic and relapsing occurrences

63. Chronic inflammatory lesion confined to the rectum and colon

64. Highly specific T-cell disorder with normal absolute number of T cells

65. Characterized by absence of tonsils, germinal centers, B cells, and serum Ig of less than 10%; cell-mediated immunity appears normal

66. Loss of adenosine deaminase enzyme in 50% of patients, resulting in accumulation of toxic deoxyadenosine triphosphate (dATP)

67. Defective neutrophil bactericidal activity resulting from depressed superoxide dismutase

68. Presence of autoantibody to the thyroid stimulating hormone receptor

69. Association with an antiacetylcholine receptor antibody

70. Soluble anti-DNA–DNA complexes result in glomerulonephritis

71. Characterized by autoantibodies against intrinsic factor

72. Characterized by absence of T cells, hypocalcemia, and tetany with lowered cell-mediated immunity

73. Characterized by a triad of thrombocytopenia, eczema, and recurrent infections

Answers and Explanations

1–E. IgE, the reagins or reaginic antibodies, mediates the allergic reaction. IgE binds allergens via their antigen-binding sites and are bound to tissue mast cells by their specialized Fc region.

2–C. IgM is the first antibody class produced in response to an antigen, and it is also the predominant antibody in a primary immune response.

3–E. IgG is the predominant immunoglobulin in serum. A normal person has approximately 73% IgG, 19% IgA, 7% IgM, 1% IgD, and 0.01% IgE. These ratios remain constant even in cases of hyperimmunization.

4–A. Secretory IgA is the predominant antibody in exocrine secretions (e.g., milk, saliva, tears), where it is usually found in the dimeric form, held together by a J chain, and with an attached secretory component to help stabilize it against proteolytic enzymes.

5–B. IgM, the first antibody to be produced after antigenic stimulation, has a very important role in the first few days of a primary immune response. The largest of the immunoglobulin molecules, it is not involved in allergic (type I hypersensitivity) reactions.

6–A. Papain splits IgG to produce two Fab (antigen-binding) fragments or fractions and a crystalliz-able fragment (Fc). Because the Fab is monovalent, antigen can be bound by the Fab but not cross-linked and precipitated. A Fab fragment contains the V region of both the heavy and light chains.

7–B. Neonatal thymectomy severely decreases the number of functional T cells throughout the body, resulting in decreased circulating blood lymphocytes (predominant T cells) and depleted T-cell areas in lymph nodes and spleen. Allograft rejection would be decreased because of decreased or depleted $CD8^+$ T cells, and antibody levels would be decreased due to decreased or depleted $CD4^+$ T helper cells.

8–C. IgG has a molecular weight of approximately 150 kilodaltons (150,000 molecular weight). IgD is similar in weight. IgA weighs 160 kilodaltons; IgE weighs approximately 200 kilodaltons, and IgM weighs 900 kilodaltons.

9–D. The transfer of immune serum is a prime example of passively acquired immunity. The immunity thus passively transferred remains as long as the antibodies persist (usually several weeks). Actively acquired immunity, which is essentially of unlimited duration, can be achieved by having the disease, by being exposed to subclinical doses of a specific organism, or by receiving the appropriate vaccina-tion.

10–D. HIV is a retrovirus containing two copies of its RNA genome within its core. It penetrates a $CD4^+$ cell, uncoats, then makes a DNA copy of its RNA via reverse transcriptase, then inserts this into the human DNA genome to form the provirion.

11–C. Anaphylactic (class I hypersensitivity) reactions occur after the release and manufacture of substances from IgE-coated mast cells. Complement activation plays no role, and C3a anaphylatoxin is not involved. C3a itself causes mast-cell content release during complement activation (class II and class III hypersensitivity reactions).

12–D. The heavy chain defines the immunoglobulin class. Gamma (γ) chains specify IgG, mu (μ) chains specify IgM, and so on. Each of the classes can contain either a kappa (κ) or lambda (λ) set of light chains. IgA and IgM can contain a J chain. Only IgA can have a secretory component, also known as a T (transport) chain.

13–D. The classic cascade consists of the sequential activation of C1, C4, C2, C3, C5, C6, C7, C8, and C9. The formation of C4b and C2a in the presence of Mg^{2+} allows for cleavage of the C3 moiety.

14–E. IL-1 plays no known role in the release of mast-cell contents. Complement activation and release of C3a and C5a cause mast-cell activity, as does cross-linking IgE bound to the mast-cell surface.

15–A. Vasculitis and antinuclear antibody are hallmarks of SLE, as is a "lumpy-bumpy" deposition of immune complexes on and behind the glomerular basement membrane. A linear deposition occurs only when the antigen is part of this membrane, as in Goodpasture's nephritis. Rheumatoid factors are frequently present in SLE.

16–D. Rheumatoid factor is an IgM molecule with a specificity for the Fc portion of endogenous IgG.

17–D. Increased IgG in the cerebrospinal fluid is a typical finding in multiple sclerosis patients, along with mononuclear infiltration in the CNS and a decrease in suppressor T-cell function. Autoanti-bodies to the intrinsic factor and a loss in vitamin B_{12} uptake characterize pernicious anemia.

18–B. Immunity to *Candida* is predominately cell-mediated; thus, susceptibility is increased in in-stances of depressed T-cell function, as in congenital thymic aplasia (DiGeorge syndrome).

19–D. In chronic granulomatous disease, the inability to kill ingested microorganisms, rather than a defect in simple phagocytosis, is the dominant malfunction. There is no evidence for a loss of complement components or immunoglobulins.

20–C. SCID is a devastating terminal disease involving a lesion in the stem-cell population, such that lymphoid tissue does not form. Fifty percent of patients with SCID exhibit a loss in adenosine deaminase activity. A loss in NADPH, on the other hand, characterizes the neutrophils in chronic granulomatous disease. The normal condition of transient hypogammaglobulinemia of infancy is characterized by a temporary low rate of synthesis of secretable immunoglobulin in newborn infants from approximately age 3 to 6 months.

21–A. Generally, suppressor cell function and cellular immunity are diminished in the elderly. As a result, IL-2 levels diminish.

22–C. Complement is the key mediator of the glomerulonephritis and vasculitis induced by immune complex (type III) hypersensitivity reactions.

23–D. Complement consists of components C1–C9 plus factors B and D, properdin, and numerous control proteins. These globulins constitute at least 10% of the total pool but are not immunoglobulins.

24–C. Calcium holds the C1 components together. Chelation of Ca^{2+} leads to the dissolution of C1 into its Clq, Clr, and Cls subunits.

25–A. IgG is the only immunoglobulin that passes the placental barrier. Anti-Rh antibody of the IgG type readily crosses the placenta and causes erythroblastosis fetalis. IgM does not pass the placenta nor do the majority of natural isohemagglutinins (IgM molecules predominately).

26–C. A heterozygous individual, by definition, would be Dd with respect to Rh. An Rh-negative female would be dd. A Dd x dd cross would allow for 50% of the offspring to be Rh positive.

27–D. Antibody molecules are composed of two identical H chains and two identical L chains held together by disulfide bonds. Each antibody molecule has a carbohydrate moiety associated with the H chain. Electrophoretically, the antibody molecules are very heterogeneous, although the majority reside in the γ-globulin fraction.

28–D. Pluripotential stem cells—cells giving rise to reticulocytes, monocytes, and lymphocytes—come from the fetal liver, embryonic yolk sac, and adult bone marrow. The adult spleen is not a hematopoietic organ in humans.

29–D. B cells, or bursal cells, are not involved in the cell-mediated immunity.

30–B. T cells arise from stem cells in the bone marrow, and they mature in the thymus. They are the main type of lymphocyte in the circulation, are involved in cell-mediated immunity, and have helping and regulatory functions in humoral immunity.

31–A. IgA is the antibody associated with secretions and mucosal surfaces. Typically, it is an IgA dimer composed of the IgA subclass associated with a J chain and a T piece.

32–B. IgG is the predominant immunoglobulin (approximately 73% of total immunoglobulin) found in the adult.

33–B. Although IgG is not produced to any great extent in utero, IgG is readily passed transplacentally. A 1-day-old infant has adult levels of maternally derived IgG.

34–E. Atopic allergic responses are the realm of IgE (reaginic) antibody.

35–C. The initial immunoglobulin produced in reaction to an antigen is IgM. IgM is also the first immunoglobulin to be synthesized in ontogeny.

36–B. IgG has the longest half-life of the immunoglobulins (21-day average). The shortest half-life is that of IgE, which is approximately 48 hours.

37–D. IL-4 is the major interleukin involved in the shift to IgE production and concomitant stimulation of mast cells. IL-4 is therefore important in the inception and maintenance of type I hypersensitivity reactions.

38–A. Macrophage and macrophage-like cells produce IL-1. (All the other interleukins listed are T-cell products.) Macrophages are also known to produce TNF-γ and several other monokines. Some researchers believe that IL-6 and IL-8 are produced by both T cells and macrophages.

39–C. IL-3 is the major hematopoiesis stimulator of the interleukins listed.

40–A. IL-1, or endogenous pyrogen, is a cytokine released from antigen-processing cells and enhances T-cell responses.

41–G. IFN-γ is a potent stimulator of NK and T-cell activity and enhances the activity of APCs by up-regulating the expression of class II histocompatibility antigens on the APC surface.

42–H. TNF-β, or tumor necrosis factor beta, is manufactured by T cells. TNF-α is a similar molecule produced by macrophages.

43–B. IL-2 was formerly called T-cell growth factor.

44–E. The synthesis of IgA is enhanced by IL-5 production.

45–A. The production of IL-1 by macrophages stimulates production of IL-2 by the targeted T cells as well as the production of IL-2 receptors on these T cells.

46–C. HIV attaches to T cells via the CD4 molecule, which is an integral part of the T helper subset and is normally the receptor for class II histocompatibility antigens. The gp120 molecule probably mimics the class II histocompatibility antigen structure.

47–B. CD3 is a five-chain entity associated with the T-cell receptor. It consists of gamma, delta, and epsilon chains and two zeta chains. After antigen binding, CD3 is probably a transducer of the signal from the T-cell receptor to the internal milieu of the cell.

48–A. CD2 is an adhesion molecule; its natural ligand is LFA-3 (CD58).

49–A. CD2 allows for T-cell rosettes of sheep red blood cells and allows T cells to bind to many other cells and surfaces.

50–E. CD25 is the IL-2 receptor.

51–D. The CD8 molecule, found on all T cytotoxic cells, binds to the class I HLA antigens found on every nucleated cell.

52–C. The CD4 molecule, found on all T helper cells, binds to the class II HLA antigens present on APCs.

53–B. CD3 is invariably part of the T-cell receptor complex. The other constituent is CD4 or CD3.

54–A. Hives, urticaria, and allergy are clinical expressions of a type I (anaphylactic) hypersensitivity reaction.

55–C. Farmer's lung, a type III hypersensitivity reaction, consists of complexes of antibody to inhaled aspergillus mold.

56–B. Addison's disease is characterized by antibody to the adrenal cells and is thus a type II (cytotoxic) hypersensitivity reaction.

57–B. Myasthenia gravis is characterized by antibody directed to muscle acetylcholine receptors and is thus a class II (cytotoxic) hypersensitivity reaction.

58–D. The Mantoux test, which measures the reaction to purified protein derivative of *Mycobacterium tuberculosis*, demonstrates a classic example of a type IV (delayed) hypersensitivity reaction.

59–C. Serum sickness occurs as a result of prophylactic treatment of a patient with foreign immune globulin injection (e.g., horse tetanus antitoxin). This can result in complexes of antibody to the horse antigen and thus an immune complex (type III hypersensitivity) reaction.

60–B. Antibodies directed to red blood cell epitopes cause hemolytic anemia. This is a classic case of a type II (cytotoxic) hypersensitivity reaction.

61–K. Dysgammaglobulinemia commonly results in depressed IgA levels. Patients have a normal number of IgA cells but the cells fail to differentiate into plasma cells.

62–B. Patients with multiple sclerosis generally have increased IgG in the cerebrospinal fluid and demyelinating lesions in the white matter of the CNS. Multiple sclerosis is a chronic relapsing disease.

63–A. Ulcerative colitis is characterized by chronic inflammatory lesions confined to the rectum and colon. The disease is of unknown etiology but patients have antibodies that are cross-reactive with *Escherichia coli*.

64–M. Patients with chronic mucocutaneous candidiasis have normal T-cell absolute numbers. This disorder is characterized by an absence of immunity to *Candida*.

65–I. Congenital agammaglobulinemia, or Bruton's disease, is diagnosed by the absence of tonsils, germinal centers, B cells, and serum Ig of less than 10%. It is a sex-linked (male) disorder characterized by recurrent pyogenic infections and digestive tract disorders that usually begin at age 5 to 6 months.

66–G. SCID is characterized by a genetic defect in stem cells, resulting in absence of the thymus and T cells and B cells. Patients are extremely susceptible to infections and have a short life span.

67–C. Chronic granulomatous disease is characterized by a genetic defect in the nicotinamide adenine dinucleotide phosphate (NADPH) oxidase system. It may be treated with interferon-γ.

68–L. Graves' disease (hyperthyroidism) is characterized by autoantibodies to the thyroid-stimulating hormone receptor and infiltration of the thyroid gland with T cells and B cells.

69–F. Myasthenia gravis is characterized by a defect in neuromuscular transmission resulting in muscle weakness and fatigue. It causes loss of the acetylcholine receptor.

70–D. SLE usually occurs in young women and is an episodic multisystem disease. It is characterized by multiple autoreactive antibodies, the most dominant being antinuclear antibody.

71–H. Pernicious anemia is characterized by autoantibodies to the gastric parietal cell and intrinsic factor. It results in inability to absorb vitamin B_{12}.

72–E. Congenital thymic aplasia, or DiGeorge syndrome, is characterized by the absence of T cells and by hypocalcemia and tetany. It results in a depressed cell-mediated immunity, which permits disease caused by opportunistic organisms.

73–J. Wiskott-Aldrich syndrome is a sex-linked (male) disease. Patients are seen with a triad of thrombocytopenia, eczema, and recurrent infections. It is characterized by a depressed cell-mediated immunity and serum IgM but normal IgG and IgA levels.

Comprehensive Examination

Directions: Each of the numbered items or incomplete statements in this section is followed by answers or by completions of the statement. Select the **one** lettered answer or completion that is **best** in each case.

1. A 72-year-old man is brought to a local homeless shelter. He is obviously underweight and alcoholic. He is complaining of chest pain, fever, shaking chills, cough, and myalgia. The cough is producing rust-colored mucoid sputa. His temperature on admission is 40°C. His white cell count of 16,000 cells/mm^3 is predominantly neutrophils with an overall left shift. An α-hemolytic, lancet-shaped, gram-positive diplococcus is isolated on blood agar. The organism is most likely

(A) *Legionella pneumophila.*
(B) *Klebsiella pneumoniae.*
(C) *Mycoplasma pneumoniae.*
(D) *Neisseria meningitidis.*
(E) *Streptococcus pneumoniae.*

2. Which of the following statements concerning skin rashes associated with virus infections is correct?

(A) They are the result of virus replication in the skin.
(B) They are found with localized virus infections.
(C) They are of little value in the diagnosis of virus infections.
(D) They result from viral replication in macrophages.

3. Stimulation of the Th$_1$ cell population with processed antigen and interleukin-1 (IL-1) can reciprocally activate macrophages if it releases

(A) complement components.
(B) IL-2.
(C) IL-6.
(D) interferon-γ (INF-γ).

4. A 7-year-old child presents with three lesions on his head that are itchy, highly erythematous, and sore to the touch. The most advanced lesion is a boggy, kerion-type lesion. The lesions fluoresce under Wood's lamp examination. Skin scrapings from lesion margins mounted in KOH demonstrate the presence of true hyphae and arthroconidia. Besides treating the infection, what other course of action needs to be taken?

(A) No action needs to be taken; the infection is most likely geophilic and could not have been prevented.
(B) The child's school should be notified because the symptoms are consistent with anthropophilic infections.
(C) Family pets need to be examined and, if lesions are found, the pet must also be treated with antifungal agents.

5. Which of the following statements regarding specialized transduction is true?

(A) The transducing phages are not defective.
(B) Antecedent lysogeny is required to produce specialized transducing particles.
(C) Any bacterial gene can be transduced.
(D) It is carried out by virulent rather than temperate phages.

6. How does *Mycoplasma pneumoniae* differ from *Rickettsia prowazekii?*

(A) It is a prokaryote.
(B) It is dimorphic.
(C) It lacks a cell wall.
(D) It has a single chromosome.

7. CD8 is a surface membrane protein on T cells with which of the following characteristics?

(A) It recognizes class I human leukocyte antigens (HLAs).
(B) It recognizes class II HLA.
(C) It characterizes T helper cells.
(D) It is strongly chemotactic.

8. Which characteristic best delineates pathogenic strains of *Corynebacterium diphtheriae?*

(A) Black to gray colonies on tellurite medium
(B) Plasmid with tox^+ genes
(C) Chromosomal inv^+ genes
(D) Lysogeny with corynebacteriophage-β

9. A 12-year-old boy receives several tick bites while on a long camping trip through the southeastern part of the United States. He develops fever, sore throat, malaise, and a rash on the lower parts of both his arms and legs. When he starts feeling worse and his wrists and ankles begin to swell, the trip chaperon takes him to an urgent care facility. The boy's temperature is 101.5°C. At the top of the differential diagnosis list should be

A. Q fever
B. streptococcal pharyngitis
C. Lyme disease
D. Rocky Mountain spotted fever
E. epidemic typhus

10. The T-cell antigen receptor is associated with which of the following characteristics?

(A) It is a monomeric IgM.
(B) It requires free antigen for triggering.
(C) It is associated with CD4 or CD8.
(D) It is nonspecific.

11. In the following pairs of organisms, which first organism is easiest to distinguish from the second listed in the pair by Gram stain?

(A) *Listeria* and *Proteus*
(B) *Clostridium* and *Lactobacillus*
(C) *Haemophilus* and *Escherichia*
(D) *Corynebacterium* and *Bacillus*
(E) *Salmonella* and *Shigella*

12. Neonatal meningitis is most likely to be caused by which one of the following pairs of organisms?

(A) *Escherichia coli* K1 and *Streptococcus pneumoniae*
(B) *Listeria monocytogenes* and *Haemophilus influenzae*
(C) *Neisseria meningitidis* and *Streptococcus agalactiae*
(D) *E. coli* K1 and group B streptococci
(E) *Listeria* and *E. coli* O157:H7

13. Which of the following statements concerning rotaviruses is true?

(A) They have a single-stranded, circular, negative-sense RNA.
(B) They cause nosocomial infections.
(C) They produce an occupational disease of poultry workers.
(D) They have an arthropod vector.

14. Which of the following statements characterizes neonatal thymectomy?

(A) It depletes the periarteriolar region of the spleen.
(B) It eliminates germinal center formation.
(C) It enhances graft rejection.
(D) It results in autoimmunity.

15. Which of the following statements regarding serodiagnosis of *Treponema pallidum* disease (syphilis) is correct?

(A) The Venereal Disease Research Laboratory (VDRL) test is highly specific and remains positive for life even if the patient is treated with antibiotics.
(B) Biologic false-positive results are more common with the microhemagglutination assay for *T. pallidum* (MHA-TP) than they are with the rapid plasma reagin (RPR) test.
(C) Congenital syphilis can be determined at birth by the IgG fluorescent treponemal antibody-absorption test (FTA-abs).
(D) If early infection or previous infection needs to be documented, the best test is the FTA-abs test.

16. Which of the following organisms is noted for crossing the placenta, resulting in a high mortality rate from disseminated granulomas and abscesses in the fetus?

(A) *Escherichia coli*
(B) *Chlamydia pneumoniae*
(C) *Listeria monocytogenes*
(D) *Mycoplasma pneumoniae*
(E) *Streptococcus agalactiae*

17. Which of the following components is a potent neutrophil chemotactic agent?

(A) C1
(B) C2
(C) C5a
(D) C789 complex

18. What does a positive tuberculin test result indicate?

(A) An antibody titer to *Mycobacterium tuberculosis*
(B) An active infection with *M. tuberculosis*
(C) Previous infection with *M. tuberculosis* or *Mycobacterium bovis*
(D) An active infection with any of the nontuberculosis mycobacteria

19. Which of the following viral oncoproteins is associated with human papillomaviruses?

(A) Large T antigen
(B) E1A protein
(C) E6 protein
(D) TAX protein

20. Which of the following processes is most likely to be inhibited by the presence of extracellular nucleases?

(A) Conjugation
(B) Generalized transduction
(C) Specialized transduction
(D) Transformation
(E) Transposition

21. A patient with acquired immune deficiency syndrome (AIDS) has headaches of increasing severity and mental lethargy. On physical examination, macronodular skin lesions are noted. The cerebrospinal fluid (CSF) is clear, and protein and glucose concentrations are within normal levels. On India ink wet mount, encapsulated yeasts can be seen. Which of the following findings permits rapid confirmation of the identity of the infective organism?

(A) Detection of specific antibodies in the CSF
(B) Detection of polysaccharide capsule in the CSF
(C) Detection of lipo-oligosaccharides in the CSF
(D) Detection of cell-wall antigens in the CSF

22. A deficiency in NADH or NADPH oxidase and increased susceptibility to organisms of low virulence is a characteristic of

(A) chronic granulomatous disease.
(B) angioneurotic edema.
(C) chronic active hepatitis.
(D) Graves' disease.

23. Which of the following statements regarding *Haemophilus* infection and immunity is correct?

(A) Antibodies to type c capsular polysaccharide will prevent most life-threatening pediatric infections with *Haemophilus influenzae*.
(B) IgA protease-producing strains of *H. influenzae* have reduced colonizing ability.
(C) Purulence is a hallmark of *Haemophilus aegyptius* pinkeye.
(D) The primary chancre of *Haemophilus ducreyi* is a hard painful chancre.

24. In which one of the following fungal scalp infections is hair loss most likely to be permanent?

(A) Anthropophilic tinea capitis
(B) Black-dot tinea capitis of adults
(C) Favus (tinea favosa)
(D) Zoophilic tinea capitis

25. Which of the following statements regarding *Neisseria meningitidis* infections is correct?

(A) Skin lesions progress from purpura to petechiae.
(B) Upper respiratory colonization generally precedes meningococcemia.
(C) Meningitis is most commonly detected with culture of cerebrospinal fluid (CSF).
(D) Jarisch-Herxheimer reaction is the fulminating form of meningococcemia with adrenal insufficiency.
(E) The septicemia rarely spreads to organs other than the meninges.

26. Assuming that route and concentration of the inocula are equivalent, which one of the following inocula would be most antigenic in a normal immunocompetent host?

(A) Homologous red blood cells
(B) Homologous serum protein
(C) Heterologous carbohydrate
(D) Heterologous serum protein
(E) 2,4 Dinitrobenzene

27. Which of the following proteins is associated with the *v-src* oncogene of Rous sarcoma virus?

(A) Protein kinase
(B) Growth factor
(C) DNA-binding protein
(D) G protein

28. The organism isolated from infected mosquito bites in a child is a gram-positive coccus that is β-hemolytic, catalase-positive, and coagulase-positive. Which organism was most likely isolated?

(A) Group A streptococcus
(B) Group B streptococcus
(C) *Staphylococcus aureus*
(D) *Staphylococcus epidermidis*

29. Immunocompromised patients are frequently given specific human gamma globulin for protection from a specific viral disease. Which of the viruses listed below is the targeted virus?

(A) Varicella-zoster virus
(B) Poliovirus
(C) Herpes simplex virus
(D) Influenza virus

30. It is assumed that the genes for pyelonephritis-associated pili and a chromosomal drug resistance and sensitivity to amikacin are located close to the origin of transfer for the F-factor and are among the first chromosomal genes transferred in the following cross. Conjugation occurs between the following two *E. coli: pap*$^+$ ami^s Hfr cell x *pap*$^-$ ami^r recA$^+$ F$^-$ cell.
Which is the most likely outcome?

(A) Both cells will be F$^+$, but there will be no change in the *pap* and *ami* genes for either cell.
(B) Both cells will be Hfr, with the possibility that both may be *pap*$^+$ ami^s.
(C) The Hfr cell will remain Hfr but may become *pap*$^+$ ami^r. The F$^-$ cell remains F$^-$ but may become *pap*$^+$ ami^r.
(D) The Hfr cell will stay Hfr and *pap*$^+$ ami^s. The F$^-$ cell remains F$^-$ but may become *pap*$^+$ ami^r.

31. Which of the following organisms is most likely to cause infection with hypovolemic shock?

(A) *Campylobacter jejuni*
(B) *Vibrio cholerae*
(C) *Salmonella typhi*
(D) *Vibrio parahaemolyticus*

32. Vascular inflammation and glomerulonephritis induced by autoantibodies are characteristic of

(A) Arthus reaction.
(B) angioneurotic edema.
(C) systemic lupus erythematosus.
(D) hemolytic anemia.

33. Which of the following terms identifies a virus infection in which the infectious virus is continuously present for an extended, perhaps lifelong, period?

(A) Congenital
(B) Persistent
(C) Latent
(D) Slow

34. In which of the following phases of growth is a gram-positive bacterium most susceptible to the action of penicillin?

(A) Lag
(B) Exponential
(C) Stationary
(D) Decline

35. Which one of the following organisms produces a blue-green pus?

(A) *Aspergillus*
(B) *Staphylococcus aureus*
(C) *Streptococcus pyogenes*
(D) *Pseudomonas aeruginosa*

36. Which one of the following pairs of toxins has similar molecular mechanisms of action but different cellular targets?

(A) Scarlet fever toxin and *Neisseria meningitidis* toxin
(B) Pertussis toxin and *Pseudomonas aeruginosa* exotoxin A
(C) Botulism toxin and tetanus toxin
(D) Shiga toxin and *Escherichia coli* LT

37. Beta-lactamase production is a major problem in which one of the following organisms?

(A) *Corynebacterium diphtheriae*
(B) *Neisseria meningitidis*
(C) *Staphylococcus aureus*
(D) *Treponema pallidum*

38. Which of the following molecules is genetically encoded on only one chromosome?

(A) IgG
(B) IgM
(C) T-cell receptor
(D) HLA-B
(E) HLA-DR

39. Which of the following statements about the prevention of clostridial infections is correct?

(A) The low incidence of spores in the environment makes prevention difficult.
(B) Tetanus vaccine should not be given to pregnant women.
(C) In developing countries, the incidence of neonatal tetanus can be minimized by ensuring the cleanliness of the umbilical stump.
(D) *Botulinum* vaccine should be given routinely to newborns to prevent infant botulism.
(E) Botulism is spread through inhalation of spores.

40. Which of the following viruses has both a live attenuated and a killed vaccine available?

(A) Measles
(B) Influenza
(C) Rabies
(D) Polio

41. Which one of the following characteristics describes interleukin-1 (IL-1)?

(A) Inhibition of T cells
(B) Initiation of the acute phase reactants
(C) Synthesis restricted to mononuclear phagocytes
(D) Suppression of tumor necrosis factor (TNF)

42. Which of the following statements about the treatment of cholera is correct?

(A) Once treatment is started, recovery is slow and the patient remains sick for a few weeks.
(B) Rice-water stools are highly contagious and provide the primary mechanism of disease spread.
(C) Vaccine should routinely be given to persons traveling to endemic areas.
(D) Treatment should be initiated immediately with oral replacement of fluid and electrolytes.
(E) Patients can be treated at home.

43. Which of the following statements concerning $\gamma_2 \kappa_2$ antibody is true?

(A) It contains a J chain.
(B) It contains a secretory piece.
(C) It contains a hypervariable region.
(D) It is the initial antibody synthesized after antigen.

44. The initial host defense mechanism that occurs at the first site of primary virus infection is

(A) inflammation.
(B) IgM antibody production.
(C) sensitized T-cell production.
(D) interferon production.

45. Which of the following genetic mechanisms is responsible for the conversion of nontoxigenic strains of *Corynebacterium diphtheriae* to toxigenic strains?

(A) Lysogenic phage conversion
(B) In vivo transformation
(C) Reciprocal genetic recombination
(D) Conjugation

46. Which one of the following characteristics concerning influenza A virus is correct?

(A) It can cause generalized infections.
(B) It has the capacity to undergo genetic reassortment.
(C) It can cause encephalitis.
(D) It has a nonsegmented, negative-sense genome.

47. Which of the following conditions is an inflammatory response (caused by antibodies reacting with parietal cells of gastric mucosa) that results in depressed acid secretion and atrophic gastritis?

(A) Serum sickness
(B) Amyloidosis
(C) Pernicious anemia
(D) Ulcerative colitis

48. Which of the following statements about Lyme disease and its prevention and treatment is correct?

(A) All three stages of this disease, like syphilis, are relatively easy to cure with appropriate antibiotic therapy.
(B) The endemic area in the United States is the West Coast.
(C) Spread to humans occurs through fleas or lice.
(D) The highest incidence of stage 1 disease occurs in the summer.

49. In a cross with an F^+ cell and an F^- cell

(A) only the chromosomal genes are transferred.
(B) only the plasmid genes are transferred.
(C) all of the plasmid and chromosomal genes are transferred.
(D) neither the plasmid nor chromosomal genes are transferred.

50. Miliary tuberculosis is most often the result of spread via

(A) the bloodstream.
(B) nerves.
(C) contiguous spread through the tissues.
(D) the lymphatics.

51. Which of the following statements characterizes the $(Fab')_2$ fragment of antibody?

(A) It cannot precipitate with antigen.
(B) It contains both light and heavy chain domains.
(C) It activates the first component of complement.
(D) It binds to mast cells to release histamine.

52. Which of the following phrases best describes a prophage?

(A) A phage that lacks receptors
(B) A cell-wall–attached phage that has released its DNA
(C) A newly assembled intracellular phage particle
(D) Intracellular temperate phage DNA

53. Which of the following statements about endogenous type C viruses is correct?

(A) They are defective viruses.
(B) They are pathogenic for their hosts.
(C) They cause tumors in their hosts.
(D) They have a provirus form.

54. Anti-A isohemagglutinins are present in persons with which one of the following blood types?

(A) Type A
(B) Type B
(C) Type AB

55. Which of the following terms best describes bacteria that can use fermentation pathways and contains superoxide dismutase?

(A) Obligate aerobe
(B) Obligate anaerobe
(C) Facultative anaerobe
(D) Aerobic heterotroph

56. Which of the following tests is the most sensitive type of serologic test?

(A) Virus neutralization
(B) Enzyme-linked immunosorbent assay (ELISA)
(C) Nucleic acid hybridization
(D) Hemadsorption

57. Division and differentiation of B cells leading to production of plasma cells require

(A) CD4 and CD8.
(B) interleukin (IL)-1 and IL-3.
(C) IL-1.
(D) IL-4 and IL-6.

58. Endotoxic activity is associated with

(A) catalase.
(B) lipid A.
(C) flagella from gram-negative bacteria.
(D) the O-specific polysaccharide side chain of gram-negative bacteria.

59. Which of the following statements correctly applies to the infectious virus particle of a naked virus?

(A) It contains lipases necessary for infection.
(B) It is called a viroid.
(C) It contains attachment (receptor) proteins.
(D) It may be inactivated by treatment with nucleases.

60. Which of the following statements about the treatment and prevention of whooping cough is correct?

(A) The catarrhal stage is highly contagious.
(B) Residual cough after antibiotic treatment indicates treatment failure; treatment with a different antibiotic should be attempted.
(C) Secondary bacterial infections are infrequent during the paroxysmal stage.
(D) Vaccine causes severe side effects in 1 of 10,000 recipients; the vaccine should not be given routinely.

61. Which of the following agents interferes with membrane structure?

(A) Phenols
(B) Detergents
(C) Soaps
(D) Organic solvents
(E) All of the above

62. A bacterial growth medium that contains penicillin is a

(A) minimal medium.
(B) differential medium.
(C) selective medium.
(D) complex medium.

63. Which of the following statements concerning *Chlamydia trachomatis* is correct?

(A) It is the most common bacterial sexually transmitted disease among college populations.
(B) It is an intracellular-dwelling virus.
(C) It rarely induces the carrier state.
(D) It is a motile one-cell animal parasite.

64. Which of the following statements concerning streptococci is correct?

(A) They are gram-negative cocci usually strung in chains.
(B) They possess an endotoxin.
(C) They are generally resistant to penicillin.
(D) They attach to mucosal surfaces via fimbriae.

65. The region containing the greatest number of antigenic epitopes in gram-negative bacteria is

(A) mucopeptide.
(B) lipid A.
(C) teichoic acids.
(D) O side chains.

66. Which of the following therapies has been demonstrated to be most effective in combating acquired immune deficiency syndrome (AIDS)?

(A) Vaccination to gp18
(B) Injection of RNase
(C) Heat-activated virus
(D) Zidovudine therapy
(E) Vaccination to gp120

67. The number of live bacteria in a sample is best determined by

(A) turbidity measurement.
(B) viable count.
(C) dry weight.
(D) protein measurement.

68. Which one of the following clinical manifestations of *Neisseria gonorrhoeae* is correct?

(A) Pharyngeal infection is always mild and mimics viral sore throat.
(B) Dermatitis involves rash over the trunk and extremities.
(C) Ophthalmia neonatorum is always mild.
(D) Both men and women can be asymptomatic.
(E) Urethral symptoms are painless.

69. Which of the following statements characterizes idiotypic determinants?

(A) They are found in the Fc fragment of immunoglobulins.
(B) They are found on protein antigens.
(C) They can be antigenic.
(D) They are responsible for rejection of transplants.

70. Which of the following would be found in the urine of patients with multiple myeloma?

(A) Bence Jones proteins
(B) Complement components
(C) Heavy chains
(D) Fc fragments

Directions: Each of the numbered items or incomplete statements in this section is negatively phrased, as indicated by a capitalized word such as NOT, LEAST, or EXCEPT. Select the **one** lettered answer that is **best** in each case.

71. All of the following statements concerning respiratory syncytial virus are correct EXCEPT

(A) it belongs to the paramyxovirus family.
(B) it is the major cause of severe pneumonia in infants.
(C) it can cause severe infections that may be treated with ribavirin.
(D) it has a large surface glycoprotein with hemagglutination and neuraminidase activity.

72. A patient with sickle cell anemia is least likely to have repeated septicemias with

(A) *Escherichia coli.*
(B) *Haemophilus influenzae.*
(C) *Neisseria meningitidis.*
(D) *Salmonella enteritidis.*
(E) *Streptococcus pneumoniae.*

73. Mononucleosis or mononucleosis-like disease may occur with infections with all of the following organisms EXCEPT

(A) Epstein-Barr virus.
(B) *Bordetella pertussis.*
(C) human immunodeficiency virus (HIV).
(D) *Listeria monocytogenes.*

74. IgA proteases play a role in colonization in all of the following organisms EXCEPT

(A) *Haemophilus influenzae.*
(B) *Chlamydia psittaci.*
(C) *Neisseria gonorrhoeae.*
(D) *Neisseria meningitidis.*
(E) *Streptococcus pneumoniae.*

75. All of the following characteristics are advantages of live attenuated virus vaccines EXCEPT they

(A) are given by the natural route of infection.
(B) induce an effective cell-mediated response.
(C) are usually administered in a single dose.
(D) are stable with no possibility to change virulence.

76. All of the following statements regarding the transfer of drug resistance in the Enterobacteriaceae are true EXCEPT

(A) only one strand of the R-factor DNA is transferred.
(B) drug resistance may be exchanged with both parents donating to the other.
(C) *tra* region genes coding for functions such as pili synthesis and conjugal DNA metabolism must be present.
(D) transfer in nature is rarely by transformation.

77. All of the following media are differential EXCEPT

(A) tellurite agar.
(B) eosin-methylene blue agar.
(C) MacConkey agar.
(D) Mueller-Hinton agar.

78. All of the following statements regarding plague transmission and progression are true EXCEPT

(A) plague patients should be considered contagious because of potential respiratory droplet transmission.
(B) hallmarks of bubonic plague include rapid elevation in temperature and erythema nodosum.
(C) death in 3 to 5 days in untreated patients is from vascular collapse and disseminated intravascular coagulation.
(D) plague is endemic in the southwestern areas of the United States where it is maintained in wild rodent populations and transmitted to humans by flea bites.

79. Capsules play important roles in all of the following diseases EXCEPT

(A) cryptococcoses.
(B) gonorrhea.
(C) *Haemophilus* meningitis.
(D) meningococcemia.
(E) pneumococcal pneumonia.

80. All of the following statements concerning acute clinical viral disease are true EXCEPT

(A) it occurs whenever a virus enters the body.
(B) its virulence depends on the size of viral inoculum.
(C) it involves specific target organs.
(D) it has relatively short incubation periods.

81. Exotoxins play the dominant role in the pathogenesis of each of the following diseases EXCEPT

(A) cholera.
(B) diphtheria.
(C) gastroenteritis caused by enterotoxigenic *Escherichia coli*.
(D) pertussis.
(E) plague.

82. All of the following are properties of INF-γ EXCEPT

(A) induction of 2′,5′-adenyl synthetase.
(B) host cell–specific gene product.
(C) direct inactivation of eIF-2.
(D) toxic side effects when used clinically.

83. Assuming that route and concentration of inocula are appropriate, an immune response is expected to all of the following EXCEPT

(A) 2,4 dinitrobenzene.
(B) heterologous red blood cells.
(C) heterologous carbohydrates.
(D) heterologous enzymes.
(E) heterologous immunoglobulins.

84. All of the following retroviruses are members of the oncovirus group EXCEPT

(A) human T-cell lymphotrophic virus II.
(B) feline sarcoma virus.
(C) human immunodeficiency virus.
(D) Friend leukemia virus.

85. All of the following statements concerning viral gastroenteritis are correct EXCEPT

(A) it is caused by enveloped viruses.
(B) it is associated with RNA viruses.
(C) it is observed to occur in epidemics.
(D) it is often diagnosed by enzyme-linked immunosorbent assay on fecal samples.

86. All of the following statements about legionnaires' disease are true EXCEPT

(A) it often occurs in epidemics.
(B) it is not contagious.
(C) smokers and nonsmokers are equally affected.
(D) it usually occurs with abrupt onset of headache, fever, chills, malaise, and unproductive cough.
(E) it can be diagnosed by direct fluorescent antibody staining of specimens.

87. All of the following molecules are within the immunoglobulin superfamily EXCEPT

(A) T-cell receptor.
(B) immunoglobulin E.
(C) HLA-A and other class I histocompatibility antigens.
(D) HLA-DR and other class II histocompatibility antigens.
(E) C4 and other class III histocompatibility antigens.

88. All of the following statements about exotoxins are true EXCEPT

(A) they are heat stable at 100°C.
(B) they are produced by both gram-positive and gram-negative bacteria.
(C) they may be neutralized by antitoxins.
(D) they are proteins.

89. The role of macrophages in the immune response includes all of the following functions EXCEPT

(A) antigen engulfment.
(B) production of IL-1.
(C) production of IL-2.
(D) production of endogenous pyrogen.
(E) presentation of antigen in context of class II histocompatibility antigens.

90. CD4 cells are involved in all of the following processes EXCEPT

(A) acting as a "helper function" for B cells.
(B) processing and presenting antigens.
(C) producing and releasing interleukin-2.
(D) regulating intensity of NK cell and null cell activity.
(E) producing and releasing IFN-γ.

91. All of the following statements about the clinical manifestations of syphilis are correct EXCEPT

(A) it is characterized by vascular involvement.
(B) *Treponema pallidum* causes soft chancre.
(C) secondary stage infects most tissues of the body.
(D) tertiary syphilis is fatal.
(E) secondary stage may recur if untreated.

92. B cells can be involved in all of the following processes EXCEPT

(A) capping and internalization of antigen bound by surface immunoglobulin receptors.
(B) antigen processing and presentation.
(C) production and release of IFN-γ.
(D) maturation to plasma cells.
(E) expression of class II histocompatibility antigens on cell surface.

93. All of the following statements about *Neisseria meningitidis* are true EXCEPT

(A) the organism ferments glucose and maltose.
(B) capsular polysaccharide is detected in serum or cerebrospinal fluid in disseminated infections.
(C) it produces meningitis, primarily in children age 6 months to 2 years.
(D) it is a hardy organism that requires no special laboratory identification procedure.
(E) the organism possesses an endotoxin and is oxidase positive.

94. All of the following statements concerning viral hepatitis are correct EXCEPT it

(A) may be caused by a circular, double-stranded DNA virus.
(B) may be diagnosed by an enzyme-linked immunosorbent assay (ELISA).
(C) is an example of a latent infection.
(D) may be caused by several distinct types of viruses.

95. All of the following statements concerning clinical manifestations of *Neisseria meningitidis* are true EXCEPT

(A) rapid progression of the disease requires prompt treatment without waiting for laboratory identification of the organism.
(B) vasculitic purpura is a key diagnostic finding.
(C) early rash may be confused with Rocky Mountain spotted fever, secondary syphilis, rubella, or rubeola.
(D) there are no severe sequelae after recovery.

96. All of the following compounds are mitogens that stimulate human T cells to proliferate EXCEPT

(A) lipopolysaccharide.
(B) concanavalin A.
(C) pokeweed mitogen.
(D) phytohemagglutinin.

97. All of the following statements about clinical manifestations of diphtheria are correct EXCEPT

(A) cutaneous infection may spread to another patient and cause pharyngeal diphtheria.
(B) bull neck appearance is characteristic.
(C) two major areas of damage due to exotoxin are the heart and nerves.
(D) early symptoms include a mild fever.
(E) after infecting the pharyngeal area, organisms enter the bloodstream and invade other tissues.

98. All of the following substances are T-independent antigens EXCEPT

(A) endotoxin.
(B) lipopolysaccharide.
(C) polymerized flagellin.
(D) phytohemagglutinin.
(E) Epstein-Barr virus.

99. The human immunodeficiency virus (HIV)-1 has been shown to be transmitted by all of the following mechanisms EXCEPT

(A) sexual contact.
(B) perinatal infection.
(C) shared needles.
(D) mosquitoes.
(E) blood transfusion.

100. All of the following substances are mediators of immediate (type I) hypersensitivity EXCEPT

(A) histamine.
(B) anaphylatoxins.
(C) slow-reacting substance of anaphylaxis.
(D) eosinophilic chemotactic factor of anaphylaxis.
(E) kinins.

101. A typical antibody molecule has all of the following characteristics EXCEPT it

(A) consists of at least two identical heavy and two identical light chains.
(B) has at least two antigen-binding sites.
(C) has only one specificity for antigen.
(D) is a glycosylated molecule.
(E) has two constant domains on each of the heavy chains.

Directions: Each group of items in this section consists of lettered options followed by a set of numbered items. For each item, select the **one** lettered option that is most closely associated with it. Each lettered option may be selected once, more than once, or not at all.

Questions 102–105

Match each pathogen with the factor that is best correlated with virulence.

(A) Adhesions
(B) Capsule
(C) Intracellular replication
(D) Exotoxin that inhibits protein synthesis through blocking EF-2
(E) Exotoxin that causes increase in cyclic adenosine monophosphate (cAMP)
(F) Exotoxin that inhibits protein synthesis through binding to the 60S ribosomal subunit
(G) V and W antigens
(H) X and V factors

102. *Yersinia pestis*

103. *Escherichia coli* (causing traveler's diarrhea)

104. *Francisella tularensis*

105. *Haemophilus influenzae* type B

Questions 106–110

Match each characteristic with the structure that is related to it.

(A) Outer membrane
(B) Mesosome
(C) Peptidoglycan
(D) Capsule
(E) Lipopolysaccharide
(F) Teichoic acid
(G) Lipoprotein

106. Is found only in gram-positive bacteria

107. Is also called endotoxin

108. Contains *N*-acetylmuramic acid

109. Contains O antigen

110. Protects bacteria from phagocytosis

Questions 111–114

Match each action with the appropriate antiviral agent.

(A) Interferon
(B) Foscarnet
(C) Acyclovir
(D) Zidovudine
(E) Cytarabine
(F) Ribavirin
(G) Amantadine
(H) Vidarabine

111. Nucleoside analogue that inhibits reverse transcriptase

112. Blocks virus penetration and uncoating of influenza A virus

113. Non-nucleoside analogue that inhibits herpesvirus DNA

114. Induces 2,5A synthetase

Questions 115–120

Match each disease with its common predisposing condition.

(A) C5–C8 deficiencies
(B) Epstein-Barr virus infection
(C) Hepatitis A infection
(D) Hepatitis B infection
(E) Hepatitis D infection
(F) Influenza infection
(G) Ketoacidotic diabetes
(H) Severe neutropenia

115. Invasive aspergillosis

116. Repeated *Neisseria meningitidis* infections

117. *Streptococcus pneumoniae* pneumonia

118. Rhinocerebral *Mucor* infection (zygomycosis)

119. Nasal carcinoma

120. Hepatocellular carcinoma

Questions 121–124

Match each of the cell types with the appropriate cell surface markers.

(A) $CD2^-$ $CD3^-$ $CD4^-$ $CD8^-$ TCR^- cell
(B) $CD2^+$ $CD3^+$ $CD4^-$ $CD8^-$ TCR^+ cell
(C) $CD2^+$ $CD3^+$ $CD4^+$ $CD8^-$ TCR^+ cell
(D) $CD2^+$ $CD3^+$ $CD4^-$ $CD8^+$ TCR^+ cell
(E) $CD2^+$ $CD3^+$ $CD4^+$ $CD8^+$ TCR^+ cell

121. Pre–T cell

122. T helper cell

123. T cytotoxic cell

124. T lymphocyte immediately before differentiation into T-helper and T-cytotoxic cells

Questions 125–128

Match the characteristic below with the gram-positive organism that is associated with it.

(A) *Enterococcus faecalis*
(B) *Staphylococcus aureus*
(C) *Staphylococcus epidermidis*
(D) *Streptococcus agalactiae*
(E) *Streptococcus pneumoniae*
(F) *Streptococcus pyogenes*
(G) *Streptococcus viridans*

125. Biofilm that adheres to intravenous catheters

126. M protein that is typeable

127. Bile solubility

128. Attachment to damaged heart valve in patients after bowel surgery

Questions 129–132

Match each distinguishing characteristic with the appropriate virus.

(A) Respiratory syncytial virus
(B) Parvovirus
(C) Reovirus
(D) Parainfluenza virus
(E) Bunyavirus
(F) Arenavirus

129. Induces characteristic giant, multinucleated cells

130. Has arthropod vectors

131. Has a segmented, ambisense genome

132. Causes croup

Questions 133–135

Match each of the following characteristics with the complement component most closely related to it.

(A) C5b
(B) C5a
(C) C1qrs
(D) C4b2a
(E) C2b

133. Anaphylatoxin

134. C3 convertase

135. Attaches to Fc of IgM

Questions 136–139

Match the characteristic with the anaerobe it best describes.

(A) *Bacteroides* species
(B) *Clostridium botulinum*
(C) *Clostridium difficile*
(D) *Clostridium perfringens*
(E) *Clostridium tetani*
(F) *Escherichia coli*

136. Most common organism in the human gastrointestinal tract

137. Most likely organism to overgrow the gastrointestinal tract during antibiotic treatment and cause gastroenteritis

138. Most likely agent to cause a flaccid paralysis, which may lead to respiratory arrest in a 5-month-old child

139. Most likely to cause urinary tract infections

Questions 140–143

For each disease, choose the most appropriate and effective method for reducing its transmission.

(A) Avoid intravenous drug abuse
(B) Avoid swimming in contaminated water
(C) Avoid using human excrement as vegetable fertilizer
(D) Cook fish and seafood thoroughly
(E) Heat all canned foods to 60°C for 10 minutes
(F) Avoid cat litter or take proper care in changing litter
(G) Wear shoes outside in endemic regions

140. Toxoplasmosis

141. Amebic meningoencephalitis

142. *Vibrio parahaemolyticus* gastroenteritis

143. Hookworm infections

Questions 144–147

Match each description with the disease that is associated with it.

(A) Infectious hepatitis
(B) Measles
(C) Serum hepatitis
(D) Infectious mononucleosis
(E) Shingles
(F) German measles

144. Is caused by a virus that uses a reverse transcriptase during replication

145. Is associated with congenital infections

146. Can occur during immunosuppression

147. Can be associated with the delta agent

Questions 148–155

Match each of the following characteristics with the cell type most closely related to it.

(A) CD4$^+$ cell
(B) CD8$^+$ cell
(C) Mature B cell
(D) Plasma cell
(E) Natural killer (NK) cell
(F) Null (K) cell
(G) Monocyte–macrophage

148. Cell involved in antibody-dependent cell cytotoxicity

149. Cell actively secreting a specific idiotype of antibody

150. Cell involved in recognition of antigen in context of class II histocompatibility antigen

151. Cell interacting directly with antigen-presenting cells (APCs)

152. Cell capable of attacking a certain tumor cell spontaneously (i.e., without prior sensitization)

153. Cell involved in antigen processing and presentation

154. Cell with surface IgM and surface IgD

155. Cell involved in recognition of antigen in context of class I histocompatibility antigen

Questions 156–159

Match the condition described below with the causative agent.

(A) *Bacillus cereus*
(B) *Giardia lamblia*
(C) Norwalk agent
(D) Rotavirus
(E) *Salmonella enteritidis*
(F) *Staphylococcus aureus*
(G) *Vibrio parahaemolyticus*

156. Prolonged (6 days) watery diarrhea with no neutrophils in a 6-month-old child; causative agent is a double-stranded RNA virus.

157. Diarrhea associated with pale greasy stools, maladsorption, and severe cramping; probably acquired from drinking untreated stream water on a recent Canadian camping trip.

158. Patient with explosive watery, noninflammatory diarrhea with headache, abdominal cramps, nausea, vomiting, and fever. Symptoms began the day after eating raw oysters in August.

159. Outbreak of watery diarrhea in 6 members of a party of 20 who ate at a Chinese restaurant the day before. Fried rice was implicated.

Questions 160–163

For each patient, select the microorganism that is most likely to have caused the illness described.

(A) *Coccidioides immitis*
(B) Coxsackie A virus
(C) *Haemophilus ducreyi*
(D) *Histoplasma capsulatum*
(E) *Neisseria gonorrhoeae*
(F) *Neisseria meningitidis*
(G) *Streptococcus pyogenes*
(H) *Rickettsia prowazekii*
(I) *Rickettsia rickettsii*
(J) *Treponema pallidum*

160. A 30-year-old male homosexual is seen with an indurated penile ulcer that he reports began as a hard nodule. It is not painful. Regional lymphadenopathy is noted.

161. A 6-year-old girl has a temperature of 38.5°C, a sore throat, difficulty swallowing, and vomiting. Examination reveals the soft palate and posterior oral cavity are reddened with vesicular lesions. No tonsillar abscesses or exudate is seen.

162. A 9-year-old boy from South Carolina is seen with fever, sore throat, malaise, and a macular rash that began on his hands and feet (palms and soles, respectively) and that is progressing inward. There is swelling of both ankles and wrists. A wood tick (*Dermacentor*) was removed 6 days earlier.

163. A 16-year-old girl, who recently moved to southern California from Montana, is seen in late August with cough, malaise, low-grade fever, myalgias, and erythema nodosum on her shins. Rales are heard and respiratory infiltrates are noted on radiograph.

Questions 164–166

Match each of the following descriptions with the appropriate viral gene or gene product.

(A) Delta hemagglutinin
(B) E1A protein
(C) Large T antigen
(D) TAT protein
(E) VCA protein
(F) TAX protein
(G) Matrix protein

164. Transactivating transcriptional activator of human T-cell lymphotrophic virus I (HTLV-I)

165. Found in infectious mononucleosis patients

166. Viral receptor of reoviruses

Questions 167–170

Match the distinguishing characteristic below with the tumor virus to which it best applies.

(A) Mouse mammary tumor virus
(B) Rous sarcoma virus
(C) Polyomavirus
(D) Human T lymphotrophic virus
(E) Hepatitis B virus
(F) Harvey sarcoma virus

167. Has an oncogene that codes for a guanine-nucleotide–binding protein

168. Does not use a reverse transcriptase during replication

169. Lacks a functional virogene

170. Is a type B RNA tumor virus

Questions 171–174

Match the characteristic to the appropriate antibiotic.

(A) Tetracycline
(B) Cephalosporin
(C) Streptomycin
(D) Erythromycin
(E) Griseofulvin
(F) Bacitracin
(G) Chloramphenicol

171. Causes misreading of mRNA

172. Has a beta-lactam ring in its structure

173. Fungistatic drug

174. Bactericidal for gram-negative bacteria

Questions 175–178

Match the following microorganisms to the vector that is responsible for its transmission.

(A) Lice—genus *Pediculus*
(B) Mites
(C) Mosquitoes—genus *Aedes*
(D) Mosquitoes—genus *Anopheles*
(E) Reduviidae bugs
(F) Sandflies
(G) Ticks—genus *Dermacentor*
(H) Ticks—genus *Ixodes*
(I) Tsetse fly

175. *Borrelia burgdorferi*

176. *Leishmania donovani*

177. Orbivirus

178. *Rickettsia prowazekii*

Questions 179–184

Match each case with the morphologic description of the causative agent.

(A) Acid-fast organism
(B) Dimorphic fungus
(C) DWA virus
(D) Filamentous fungus
(E) Gram-positive coccus
(F) Gram-negative coccus
(G) Gram-negative rod
(H) Helminth
(I) Mycoplasma
(J) Prion
(K) Protozoan
(L) Viroid

179. A 45-year-old man has mental degeneration after a prolonged but inapparent infection; at autopsy, a subacute spongiform encephalopathy is found.

180. A patient in the terminal stage of acquired immune deficiency syndrome (AIDS) has a pulmonary infection caused by an organism that requires 4 weeks to grow on Löwenstein-Jensen medium.

181. Symptoms of liver damage and a blocked bile duct develop in a patient who has just received general anesthesia.

182. A 27-year-old South African gold miner is seen with subcutaneous nodular lesions along the lymphatics from the initial site of trauma caused by a mine timber sliver.

183. A 14-year-old boy has pneumonia with a severe, prolonged hacking cough; Stevens-Johnson syndrome develops during treatment; cold agglutinins develop; the boy is treated appropriately and successfully with erythromycin.

184. A patient with acquired immune deficiency syndrome (AIDS) has severe, nonresolving diarrhea.

Answers and Explanations

1–E. *S. pneumoniae* is the most common causative agent of pneumonia in alcoholics. *K. pneumoniae* is less common (and more deadly). Almost all of the small percentage of patients who do have pneumonia caused by *K. pneumoniae* suffer from chronic lung disease or alcoholism. *Legionella* and *Klebsiella* are both gram-negative rods. *N. meningitidis* is a gram-negative diplococcus. Neither *Legionella* nor *Mycoplasma* would have grown on blood agar.

2–A. Characteristic skin rashes are frequently associated with some generalized or systemic viral infections and result from viral replication in the cells composing the skin.

3–D. INF-γ is the only potent activator of the macrophages listed.

4–C. The highly inflamed nature of the lesion is strongly suggestive of a dermatophyte that was acquired from a family pet. The pet and the child must be treated with antifungal agents such as griseofulvin or oral ketoconazole.

5–B. Temperate phages that can integrate their DNA into the bacterial DNA are the only type of viruses that can carry out specialized transduction. When a state of lysogeny is established, it inserts its DNA into a specific gene region of the bacterial DNA. If the excision process is not perfect, bacterial genes on either side of the integration site can be excised out, replicated with the phage DNA, and integrated into the phage progeny. The progeny, having lost some of their own genes and having picked up bacterial genes, are then capable of specialized transduction. These bacterial genes are then transferred to the next cell which that virus infects (but cannot replicate in). In generalized transduction, which is carried out most commonly by virulent phages, any bacterial gene can be transduced. All transducing phages are defective.

6–C. Both *M. pneumoniae* and *R. prowazekii* are prokaryotic microorganisms, but *M. pneumoniae* lacks a cell wall.

7–A. CD8 recognizes class I HLA selectively. It is found on T suppressor and T cytotoxic cells. CD4 characterizes T helper cells.

8–D. Only toxin-producing strains of *C. diphtheriae* cause diphtheria. The genes directing the production of the toxin are located on molecules of corynebacteriophage-β DNA, which are stable in *C. diphtheriae*. Neither plasmids nor the chromosome contain the genes to direct the synthesis of the toxin. Repressor molecules for the *tox*$^+$ gene are on the chromosome, however. Both toxigenic and nontoxigenic strains of *C. diphtheriae* will be gray to black on tellurite medium.

9–A. The rash associated with *R. rickettsii* originates on the ankles or wrists and spreads to the body trunk.

10–C. The T-cell antigen receptor is specific for antigen bound to an antigen-presenting cell. It is a multicomponent molecule associated with CD3. Transmission of the signal also involves association with major histocompatibility complex (MHC) class II molecules via CD4 and with MHC class I molecules via CD8.

11–A. *Listeria* is a gram-positive rod, whereas *Proteus* is a gram-negative rod. *Clostridium, Lactobacillus, Corynebacterium,* and *Bacillus* are gram-positive rods, whereas *Haemophilus, Escherichia, Salmonella,* and *Shigella* are gram-negative rods.

12–D. *E. coli* (the encapsulated K1 strains) and *S. agalactiae* (group B streptococcus) are the most common causative agents of neonatal meningitis. *Listeria* is a less frequent causative agent of neonatal meningitis and other severe disease in newborns. *H. influenzae* and *N. meningitidis* rarely cause neonatal meningitis. Most pneumococcal pneumonia is in adults, particularly the elderly.

13–B. Rotaviruses are frequently involved in nosocomial infantile diarrhea observed in hospital nurseries. Rotaviruses have 11 segments of double-stranded RNA and are positive-sense viruses, which are not spread by arthropods. Newcastle disease virus, a paramyxovirus, causes an occupational disease of poultry workers.

14–A. A thymic-dependent area of the spleen is the periarteriolar region, whereas the germinal center contains predominantly B lymphocytes. Removal of the thymus aids in graft retention, because the effector T cells would then be missing. It does not result in autoimmunity.

15–D. The FTA-abs test detects the specific antibody that is positive slightly earlier than the reaginic antibody and remains positive with or without antibiotic therapy. VDRL detects the less specific reaginic antibodies, which sometimes decline without treatment. The MHA-TP (like the FTA-abs test) is more specific, whereas the PRP detects the less specific reaginic antibodies. Because IgG can cross the placenta, IgG FTA-abs is not a good indicator of congenital syphilis. However, the test can be modified to measure IgM antibody, which is a better predictor of congenital infection.

16–C. *Listeria* may cause in utero infections or may infect the baby during delivery. In utero infections are generally severe and are characterized by multiple granulomas and abscesses. Except for *M. pneumoniae*, the other organisms listed cause infections acquired during birth.

17–C. C5a promotes chemotaxis. The complement components C1, C2, and the C789 complex do not promote chemotaxis.

18–C. The tuberculin test indicates previous infection with *M. tuberculosis* or *M. bovis* from between several weeks to 5 years. It does not provide proof of current active infection with *M. tuberculosis*. The tuberculin test detects cell-mediated immunity and not antibody. Skin testing for specific antigens for nontuberculous mycobacteria is available.

19–C. The early protein E6 is associated with the oncogenic potential of human papillomavirus.

20–D. In transformation, the DNA is extracellular before it is picked up by the competent cells; during this period, the DNA is subject to the extracellular endonucleases. Because the DNA in generalized and specialized transductions is protected extracellularly by the virus capsid, it is not subject to extracellular endonucleases. In conjugation, the DNA is never outside of a cell. Transposition is a mechanism of inserting a transposon into another molecule of DNA and has no extracellular transport mechanism associated with it.

21–B. *Cryptococcus* is the only medically important yeast with a capsule. The capsule consists of polysaccharide, is antigenic, and diffuses away from the cell in fluids. Antigenic tests used to detect capsules are twice as likely to be positive in cryptococcal meningitis than are the India ink mounts, but some nonencapsulated strains have been isolated from AIDS patients.

22–A. Only patients with chronic granulomatous disease exhibit a deficiency in NADH or NADPH oxidase and increased susceptibility to organisms of low virulence. Chronic granulomatous disease is an inherited condition.

23–C. Purulence is characteristic of acute conjunctivitis. Although most invasive *H. influenzae* disease is caused by type b strains (and therefore not protected for by type c antibodies), the chronic ear infections are usually nontypeable. IgA protease production increases the colonizing ability of *H. influenzae*. The primary chancre of *H. ducreyi* is soft, not hard. It is, however, painful.

24–C. Scarring and permanent hair loss are most likely to occur with favus.

25–B. *Neisseria meningitidis* is an IgA protease producer with a capsule; these virulence factors play a role in the upper respiratory colonization that precedes either meningitis or meningococcemia. Skin lesions develop from petechiae to frank purpura. A presumptive diagnosis of meningitis is almost always made by finding polysaccharide capsule antigens present in the CSF (by some rapid test like latex particle agglutination) or by finding the organisms on Gram stain of the CSF sediment. Definitive diagnosis is made with the growth on chocolate agar of gram-negative, encapsulated diplococci that are oxidase-positive and ferment maltose. The Waterhouse-Friderichsen syndrome, not the Jarisch-Herxheimer reaction, is the fulminating form of meningococcemia.

26–D. Heterologous serum protein would have the greatest antigenicity of the structures listed. It is "foreign," is usually of appropriate weight, and has a very well-defined tertiary and quaternary structure.

27–A. The *v-src* oncogene associated with the Rous sarcoma virus codes for a tyrosine protein kinase with a biologic activity that results in cellular transformation.

28–C. Although groups A and B streptococci and *S. aureus* are β-hemolytic, only the streptococci are catalase-negative. Only *S. aureus* is both β-hemolytic and coagulase-positive.

29–A. Pooled human gamma globulin fractions with specific activity against varicella-zoster virus (varicella-zoster immune globulin) are used for passive immunization of immunocompromised individuals.

30–D. In any conjugal cross, the donor cell does not take up DNA and thus remains as it originally was. The *tra* gene segment (controlling such essential functions as sex pili formation and conjugal DNA metabolism) is essential for a cell to be F$^+$ or Hfr. In any Hfr cross, this region would be transferred last (after all of the chromosomal genes), so it is virtually never transferred. Thus, in an Hfr$^-$ x F$^-$ cross, the F$^-$ cell remains F$^-$. However, a few chromosomal genes are transferred; and because the F$^-$ cell is *recA*$^+$, it may result in new gene combinations, such as *pap*$^+$ *ami*^{r}. This organism is then amikacin-resistant and can cause ascending urinary tract infections.

31–B. The loss of fluids and electrolytes is rapid and most severe with *V. cholerae*. If untreated, this infection may lead to dehydration, hemoconcentration, and hypovolemic shock.

32–C. Glomerulonephritis is a hallmark of patients with systemic lupus erythematosus, which is a vascular inflammation induced by autoantibodies produced by a variety of cellular antigens.

33–B. Persistent virus infections involve the continuous presence of infectious virus for an extended time, which may result in "carrier" individuals. Latent infections persist in the body in a noninfectious form and, unlike persistent infections, are difficult to detect in cells. Slow infections have a prolonged incubation period in which infectious viruses are sometimes produced.

34–B. Gram-positive bacteria would be most susceptible to penicillin in the exponential phase, because this is the phase in which cell-wall synthesis is greatest.

35–D. *P. aeruginosa* produces a blue-green pigment, which is particularly notable in burn wounds infected with *Pseudomonas*.

36–B. Pertussis toxin and *Pseudomonas* exotoxin A are both ADP-ribosylating toxins that irreversibly inactivate EF-2 and inhibit protein synthesis. Although they have similar modes of action, they differ in their target and antigenicity.

37–C. Production of beta-lactamases has become a major problem in *S. aureus* infections. Until antimicrobial susceptibilities are accomplished, treatment should be started with a penicillinase-resistant antibiotic. Because there is little beta-lactam resistance, penicillin G or erythromycin is the accepted drug of choice (along with antitoxin) for *Corynebacterium* diphtherial infections. Penicillin G is the drug of choice for both *N. meningitidis* and *T. pallidum*.

38–E. Of the molecules listed, only the class II histocompatibility antigens (which include HLA-DR, HLA-DQ, and HLA-DS) are totally encoded on one chromosome (chromosome 6). IgG and IgM are encoded on the H chain of chromosome 14 and the kappa chain of chromosome 2 or the lambda chain of chromosome 22. The T-cell receptor is encoded on the alpha chain of chromosome 7 and the beta chain of chromosome 14. The class I histocompatibility antigens are encoded on the alpha chain of chromosome 6 and on the β_2-microglobulin of chromosome 2.

39–C. In developing countries, the incidence of neonatal tetanus can be minimized by ensuring the cleanliness of the umbilical stump. The high incidence of clostridial spores makes prevention extremely difficult. Tetanus vaccine should be given to pregnant women to boost maternal antibodies. A botulism vaccine that seems to be somewhat effective is available for laboratory workers investigating *C. botulinum*, but not for other populations. Botulism is spread in infants by the ingestion of spores and in adults by the ingestion of contaminated food containing the exotoxin.

40–D. Active immunization for poliovirus may involve the use of live attenuated trivalent Sabin vaccine or killed Salk vaccine.

41–B. IL-1 aids in the initiation of the acute phase response to bacterial invasion. It is synthesized by many cell types, activates T cells, and can act synergistically with TNF.

42–B. Rice-water stools are highly contagious and provide the primary mechanism of disease spread. As soon as intravenous fluids and electrolytes are administered, recovery should take place within hours. No effective vaccine is generally available; the choleragen toxin is so potent and fast-acting that vaccine-induced immunity is not helpful. Immediate treatment is by the intravenous route. Patients should be hospitalized.

43–C. All antibodies contain a hypervariable region at which antigen is bound. IgG does not contain a J chain because it is a singular entity. It is preceded in synthesis by IgM. Only IgA contains a secretory piece because it needs to be transported across mucosal surfaces.

44–D. Because interferon is produced in the first cell infected by the virus, it is the first host defense mechanism that occurs in response to a primary virus infection.

45–A. A toxigenic strain of *C. diphtheriae* is produced as a result of lysogenic phage conversion after injection of a temperate bacteriophage into a nontoxigenic strain of the organism.

46–B. Influenza A virus, which causes a localized respiratory infection, has a segmented genome composed of eight pieces of negative-sense, single-stranded RNA, which can "reassort" when two different strains infect the same cell.

47–C. This syndrome is exhibited by patients with pernicious anemia and is not characteristic of the other diseases.

48–D. The highest incidence of Lyme disease correlates with tick season—summer. Spread to humans is primarily by tick bites. Stage 3 can be difficult to eradicate. Lyme disease is endemic in Minnesota, Wisconsin, and the northeastern seaboard of the United States.

49–B. An F^+ cell contains the fertility factor in the free plasmid state. In the cross between an F^+ cell and an F^- cell, chromosomal genes are not transferred because they are not covalently linked to the plasmid. Only the plasmid genes are transferred.

50–A. Miliary tuberculosis results from hematogenous spread of *Mycobacterium tuberculosis*.

51–B. The variable region binding with antigen is comprised of amino acids from both the light and heavy chain domains. Because the $(Fab')_2$ fragment of antibody is bivalent, it can form a lattice with and precipitate antigen. The Fc fragment contains the binding site to the membranes of other cells as well as the site-activating complement.

52–D. The integrated intracellular form of the DNA of a temperate phage is called a prophage.

53–D. Endogenous type C viruses are retroviruses that are not pathogenic for their hosts and often replicate when cells harboring them are placed in culture. Their genetic material exists in a provirus form in host cells.

54–B. The isohemagglutinins (anti-A and anti-B) are found only in individuals who do not possess the homologous antigenic determinant.

55–C. Facultative anaerobes grow in the presence or absence of oxygen; a respiratory mode is used when oxygen is present, and fermentation occurs when it is not. Facultative anaerobes contain the enzyme superoxide dismutase, which aids aerobic growth by preventing the accumulation of the superoxide ion. Obligate aerobes do not have fermentative pathways and require oxygen for growth; obligate anaerobes lack superoxide dismutase. The heterotrophs require preformed organic compounds for growth.

56–B. ELISA tests are approximately 1000-fold more sensitive than the other serologic tests listed. Nucleic acid hybridization is not a type of serologic test.

57–D. Amplification of pre–B cells along the pathway leading to the terminal plasma cell requires IL-4 and IL-6. IL-1 is involved mainly in T-cell activation, and CD4 and CD8 function during interaction of the T cell with antigen-presenting cells.

58–B. Endotoxic activity is associated with lipid A. No toxicity is associated with the O polysaccharides, the flagella from gram-negative bacteria, or catalase.

59–C. The infectious virus particle, which is called a virion, not a viroid, contains viral-specific proteins responsible for attachment to the host cell. It may be inactivated by proteases, not nucleases, and there is no indication that lipases are part of naked virions.

60–A. The catarrhal stage is highly contagious. Residual cough occurs even after successful antibiotic therapy. Severe side effects to the vaccine occur in a low percentage of recipients (1 in more than 300,000 cases); routine immunization of all young children is recommended.

61–E. Phenols, detergents, soaps, and organic solvents all interfere with membrane structure.

62–C. A selective medium permits growth in the presence of agents inhibiting other bacteria. A minimal medium contains the minimum quantity and number of nutrients capable of sustaining growth of the organism, whereas a differential medium differentiates among organisms on the basis of color due to differential fermentation or pH.

63–A. Of the bacteria causing sexually transmitted diseases, the bacterium found most prevalently in college-age students is *C. trachomatis*. It is a small intracellular-dwelling bacterium that often induces the carrier state. *Trichomonas vaginalis* is a motile one-cell parasite.

64–D. Streptococci attach to mucosal surfaces via fimbriae. They are gram-positive cocci that do not possess an endotoxin. Although most are sensitive to penicillin, resistant strains are beginning to emerge, especially *S. pneumoniae*.

65–D. O side chains contain the greatest number of antigenic epitopes in gram-negative bacteria. The mucopeptide, lipid A, and teichoic acids are poorly antigenic because they have few antigenic epitopes.

66–D. Of the treatment methods listed, zidovudine (azidothymidine, AZT) therapy has the best therapeutic value.

67–B. Turbidity, dry weight, and protein are all indirect indexes of the true number of bacteria in a sample. Even viable counts, which measure live bacteria, do not always give a true count because bacteria may clump and aggregate, thus appearing as a single entity.

68–D. Both men and women can be asymptomatic, thus facilitating spread of gonorrhea. Pharyngeal infection can be severe with manifestations similar to a streptococcal sore throat. Dermatitis usually occurs as a simple pustule over the inflamed joint. Ophthalmia neonatorum can be severe and cause blindness. Chlamydial eye infections of newborns are relatively mild and do not impair sight.

69–C. Because idiotypic determinants on antibodies contain amino acid sequences in the $(Fab')_2$ variable regions that are unique to the respondent, they can be antigenic.

70–A. The Bence Jones proteins are dimers of free light chains found in the urine of some patients with multiple myeloma (plasma cell tumors).

71–D. Respiratory syncytial virus is the only member of the paramyxovirus family that lacks the envelope glycoprotein hemagglutinin–neuraminidase.

72–A. Of the organisms listed, all but *E. coli* are noted for causing repeated infections in sickle cell anemia.

73–B. *B. pertussis* is unusual among bacterial infections in that it causes a lymphocytosis. A mononucleosis-like presentation may occur during the first year of HIV infection.

74–B. *C. psittaci*, which is an intracellular organism, does not have to colonize the outer epithelial surfaces to cause disease. All of the other organisms produce an IgA protease for colonization.

75–D. One disadvantage of live attenuated virus vaccines is that they have the genetic potential to mutate to a virulent form.

76–B. The DNA in bacterial conjugation (a single strand) goes only from the donor parent to the recipient and not vice versa. This special mechanism requires the genes for conjugal DNA metabolism. Transformation occurs naturally only with gram-positive bacteria; in the laboratory, transformation of gram-negative cells can be carried out with manipulation of the bacterial envelope.

77–D. A differential medium allows differentiation of two different kinds of bacteria, whereas an enrichment medium contains added growth factors to encourage the growth of certain bacteria. A selective medium may have inhibitors to prevent the growth of certain bacteria. Mueller-Hinton agar is widely used for drug susceptibility testing because a wide range of organisms grow on it; however, it is not a differential medium.

78–B. The hallmarks of plague are a rapid elevation in temperature and regional buboes, rather than erythema nodosum.

79–B. *Neisseria gonorrhoeae* lacks a significant capsule; the pili are the best correlate with virulence. Meningitis-causing strains of *Haemophilus influenzae* with their type b capsule, *Cryptococcus*, *Neisseria meningitidis*, and *Streptococcus pneumoniae* all have polysaccharide capsules that play an important role in virulence.

80–A. Most viral infections result in inapparent or subclinical disease rather than acute clinical disease.

81–E. The virulence of *Yersinia pestis* does not depend on exotoxins. Instead, it depends on a variety of other factors, the most important of which is its ability to proliferate intracellularly. Associated with this ability and virulence are Ca^{2+} dependence; V and W antigens; *Yersinia* outer membrane proteins; F-1cr envelope antigen; coagulase, pesticin, and fibrinolysin production; and pigment absorption.

82–C. INF-γ does not directly inactivate eIF-2 but induces a protein kinase that phosphorylates it, thus rendering it inactive.

83–A. All heterologous compounds may elicit some antibody response. Dinitrobenzene is a hapten by definition and, under normal circumstances, should not elicit an immune response.

84–C. HIV is a member of the lentivirus group of the retrovirus family.

85–A. Enveloped viruses cannot survive the environment of the gastrointestinal tract and therefore are not involved in viral gastroenteritis.

86–C. Smokers are clinically infected at a higher rate than nonsmokers during an epidemic of legionnaires' disease. They also have more serious cases than nonsmokers.

87–E. Of the molecules listed, only the complement components are outside the basic structure of the immunoglobulin superfamily.

88–A. Exotoxins are heat-labile proteins that are released or secreted by certain gram-positive and gram-negative bacteria. Antitoxins are antibodies that neutralize toxins.

89–C. Macrophages have all the functions listed except IL-2 production. IL-2 is produced by activated T cells.

90–B. CD4 cells, or T cells, have all the functions listed except for processing and presenting antigen.

91–B. The characteristic lesion of primary syphilis is a hard, not a soft chancre. Vascular involvement is highly characteristic of the disease. Secondary infection involves most tissues of the body, but is not fatal; however, tertiary syphilis is fatal.

92–C. B cells are not known to produce IFN-γ.

93–D. *N. meningitidis* is a delicate organism. It must be processed quickly in the laboratory and requires enriched media for growth.

94–C. Viral hepatitis is not a latent infection. Several RNA viruses, including hepatitis A virus (HAV), non-A, non-B hepatitis virus, the delta agent, yellow fever virus, and hepatitis B virus (HBV)—a circular double-stranded DNA virus—cause viral hepatitis (a classic chronic virus infection). ELISA tests are available for the diagnosis of hepatitis caused by HAV, HBV, non-A, non-B hepatitis virus, and the delta agent.

95–D. Severe sequelae are common in treated patients.

96–A. All of the listed compounds are T-cell mitogens except lipopolysaccharide, which is a B-cell mitogen.

97–E. Organisms do not invade tissues; rather, the exotoxin enters the bloodstream and affects other tissues.

98–D. All of the listed compounds are both T-independent antigens and B-cell mitogens except for phytohemagglutinin, which is a T-cell mitogen.

99–D. No transmission of HIV-1 by mosquitoes has been documented.

100–B. Complement is not directly involved in the type I anaphylactic reaction, and the anaphylatoxins C3a and C5a would not be mediators. Both C3a and C5a, however, do cause mast cells to release many of the mediators important in anaphylaxis.

101–E. There are at least three constant domains on the heavy chains of an immunoglobulin, or antibody, molecule. There may be as many as four (as in IgE and IgM).

102–G. Pathogenicity factors important in plague are calcium dependency, V and W antigens, outer membrane proteins, the F-1 envelope antigen, pesticin, coagulase, and fibrinolysin.

103–E. Traveler's diarrhea is frequently caused by enterotoxigenic strains of *E. coli* that produce the heat-labile (LT) and heat-stable (ST) toxin. LT is an exotoxin that causes an increase in cAMP.

104–C. The ability of *F. tularensis* to survive intracellular killing and to replicate intracellularly are the most important known virulence factors.

105–B. Capsule is the major antigenic determinant and virulence factor in strains causing meningitis.

106–F. Teichoic and teichuronic acids, which are polymers containing ribitol or glycerol, are found in gram-positive cell walls or cell-wall membranes.

107–E. Endotoxin activity is associated with the lipid A component of lipopolysaccharide.

108–C. Peptidoglycan (mucopeptide and murein) is a complex cell-wall polymer containing *N*-acetylglucosamine and *N*-acetylmuramic acid and associated peptides.

109–E. O antigen or O-specific side chains are major surface antigens in the polysaccharide component of lipopolysaccharide.

110–D. The capsule is a well-defined structure usually composed of polysaccharide that is external to the cell wall and protects the bacteria from phagocytosis.

111–D. Zidovudine is an analogue of thymidine, which, when converted to a triphosphate form by cellular enzymes, inhibits reverse transcriptase in human immunodeficiency virus.

112–G. Amantadine blocks the penetration and uncoating of influenza A viruses and may be used prophylactically.

113–B. Foscarnet inhibits herpesvirus DNA polymerase directly.

114–A. Interferon, a host-encoded glycoprotein that is produced in response to virus infection, induces the synthesis of several antiviral proteins, including 2,5A synthetase.

115–H. Invasive aspergillosis is found primarily in patients with neutrophil counts less than 500/mm^3. Patients with cystic fibrosis or chronic granulomatous disease may also have invasive aspergillosis.

116–A. The killing of *N. meningitidis* organisms is primarily dependent on complement-mediated cell lysis. Patients with genetic deficiencies in C5–C8 cannot carry out complement-mediated lysis of bacterial cells.

117–F. Pneumococcal pneumonia is most frequent in patients with some damage to mucociliary elevators in the upper respiratory tracts. Antecedent measles, influenza infections, or alcoholism predispose the patient to pneumococcal pneumonia.

118–G. Ketoacidotic diabetes is a major predisposing condition for zygomycosis, although lymphoma or leukemia may also predispose the patient to it.

119–B. Antecedent Epstein-Barr virus infection is associated with nasal carcinoma.

120–D. Persons with hepatitis B infection (particularly chronic infection) have an increased risk of hepatocellular carcinoma.

121–A. A pre–T cell would be a lymphocyte with no discernible T cell markers.

122–C. A T helper cell would have all the listed markers except for CD8.

123–D. A T cytotoxic cell would have all the listed markers except for CD4.

124–E. Maturing T cells have both CD4 and CD8 markers before differentiation into T helper (CD4$^+$) and T cytotoxic (CD8$^+$) cells.

125–C. *S. epidermidis* is noted for its ability to secrete biofilms and adhere to intravenous lines. *Streptococcus mutans* (a *viridans* streptococci) is also noted for the production of a dextran biofilm that adheres these organisms to dental surfaces and causes dental plaque.

126–F. *S. pyogenes* is a group A streptococci that has an M protein on its outer cell walls, which interferes with phagocytosis in the immunologically naive individual. It can be serotyped on the basis of this protein.

127–E. *S. pneumoniae* is noted for its solubility in bile.

128–A. *E. faecalis*, which is part of the normal colon flora in humans, is noted for its ability to attach to damaged heart valves when it enters the circulation after bowel surgery.

129–A. Respiratory syncytial virus causes the formation of characteristic giant cells that can be observed in nasal secretions.

130–E. The California and LaCrosse encephalitis viruses, which have mosquito vectors, are bunyaviruses.

131–F. The short genome RNA molecule of arenavirus is ambisense—that is, the 3′ half has negative sense and the 5′ half has positive sense.

132–D. Croup, an early childhood upper respiratory tract infection, is caused by type 2 parainfluenza viruses.

133–B. C5a (anaphylatoxin II) is analogous to C3a (anaphylatoxin I). C5a binds to a specific receptor on the mast cell and causes histamine release during complement activation.

134–D. The C4b2a moiety, formed sequentially after the attachment of C1 to antibody, will cleave C3 and is thus called C3 convertase.

135–C. C1qrs is the functional link between antibody on a cell surface and activation of the classic complement cascade.

136–A. *Bacteroides* is the most common organism in the human gastrointestinal tract, greatly outnumbering *E. coli* and *C. perfringens* or *C. difficile*, which are also part of the normal flora.

137–C. *C. difficile* is overwhelmingly the causative agent of pseudomembranous colitis associated with antibiotic treatment in hospitalized patients.

138–B. *C. botulinum* is the anaerobe causing infant botulism.

139–F. *E. coli* is a common causative agent of urinary tract infection. The strict anaerobes do not cause urinary tract infections.

140–F. One route of spread of toxoplasmosis is through contaminated cat litter. The other is through the ingestion of undercooked meat.

141–B. Swimming in contaminated waters may cause infection with *Acanthamoeba* or *Naegleria*, which may develop into meningoencephalitis.

142–D. *V. parahaemolyticus* is a marine organism that is transmitted through ingestion of raw or undercooked seafood.

143–G. Hookworm filariform larvae may grow in the soil in endemic regions and can penetrate skin. Wearing shoes has been shown to greatly reduce the transmission of hookworm.

144–C. The hepatitis B virus, the hepadnavirus that causes serum hepatitis, uses a virus-encoded reverse transcriptase during replication.

145–F. The rubella virus, which causes German measles, can cause a congenital rubella syndrome if the fetus is infected during the first 10 weeks of pregnancy.

146–E. Immunosuppression can cause the reactivation of varicella-zoster virus from neurons, which results in shingles.

147–C. The delta agent, a defective virus, causes a more severe form of serum hepatitis than observed with hepatitis B virus alone.

148–F. The null, or K, cell is the predominant cell involved in antibody-dependent cell cytotoxicity.

149–D. The plasma cell, with its well-developed rough endoplasmic reticulum, is the producer of specific, secreted antibody.

150–A. CD4$^+$ cells, or T helper cells, recognize antigen in the context of class II histocompatibility antigens on the surface of macrophages and other antigen-presenting cells. The natural ligand for CD4 is the class II molecule.

151–A. CD4$^+$ cells directly interact with APCs.

152–E. The NK cell is capable of spontaneously attacking and destroying certain tumor cells.

153–G. The monocyte–macrophage is the classic example of an antigen-presenting cell (APC). Other macrophage-like cells (e.g., Kupffer's cells, Langerhans' cells of the skin) probably share this APC function.

154–C. Possession of multiple classes of surface immunoglobulin is a hallmark of the mature B cell. This cell can be driven to plasma cell formation and subsequent antibody secretion by exposure to the appropriate antigen.

155–B. CD8$^+$ cells, or T-cytotoxic cells, recognize antigen in the context of class I histocompatibility antigens on the surface of all nucleated cells. The natural ligand for CD8 is the class I molecule.

156–D. The patient's age and symptoms indicate that rotavirus is the primary suspect.

157–B. Pale, greasy, malodorous stools with maladsorption are unique to *Giardia* infections.

158–G. *V. parahaemolyticus*, found in raw oysters, is the most likely causative agent.

159–A. *B. cereus*, found in rice, is not killed by steaming. The addition of eggs and other ingredients to make fried rice encourages growth if the fried rice is not held at a high temperature. Onset of watery diarrhea may occur within 2 hours or as long as 18 hours after consumption and is in response to the presence of toxin.

160–J. Only *T. pallidum* and *H. ducreyi* produce nodular penile ulcers. Major clues leading to the diagnosis of *T. pallidum* are the hard nodule or chancre and the lack of pain. *H. ducreyi* produces soft, painful chancres.

161–B. Symptoms of coxsackievirus herpangina include sore throat such as that caused by *Streptococcus;* however, vesicular lesions on the soft palate are present but tonsillar abscesses are not seen. Generally, the patient's temperature is lower in herpangina, and no left shift is noted in a white cell count.

162–H. Several organisms produce exanthems. The tick, the locale (both North Carolina and South Carolina are high endemic areas), wrist and ankle swelling, macular nature of the rash, and the progression of the rash are most suggestive of Rocky Mountain spotted fever caused by *R. prowazekii.* *N. meningitidis* may occur with sore throat and a scattered macular rash, but it usually develops into petechiae and ecchymoses. Meningeal signs, normally present, may be absent.

163–A. The most likely causative agent is *C. immitis* because the young woman has just moved to the endemic area and there are pulmonary symptoms and erythema nodosum (a good prognostic sign). Possibly, the microorganism could be *H. capsulatum,* but no indication is given as to travel to a high endemic area or exposure to bat guano in a place such as a cave. Erythema nodosum is more common in coccidioidomycosis.

164–F. TAX is an HTLV-I transcriptional activator thought to be involved in cellular transformation.

165–E. The VCA protein, or viral capsid antigen, is the main component of the Epstein-Barr virus (EBV) capsid. EBV is the causative agent of infectious mononucleosis.

166–A. The viral receptor that confers tissue trophism to reovirus types 1, 2, and 3 is delta hemagglutinin.

167–F. The *ras* gene of the Harvey sarcoma virus codes for a guanine-nucleotide–binding protein, which has biologic activity that causes cellular transformation.

168–C. Although hepatitis B virus is a DNA virus, it needs a reverse transcriptase to replicate and, therefore, only polyomavirus is not dependent on this enzyme activity for replication.

169–F. Harvey sarcoma virus, like most viruses with high oncogenic potential, is a defective virus that lacks at least one functional virogene.

170–A. Mouse mammary tumor virus (the Bittner virus) is a type B RNA tumor virus.

171–C. Streptomycin binds to the 30S ribosomal subunit, thereby causing misreading of mRNA.

172–B. Cephalosporin drugs are similar to penicillin in that they inhibit cell-wall biosynthesis and are inactivated by beta-lactamases.

173–E. Griseofulvin is a fungistatic drug that interferes with the mitotic spindle and cytoplasmic microtubule assembly, thus inhibiting cell division.

174–C. Streptomycin is an aminoglycoside antibiotic that is bactericidal for gram-negative bacteria.

175–H. *B. burgdorferi* causes Lyme disease. The reservoirs are deer and white-footed mice. The vector carrying the bacterium to humans and dogs is the *Ixodes* tick.

176–F. *L. donovani* causes visceral leishmaniasis. Nonhuman reservoirs include dogs and rodents. Sandflies carry the infection to humans.

177–G. Orbivirus is the causative agent of Colorado tick fever, which is endemic to the western United States and Canada. It is transmitted to humans via the *Dermacentor* tick.

178–A. *R. prowazekii* is the causative agent of epidemic typhus, which is transmitted via the body louse.

179–J. Creutzfeldt-Jakob disease is an unconventional slow virus, or prion disease.

180–A. *Mycobacterium avium-intracellulare* or *Mycobacterium tuberculosis*, both acid-fast organisms, are the most likely causes of this pulmonary infection in a patient with AIDS.

181–H. *Ascaris*, a helminth, may migrate into the bile duct, gallbladder, and liver, producing severe tissue damage. This process may be exacerbated by fever, antiparasitic drugs, and anesthetics.

182–B. *Sporothrix schenckii*, a dimorphic fungus, is found in the environment on various plant materials. Subcutaneous infections begin with traumatic implantation of contaminated plant material such as mine timber slivers, rose thorns, or sphagnum moss. The resulting sporotrichosis is characterized by a fixed, subcutaneous, nodular lesion (or lesions) along the lymphatics from the initial trauma site. When found in tissues, it is in the form of a cigar-shaped yeast.

183–I. Mycoplasma is a common cause of pneumonia in teenagers and young adults. During the course of the infection, some autoagglutinating antibodies (cold agglutinins) are formed against red cells. The antibodies are inactive at normal body temperature, but agglutinate red blood cells at 4°C.

184–K. *Cryptosporidium*, a protozoan, causes severe, nonresolving diarrhea in a patient with AIDS. In general, the bacterial causative agents are more responsive to treatment.

Index